# Neurogenic Communication Disorders: A Functional Approach

Edited by

**Linda E. Worrall, Ph.D.**
*Department of Speech Pathology and Audiology*
*The University of Queensland*
*Australia*

and

**Carol M. Frattali, Ph.D.**
*Research Coordinator*
*Speech-Language Pathology Section*
*W.G. Magnuson Clinical Center*
*National Institutes of Health*
*Bethesda, Maryland*

**2000**
**Thieme**
**New York • Stuttgart**

Thieme New York
333 Seventh Avenue
New York, NY 10001

Editor: Andrea Seils
Editorial Director: Ave McCracken
Editorial Assistant: Michelle Carini
Developmental Manager: Kathleen P. Lyons
Director, Production & Manufacturing:
   Anne Vinnicombe
Production Editor: Janice G. Stangel
Marketing Director: Phyllis Gold

Sales Manager: Ross Lumpkin
Chief Financial Officer: Seth S. Fishman
President: Brian D. Scanlan
Cover Designer: Michael Mendelsohn at MM
   Design 2000, Inc.
Compositor: Compset Inc.
Printer: Hamilton Printing Company

Library of Congress Cataloging-in-Publication Data
Neurogenic communication disorders: a functional approach/edited by Linda E.
Worrall and Carol M. Frattali.
      p. ; cm.
   Includes bibliographical references and index.
   ISBN 0-86577-868-X
      1. Speech therapy. 2. Communicative disorders. 3. Deglutition disorders. I. Worrall,
Linda. II. Frattali, Carol.
      [DNLM:   1. Communication Disorders—rehabilitation. 2. Deglutition
Disorders—rehabilitation. WL 340.2 N4935 2000]
   RC423 .N37 2000
   616.85'5—dc21                                                                    99-048698

**Important note:** Medical knowledge is ever-changing. As new research and clinical experience
broaden our knowledge, changes in treatment and drug therapy may be required. The authors and
editors of the material herein have consulted sources believed to be reliable in their efforts to provide
information that is complete and in accord with the standards accepted at the time of publication.
However, in view of the possibility of human error by the authors, editors, or publisher of the work
herein, or changes in medical knowledge, neither the authors, editors, publisher, nor any other party
who has been involved in the preparation of this work, warrants that the information contained
herein is in every respect accurate or complete, and they are not responsible for any errors or omissions or for the results obtained from use of such information. Readers are encouraged to confirm the
information contained herein with other sources. For example, readers are advised to check the product information sheet included in the package of each drug they plan to administer to be certain that .
the information contained in this publication is accurate and that changes have not been made in the
recommended dose or in the contraindications for administration. This recommendation is of particular importance in connection with new or infrequently used drugs.

Some of the product names, patents, and registered designs referred to in this book are in fact registered trademarks or proprietary names even though specific reference to this fact is not always made
in the text. Therefore, the appearance of a name without designation as proprietary is not to be con-
strued as a representation by the publisher that it is in the public domain.

Printed in the United States of America

5 4 3 2 1

TNY ISBN 0-86577-868-X
GTV ISBN 3-13-124471-2

*To Martha Taylor Sarno and Audrey Holland*
*and our clients who have taught us that communication is more than words.*

# Contents

# Contributors

**Rosemary Baker, Ph.D.**
*Senior Research Officer*
*Centre for Applied Linguistics and*
*    Languages (CALL)*
*Griffith University*
*Nathan Street*
*Queensland*
*Australia*

**Sally C. Byng, Ph.D.**
*Professor of Communication Disability*
*Department of Language and*
*    Communication Science*
*City University*
*Northampton Square*
*London*
*United Kingdom*

**Leora R. Cherney, Ph.D., BC-NCD**
*Associate Professor of Physical*
*    Medicine and Rehabilitation*
*Adjunct Associate Professor of*
*    Communication Sciences and*
*    Disorders*
*Northwestern University Medical*
*    School*
*Clinical Educator*
*Rehabilitation Institute of Chicago*
*Chicago, Illinois*
*United States*

**Chris Code, Ph.D.**
*Professor*
*School of Psychology*
*Washington Singer Laboratories*
*Exeter University*
*United Kingdom; and*
*Brain Damage and Communication*
*    Research*
*School of Communication Sciences*
*    and Disorders*
*University of Sydney*
*New South Wales*

*Australia*

**Bronwyn J. Davidson, B.Sp.Thy.**
*Lecturer*
*Department of Speech Pathology and*
*    Audiology*
*The University of Queensland*
*Conjoint Clinical Position*
*Royal Brisbane Hospital and the*
*    University of Queensland*
*Brisbane, Queensland*
*Australia*

**Pamela M. Enderby, Ph.D.**
*Professor of Community*
*    Rehabilitation*
*General Practice and Primary Care*
*University of Sheffield*
*Community Sciences*
*Northern General Hospital*
*Sheffield*
*United Kingdom*

**Carol M. Frattali, Ph.D.**
*Research Coordinator*
*Speech-Language Pathology Section*
*W.G. Magnuson Clinical Center*
*National Institutes of Health*
*Bethesda, Maryland*
*United States*

**Anita S. Halper, M.A., BC-NCD**
*Academic Development Coordinator*
*Rehabilitation Institute of Chicago*
*Associate Professor of Physical*
*    Medicine and Rehabilitation*
*Clinical Associate Professor of*
*    Communication Sciences and*
*    Disorders*
*Northwestern University Medical*
*    School*
*Chicago, Illinois*
*United States*

**Louise M.H. Hickson, Ph.D.**
Senior Lecturer in Audiology
Department of Speech Pathology and
    Audiology
The University of Queensland
Brisbane, Queensland
Australia

**Fabiane M. Hirsch, M.Sc.**
Speech-Language Pathologist
Speech and Hearing Sciences
University of Arizona
Tucson, Arizona
United States

**Audrey L. Holland, Ph.D.**
Regents Professor of Speech and
    Hearing Sciences
Department of Speech and Hearing
    Sciences
University of Arizona
Tucson, Arizona
United States

**Dilys Jones, B.A.**
Department of Speech Pathology and
    Audiology
University of Witswatersrand
Johannesburg
South Africa

**Brigette M. Larkins, M.Ed.**
Department of Speech Pathology and
    Audiology
The University of Queensland and
National Manager Serious Injury
Accident Rehabilitation and
    Compensation Insurance
    Company (ACC)
Wellington
New Zealand

**Jon G. Lyon, Ph.D.**
Director
Living with Aphasia, Inc.
6344 Hiusandwood Road

Mazomanie, Wisconsin
United States

**Rosemary Lubinski, Ed.D.**
Professor
Department of Communicative
    Disorders and Sciences
University at Buffalo
Amherst, New York
United States

**Robyn T. McCooey, B.App. Sc.**
Department of Speech Pathology
The Geelong Hospital
Victoria
Department of Speech
    Pathology and Audiology
The University of Queensland
Brisbane
Australia

**J.B. Orange, Ph.D.**
Associate Professor
School of Communication Sciences
    and Disorders
University of Western Ontario
Elborn College
London, Ontario
Canada

**Susan P. Parr, Ph.D.**
Research Fellow
Department of Language and
    Communication Sciences
City University
Northampton Square
London
United Kingdom

**Claire Penn, Ph.D.**
Professor
Department of Speech Pathology and
    Audiology
University of Witswatersrand
Johannesburg
South Africa

**Deborah J. Pye, B. Sp. Path. (Hons)**
*Department of Speech Pathology*
*Eventide Nursing Home*
*Brighton*
*Australia*

**Nina N. Simmons-Mackie, Ph.D.**
*Professor*
*Department of Communication*
  *Sciences and Disorders*
*Southeastern Louisiana University*
*Hammond, Louisiana*
*United States*

**Barbara C. Sonies, Ph.D.**
*Chief, Speech Language Pathology*
  *Section*
*Adjunct Professor of Speech-*
  *Language Pathology*
*Department of Hearing and Speech*
  *Sciences*
*University of Maryland*
*Department of Rehabilitation*
  *Medicine*
*National Institutes of Health*

*Bethesda, Maryland*
*United States*

**Deborah Toffolo, M.App.Sc**
*Director*
*Access Brain Injury Services*
*Riverwood*
*New South Wales*
*Australia*

**Linda E. Worrall, Ph.D.**
*Director and Senior Lecturer*
*Communication Disability in Ageing*
  *Research Unit*
*Department of Speech Pathology and*
  *Audiology*
*The University of Queensland*
*Brisbane*
*Australia*

**Edwin Yiu, Ph.D.**
*Associate Professor*
*Department of Speech and Hearing*
  *Sciences*
*The University of Hong Kong*
*Hong Kong*

# Preface

The field of speech-language pathology has witnessed a recent explosion of interest in functional approaches to communication and swallowing disorders. The growing interest in functional approaches may have occurred for a number of reasons. The profession's unprecedented interest in functional communication and swallowing has developed due to the demand for reliable, valid, and sensitive functional outcome measures. In the scientific literature, the recent increase in interest in functional approaches may reflect the growth of the discipline's research base that is exploring the complexities of measuring and treating the long-term consequences of speech, language, and swallowing impairments. Debates in the literature are moving away from whether functional communication should be assessed at all, to the present situation of exploring ways in which a balance between functional approaches and impairment based approaches can be achieved. Models of disablement are leading the way in conceptualizing the consequences of impairment in terms of everyday functioning and participation in society. Models of disablement also have the potential to act as a framework for rehabilitation efforts.

The aim of this book is to describe functional approaches to neurogenic communication and swallowing disorders in a range of populations and settings. To do this, a definition of "functional approach" was required. The World Health Organization's most recent model of disablement, the Beta-2 draft of the International Classification of Impairments, Activities and Participation (the ICIDH-2) was used to describe the approach. Within this framework, it was described as focusing on the Activity level and extending into the Participation level of the model. This description was used as a framework that is reflected across the chapters of this text.

The book is organised into four sections. The first section describes the assessment of functional communication. The first chapter provides an overview of the conceptual framework for the book while Chapters 2 and 3 describe the functional approach in more detail at the Activity and Participation levels of the WHO model. The next two chapters provide a consumer's and payer's perspective while the final chapter in this section suggests some ways in which the functional communication of linguistically and culturally diverse populations can be assessed. The next section focuses on functional therapy approaches. Chapters addressing return to work, the role of volunteers in the functional approach, real-life functionality and the social approach in aphasia exemplify the diversity of approaches within the functional perspective. The next section describes the assessment and treatment of functional communication in the specific populations of aphasia, dementia, dysarthria, dysphagia and the cognitive communication disorders following traumatic brain injury and right hemisphere damage. The next section describes functional approaches in the acute hospital setting and extended care facility while the final section discusses future directions in the functional approach.

The book was primarily written for speech-language pathologists practicing in the field of neurogenic communication disorders. The book could also be used as a text for university courses in neurogenic communication disorders in order to introduce students to this both vital and necessary aspect of treatment and clinical management.

We chose a group of contributors who were recognised leaders in their specific field and/or who were active researchers in the area. We thank them for their considerable efforts in allowing this book to become a reality. We also thank them for their efforts to overcome cross-cultural communication barriers and the tyranny of distance that proudly has contributors from Australia, Canada, Hong Kong, New Zealand, South Africa, the United Kingdom, and the United States.

**Linda E. Worrall, Ph.D.**
**Carol M. Frattali, Ph.D.**

# SECTION 1

# Assessment of Functional Communication

# A Conceptual Framework for a Functional Approach to Acquired Neurogenic Disorders of Communication and Swallowing

## Linda E. Worrall

**This introductory chapter establishes the conceptual framework for the book. Definitions of functional communication are discussed followed by an examination of how functional communication fits within the conceptual framework of the World Health Organization's International Classification of Impairments, Disabilities and Handicaps (ICIDH). The more recent version of the classification scheme, The International Classification of Impairments, Activities and Participation (ICIDH-2) is then described as a basis for refining the definition of the functional approach in neurogenic communication disorders. It is concluded that functional communication encompasses both the Activity and Participation dimensions of the ICIDH-2.**

## Introduction

Speech-language pathologists have long recognized the importance of a functional approach to neurogenic communication disorders because the functional approach considers how clients perform in natural contexts. However, the functional approach has received greater attention in recent years following healthcare restructuring and subsequent reliance on data yielded from functional assessment to decide who receives care, at what cost, and by whom (Frattali, 1993). This greater emphasis on a functional approach has highlighted the clinical inadequacies and theoretical weaknesses of the approach (Parr, 1996a).

The aim of this chapter is to establish a framework within which the functional approach to communication and swallowing can be discussed. The diversity of perspectives encompassed within a functional approach are described and more specific terminology for the dimensions within the functional approach are presented.

Much of the speech-language pathology literature on the functional approach has centered on the notion of functional communication, particularly as it applies to aphasia. While this chapter is based predominantly within the literature on functional communication in aphasia with some examples drawn from related disorders, a distinction needs to be made between the broad concept of a functional approach to neurogenic communication disorders and the narrower concept of functional communication. The use of the term "communication" in functional communication already infers some form of integrated behavior. Nevertheless, many speech-language pathologists use the terms interchangeably and this will be the case in this chapter.

First, this chapter examines the definitions of functional communication before embarking on a discussion of the relationship between functional communication and the conceptual framework of the International Classification of Impairments, Disabilities and Handicaps [ICDH; World Health Organization (WHO), 1980, 1997]. A critical review of the literature will discuss whether functional communication is a concept that is embedded in the impairment realm, disability realm, or handicap realm. Most literature to date has been based on the original ICIDH conceptual framework. The revised version of the International Classification of Impairments, Disabilities and Handicaps, the International Classification of Impairments, Activities and Participation, or ICIDH-2 (WHO, 1997) is then described and the implications for defining functional communication extracted. Finally it is suggested that the ICIDH-2 framework be used for describing concepts within the functional approach. This serves as the conceptual and terminological bases for this book.

## Definitions

There have been several attempts to define functional communication. There have also been other attempts to define functional communication in relation to conceptual frameworks in related disciplines.

Some of the first definitions of functional communication were offered by the pioneers of the area. Within the context of functional communication, Sarno (1983) described communicative effectiveness as "the total of the myriad of factors which contribute to the transmission of information" (p. 77), while Holland (1982) defined functional communication for the purposes of her observational study of functional communication in aphasia as "getting the message across in a variety of ways ranging from fully formed grammatical sentences to appropriate gestures, rather than being limited to the use of grammatically correct utterances" (p. 50).

In 1990, an advisory panel of the American Speech-Language-Hearing Association (ASHA) defined functional communication as the "ability to receive or convey a message, regardless of the mode, to communicate effectively and independently in a given environment" (ASHA, 1990, p. 2). Since this definition was published, there have been debates within the literature about some of the concepts addressed in the definition.

Simmons-Mackie and Damico (1995) have queried whether the communication that occurs in everyday life is merely receiving or conveying messages. In an ethnographic study, Simmons-Mackie and Damico found a high degree of interactional communication which serves to establish and maintain social relationships as well as transactional communication which is used to exchange information.

The inclusion of the term "independently" in the ASHA definition could also be questioned. Parr (1996a) has challenged the emphasis on the concept of "independence" in rehabilitation. The term has been criticized by the disability movement who prefer the term "autonomy." Autonomy essentially means having control over what happens and Parr supports this contention with the illustration that many people with aphasia in her studies of literacy, delegated activities and preferred to do this than struggle to do it themselves.

Two other definitions of functional communication place greater emphasis on the individual's own environment. In relation to traumatic brain injury (TBI), Hartley (1992) states that functional communication is defined as the "communication skills necessary for communicating adequately and appropriately within an individual's own environment, including independent living and consumer activities, interpersonal relationships, academic endeavors and work-related activities" (p. 265). Apart from emphasizing the individual's own environment, this definition reflects the importance of appropriateness of communication in TBI rather than just effectiveness of communication. It also illustrates the communicative environments of people with TBI (e.g., work, academic), which might be different to people with aphasia who are mostly older than the TBI population. The need for greater emphasis on the individual's own environment in a definition of functional communication is also stated by Worrall (1995) who suggested that the assessment of functional communication should assess "the ability of an individual to communicate in his or her *own everyday* environment."

Frattali (1994) states that functional assessment in speech-language pathology and audiology describes a "person's ability to communicate despite the presence of impairments such as aphasia, dysarthria, or hearing loss" (p. 306). Frattali (1992b, 1994) and others (e.g., Holland, 1994; Parr, 1996a; Ramsberger, 1994; Worrall, 1992, 1995) have thus argued that functional communication fits within the conceptual frameworks used in rehabilitation. The generic term used for these conceptual frameworks is models of disablement.

There are two main advantages of using models of disablement as a framework for the discussion of functional communication. First, these theoretical models may help to describe the process of disablement or functioning following acquired neurogenic communication and swallowing deficits. The theoretical models may also help to describe the effect of different environments such as acute hospital, extended care facilities, and community settings on the communicative ability of the person. Second, the consistency of terminology across disciplines and the specificity of definitions of the concepts within the frameworks may be useful to speech-language pathologists. There is a need for clear communication when coordinating individual cases and also a need when outcomes of groups and populations are reported. The need for unequivocal terminology also exists when communicating with the payers of health care, for example, health insurance agencies. In addition, epidemiologists who compile public health statistics for policy makers need to use an accepted and commonly used set of terminology so that the size of the problem is known. These are strong reasons why speech-language pathologists, like other rehabilitationists, should relate their work to models of disablement.

A number of models of disablement have been proposed (Jette, 1984; Nagi, 1965; WHO, 1980) and there have been several attempts to integrate some of the features of these earlier models (Verbrugge & Jette, 1994; Wilson & Cleary, 1995). However, the framework that has been most widely accepted has been the WHO's ICIDH (1980).

## The ICIDH

The WHO's model used in the ICIDH (WHO, 1980) was one of the first and has remained a universally applied framework. A revision process is under way (Thuriaux, 1995; WHO, 1997), which should culminate in the formal issue of the revised ICIDH in 2000 (WHO, 1997). The impact that these revisions will have on the definition of functional communication is discussed in some detail later in this chapter, however, the model essentially remains the same.

The ICIDH is a classification system relating to the consequences of disease at three levels: the body (impairment), the person (disability), and the person as a social being (handicap).

In the context of health experience, the definition of impairment is:

> *"any loss or abnormality of psychological, physiological or anatomical structure or function"*

Disability is defined as:

> *"any restriction or lack (resulting from an impairment) of ability to perform an activity in the manner or within the range considered normal for a human being"*

Handicap is defined as:

> *"a disadvantage for a given individual, resulting from an impairment or a disability, that limits or prevents the fulfilment of a role that is normal (depending on age, sex, and social and cultural factors) for that individual" (WHO, 1980)*

As Wyller (1997) notes, the ICIDH can be considered in two ways: as a precise coding of impairments, disabilities, and handicaps; and, as a conceptual framework for understanding disablement. Despite its widespread acceptance, the WHO model and classification scheme has received its share of criticism: criticisms about the structure and content of the classification scheme (e.g., poor clinical applicability of the classification scheme), and criticism of the conceptual framework itself (e.g., the lack of recognition of social models of disablement within the ICIDH) (see Dickson, 1996; Johnston, 1996; Marks, 1997; WCC, 1994) Nevertheless, the ICIDH is used for many purposes, for example, to determine prevalence of disability, to assist with policy formulation, and to direct care in individuals (Thuriaux, 1995). The Dutch Collaborating Center for the ICIDH (WCC,

June, 1989) states that it is being used at the micro-organizational level (in the field of health care), the meso-organizational level (at the institutional level), and the macro level ("super" organizational level, nationally and internationally). Therefore, the ICIDH is in widespread use at many different levels of health care.

One of the difficulties of a universal scheme such as this, is that it needs to be accepted in a wide variety of domains, where a domain is defined as a set of individuals given a specific purpose (WCC, May, 1989). For the most part, speech-language pathologists as a domain have not been concerned about the detail of the classification scheme per se. The profession is still coming to terms with the conceptual framework and attempting to translate it into a useful application. It is the conceptual framework that has been the focus of interest for speech-language pathologists, although with the recent revisions of the ICIDH (WHO, 1997), the classification scheme may become more useful.

There is a need to translate the definitions and classifications of the ICIDH into terms that are relevant for speech-language pathologists. It is also timely to consider the statement of Ustan et al. (1995) that "a classification in itself is not easily applied in practice unless it is supported with assessment instruments which will translate the concepts of the classification into operational questions" (p. 207). Frattali et al. (1995) have suggested a broad framework for assessing impairments, disabilities, and handicaps in speech-language pathology. Impairment is measured by traditional assessment tools that evaluate areas such as auditory comprehension, reading comprehension, speech production, and written language. Disability is measured by functional assessment tools that evaluate areas such as understanding a telephone message, understanding one-on-one or group conversations, or completing forms. Measures of handicap include handicap inventories and quality-of-life scales and may assess areas such as holding a job that requires understanding conversations or written material, or level of self-esteem.

Enderby (1997) provided outlines of two case studies in which impairment, disability, and handicap were described. The first case was a man with a mild expressive and receptive language disorder resulting from aphasia (the impairment). He had difficulty making himself understood quickly in a group of people, had stopped using the telephone, occasionally misunderstood meanings, and was dependent on others being attentive and patient listeners (the disability). As a result, he was unable to be employed, was withdrawn from social situations, had given up all hobbies, and no longer contributed to decision making (the handicap). Hence, this man was described as having a mild impairment, moderate disability, and quite severe handicap. The other case was the reverse in terms of severity. The man had a severe level of impairment (severe athetoid cerebral palsy, quadriplegia, dysarthria), little disability (totally independent with adapted wheelchair, lived in adapted accommodation, communicated in all situations with a communication aid and a special adapted telephone), and no handicap (employed as a solicitor, active member of disability movement, with full work and social life).

Despite these broad frameworks, there remains a lack of clear definition of how the various dimensions (e.g., language impairment, disability, and handicap; speech impairment, disability, and handicap; swallowing impairment, disability, and handicap) should be measured. One of the complicating factors in this process is the use of the term functional communication assessments—a term that has grown out of the medical model and one that seemingly encompasses impairments, disabilities, and handicaps. The next section reviews the literature relating to the functional approach at the impairment, disability, and handicap level.

## Functional Approach at the Impairment Level

Within the general rehabilitation literature, there has been some debate about whether "functional limitations" are an impairment level or disability concept. Traditionally in both the literature on models of disablement and in the speech-language pathology literature, the term "functional" is predominantly associated with the disability level, however, some aspects of functional have been conceptualized at the impairment level. Jette (1984) states that the term function has been used to describe the characteristic action of body parts (the function of the shoulder), the performance of bodily organs (kidney function), as well as the performance of an individual (to function in activities of daily living). This leads to the conclusion that the term "functional" can be associated with both levels of impairment and disability. Chamie (1990), however, proposes that functional limitations are a type of disability. Chamie suggests that there are two levels or types of disability—*functional limitations* (e.g., seeing, hearing, moving, grasping, climbing) and *activity restriction* (e.g., getting dressed, setting the table). Functional limitations are sometimes referred to as *simple* or basic skills (e.g., hearing) and these are prerequisites for the more *complex* activities that are used in assessing activity restriction (e.g., using the telephone) (WCC, 1994). Interestingly, Wood (1980), the author of the ICIDH, placed functional limitations in the impairment realm. In the Nagi (1965) model, functional limitations were an intermediate level between impairment and disability, although disability in the Nagi model was synonymous with the ICIDH concept of handicap. Hence, the models of disablement have not produced a clear definition of the concept of functional limitations.

While there has been some consensus that functional communication certainly occurs mainly at the level of disability, probably also at the level of handicap, and possibly at the level of impairment, Ramsberger (1994) suggests that functional relates directly to all levels. Ramsberger describes the development of the entire impairment, disability, and handicap continuum as the genesis of the functional perspective as opposed to the medical model that is concerned with etiology, pathology, and manifestations of disease. A model by Wilkerson is cited by Ramsberger (1994), which supports this view. In Wilkerson's model, there are three levels of function: micro, middle, and macro and these relate directly to impairments, disabilities, and handicaps. The micro level of assessment measures "basic functional abilities such as range of motion, strength, motor sequencing, naming, production of simple declaratives, or articulation accuracy" (p. 2). The middle level of functioning addresses "individual applied skills such as ambulation, cooking, speech intelligibility, expressing needs, reading, or following directions" (p. 2). The macro-level functions include "integrated functions such as returning to work, living independently, and resuming roles as parent, wage earner, or head of the household" (p. 3).

In summary, there has been confusion about whether the functional approach extends into the impairment level. The disablement models to date suggest that "functional limitations" are either at the impairment or disability level. It is suggested, however, that the functional approach, as used by speech-language pathologists, particularly when the term functional communication is used, does not extend into the impairment realm.

### Functional Approach at the Disability Level

The strongest proponent of functional communication assessment being a disability level measure is Frattali (1992b, 1993, 1994) in association with colleagues (Frattali et al., 1995a, 1995b). The American Speech-Language-Hearing Association Functional Assessment of Communication Skills (ASHA FACS) was developed specifically as a measure of disability and included the domains of social communication, communication of basic needs, daily planning, and reading, writing, and number concepts. It was designed to supplement measures of impairment and measures of handicap (Frattali et al., 1995a). Other measures of communicative disability include the Communicative Abilities in Daily Living—CADL (Holland, 1980) and its successor, the CADL-2 (Holland et al., 1998), the Functional Communication Profile—FCP (Sarno, 1969), the Amsterdam-Nijmegan Everyday Language Test—ANELT (Blomert et al., 1994) and possibly the Communicative Effective Index—CETI (Lomas et al., 1989).

Many other researchers (e.g., Kagan & Gailey, 1993; Worrall, 1992, 1995; Parr, 1996a) essentially agree that the concept of functional communication is predominantly based in the disability realm. Worrall (1992, 1995) and Parr (1996a), however, suggest that some modification to this concept of functional communication at the disability level is required. The major shift of emphasis is in relation to the relevancy of the activities to the individual. While Beukelman et al. (1984), Elman and Bernstein-Ellis (1995), Pierce (1996), and Smith (1985) acknowledge that the functional needs of people differ, currently there is little recognition of the specific needs of individuals in existing functional communication assessments, although Payne (1994) has developed a method of establishing the importance of functional activities for individuals. Both Parr (1996a) and Worrall (1995) suggest that this flexibility cannot be gained through standardized assessments: functional needs must be established collaboratively with the client and then assessed.

There are a number of other issues in developing functional communication assessments in the disability realm that still challenge test developers. The relationship between pragmatics and functional communication remains unclear. Parr (1996a) describes Fairclough's (1989) theory of social and asocial constructions of language and suggests that fields of study such as conversation analysis, pragmatics, and even sociolinguistics adhere to the "asocial" model. On the other hand, authors such as Davis and Wilcox (1985), Ferguson (1994), Penn (1985), and Ulatowska et al. (1992) consider that pragmatic profiles, conversational analyses, and discourse analysis are measures of everyday communicative ability and hence may be seen as measures of functional communication at the disability level. There is therefore a lack of clarity in the speech-language pathology literature about the nature of functional communication when it is placed within the ICIDH framework, particularly when it uses approaches derived from linguistics.

The distinction between functional communication and pragmatics is blurred and many speech-language pathologists use the terms interchangeably. As Worrall (1995) states, the concept of functional communication stemmed from the medical rehabilitation setting while pragmatics is an area of linguistics that has been applied to disordered communication. Hence, the two terms have their bases in different theoretical models. Some authors have used pragmatic theory to develop functional communication tests [e.g., Holland (1980) used speech act theory in the development of the CADL]; others used the same theory to develop observational profiles of "functional communication" [e.g., Skinner et al. (1984) in the development of the Edinburgh Functional Communication Profile—EFCP]. Still others have used pragmatics as a basis for their discussions of functional communication (Chapey, 1992; Hartley, 1992; Ramsberger, 1994). In a review of pragmatic assessments in adult aphasia, Manochiopinig et al. (1992) made a distinction between pragmatic and functional assessment on the basis of the purpose that they serve. They suggested that observational profiles which identify specific pragmatic behaviors (Gurland et al., 1982; Prutting & Kirchner, 1987; Skinner et al., 1984) are the *components* necessary to achieve functional communication whereas assessments such as the CADL, CETI, and FCP are *end measures* of a person's functional ability in real-life situations. However, the key argument for placing pragmatics firmly in the realm of disability is that it is not an abnormality of a body structure or body function (an impairment). It is at the level of the person and therefore must be placed within the disability dimension.

While it is important that an assessment reflects the individual everyday communicative needs of clients, it also should be culturally sensitive. Culturally diverse nations need to be aware that clients will have differing communicative needs as a result of their cultural background. Baker (1995) notes that it is characteristic of bilingual and multilingual speakers to use their different languages with different people, for different purposes, and in different domains of life and this must be taken into account when assessing the functional communication of people with a communication disorder from ethnic backgrounds. Baker studied the communicative needs of 72 people aged 65 years and over from the language background groups of Croatian, Dutch, Italian, Latvian, Polish, and Vietnamese and who were now residing in Australia. Not only did Baker find that communicative needs centered around maintaining contact with family, friends, and neighbors, and obtaining requirements such as food and medical attention, but the study also highlighted the importance of obtaining information on patterns of bilingual language use prior to assessment.

There is also a need to recognize the effect of different impairments on disability (e.g., right hemisphere damage, TBI, dementia, and dysarthria) and the effect of different environments (extended care facilities, acute hospital setting, school, home, or community setting) on the disability. ASHA has recognized these issues and is currently developing a supplemental measure to the ASHA FACS. It is also seeking to validate the ASHA FACS with various communication-disordered populations, multicultural groups within the United States, and other English-speaking countries (ASHA, personal communication).

Another major issue is whether the performance of clients is rated by others (e.g., CETI) or whether the clinician rates the performance of the client based on observation in real-life (e.g., EFCP) or simulated activities (e.g., CADL). The ASHA FACS allows the examiner to use the two sources of observation and report by significant other, and therefore infers that these methods can be used interchangeably.

Frattali (1993) cites Carey (1990). who said that it is unlikely that someone will invent a car that has the luxury of a big car, the fuel efficiency of a small car, or the flexibility of a truck used for hauling different farm machinery. It is therefore unlikely that one measure of functional communication in the disability realm will suit all clients, all impairments, all cultures, and all settings. There may also be a need in the future for functional communication assessments that suit the requirements of clinicians. Clinicians may wish to screen clients, measure a baseline for therapy, plan therapy, or measure the outcome of therapy. Again, it may be that a portfolio of tools need to be at the disposal of clinicians.

It can therefore be concluded that there is considerable diversity in the interpretation of communicative disability. Certainly, there are several measures that have been published that purport to assess at this level (see Frattali et al., 1995b), each taking a slightly different perspective or using a slightly different methodology. The diversity of functional approaches at the disability level requires a diversity of measures. There is a general consensus though that "functional communication" is firmly routed in the disability dimension.

## Functional Approach at the Handicap Level

Frattali (1992b, 1993, 1994) noted that while functional communication should be firmly centered in the disability realm, it could extend into the handicap realm. Frattali also suggested that handicap is the least well-defined concept.

Holland (1994) suggests that because the medical model was adopted by speech-language pathologists, most clinical techniques have focussed on the impairment and disability associated with neurogenic communication disorders. This has left obscure generalization processes to reduce handicap. Holland suggests therefore that adopting a handicap model means "developing interpersonally directed measures of functional ability and functional outcome and then working directly within the *social context* of communication" (p. 35). Holland offers the program at the North York Aphasia Center in Ontario (Kagan & Gailey, 1993) as a model of how a handicap approach might work in practice.

Kagan and Gailey (1993) state that the program at the North York Aphasia Center is specifically directed at reducing the handicap of aphasia by providing opportunities for conversation with skilled partners. Apart from training volunteers to act as skilled conversation partners, the Center offers the opportunity for discussion and socialization through discussion and recreational groups and if needed, individual and group counselling. As opposed to other schemes that utilize volunteers, Kagan and Gailey propose that the Aphasia Center uses volunteers to facilitate participation in the many roles of life. Kagan and Gailey ascribe to the view that functional communication skills do not include the psychosocial well-being perspective and hence contend that functional communication should not be the final goal or end point of the treatment continuum. The validation of the role of speech-language pathologists and this model of service within the ICIDH framework is an exciting development in the profession of speech-language pathology.

Again, in the context of aphasia, Lyon (1996) states that handicap refers to the personal and social consequences brought about by the disability. Lyon uses Simmons-Mackie and Damico's (1995) classification of the purposes of communication as the rationale for the treatment offered. Lyon states that the interactional nature of communication (communication that maintains and creates personal bonds) has been ignored by speech-language pathologists who tend to focus on transactional communication (information exchange). Hence, Lyon's treatment targets the social connections between spouses and hence targets the handicap of aphasia.

Parr (1996a) also argues for a move to embrace more social models of communication. One of Parr's major arguments is that there must be a power shift from the health professional to the person with a communication disability. An agenda of collaboration is suggested in which the person with a communication disability becomes the expert. This paradigm shift has happened in other disciplines such as social work and suggests that the social model should be explored in greater detail by speech-language pathologists.

In summary, while there has been a growing body of literature that suggests that speech-language pathologists should adopt a social model in the rehabilitation of acquired neurogenic communication disorders focused on the level of handicap, this has yet to be operationalized. Educated within a predominantly medical model, this is new territory for speech-language pathologists.

## ICIDH—2

In 1993, a revision process of the 1980 ICIDH was begun in response to considerable amount of critical literature about the ICIDH (see WCC, 1994). The revision process was largely undertaken by ICIDH Collaborating Centers around the world and an "Alpha" draft of the revisions was collated in May 1996. After comment by all Collaborating Centers and task forces, the "Beta-1" draft was released on the Internet for public comment and field trials. The formal release of the new ICIDH-2 is due in 1999 (Madden & Hogan, 1997; WHO, 1997).

The new draft of the ICIDH-2 proposes three dimensions:

> *In the context of a health condition:*
>
> > *Impairment is a loss or abnormality of body structure or of a physiological or psychological function.*
> >
> > *An activity is the nature and extent of functioning at the level of the person. Activities may be limited in nature, duration and quality.*
> >
> > *Participation is the nature and extent of a person's involvement in life situations in relation to impairments, activities, health conditions and contextual factors.*
>
> *(WHO, 1997)*

The major change has therefore been that the negative term "disability" has been replaced by the neutral term "activity" and similarly "handicap" by "participation." Speech-language pathologists mostly work with people who have a limitation and are therefore often concerned with the negative aspects of the dimensions, and the terms "activity limitation" and "participation restriction" have been proposed to replace disability and handicap directly.

The revisions were intended to clarify the concepts of impairments, disabilities and handicaps, so it is important to determine if the revisions will clarify the notion of functional communication. To this end, the new terms and concepts are first described and an evaluation of the merit of these revisions is then provided. The details of the revised classification scheme are provided because they offer additional insight into the nature of the concepts and may prove useful for speech-language pathologists in the future. Finally, there is a discussion of the implications that the revisions may have for functional communication.

*Impairments* relate to either body functions or body structures. The WHO (1997) has stated that limitations in certain functions such as basic functions of the body, are impairments whereas previously they might have been considered as disabilities under the term "functional limitations."

In the classification scheme, the impairments of function that are relevant to speech-language pathologists and acquired neurogenic disorders are: impairments of language (code i01600) as in the comprehension and expression of spoken and unspoken language; voice (i10100); articulation (i10200) in which dysarthria has its own code; chewing/swallowing and related functions (i50200) such as chewing/mastication, salivation, swallowing (including aspiration), regurgitation, and vomiting. There are also separate codes for impairments of structure and each area of the central nervous system (temporal lobe, brain stem, cranial nerves) and other structures of the speech and swallowing mechanism are identified.

WHO (1997) states that the *activity* dimension deals with a person's everyday life activities, that is, they are integrated activities. The activities include simple and complex activities. The activity dimension is performance based rather than aptitude or potential based and can be used in self-evaluation, clinical assessment, functional tests, or questionnaires. The inclusion of questionnaires and self-evaluation might suggest that the CETI may still be considered an activity dimension assessment. Activities are scaled by difficulties and whether assistance (personal and nonpersonal) is needed. In addition, it is recommended that performance of activities be assessed with the use of the assistive devices that the person uses in everyday life.

The classification scheme includes essentially two sections or chapters that are relevant to speech-language pathologists: communication activities (Chapter 3) and interpersonal behaviors (Chapter 8). Communication activities include understanding messages (e.g., understanding the description of a single object, understanding a phrase of two or more words), communicating messages (e.g., asking questions, making eye contact, expressing ideas in writing), and using communication devices (e.g., using a telephone, lip reading, using a typewriter or computer). Interpersonal behaviors include initiating social contact, relating to a spouse or partner, and maintaining relationships with friends and peers. There are, however, activities interspersed in other chapters that are relevant to people with acquired speech, language, and swallowing impairments (e.g., a50500, Eating and drinking; a60100, Procuring and taking care of daily necessities, including shopping and clothing; a80710, Recognizing the concept of money; a90100, Using aids for therapy and training; a90700, Using aids for communication, information, and signaling). This is consistent with the notion that the activities are to document the difficulties experienced by the individual in these day-to-day activities, whatever the cause. Hence, a person may have a limitation in drinking from a cup or glass without spilling (a50561) caused by different impairments such as a paresis of the arm or poor lip seal following a facial paresis.

The *participation* dimension deals with societal phenomena. It represents the person's degree of participation and society's response to either facilitating or hindering that participation. A fundamental feature of participation is the complex interaction between the person with the impairment or activity limitation and the context. There are seven domains of participation—participation in personal maintenance; mobility; exchange of information; social relationships; areas of education, work, leisure, and spirituality; economic life; and civic and community life. These seven life situations are slightly different to the seven survival roles included in the 1980 WHO handicap dimension.

The similarity between the participation dimension and the activity dimension is noted. There is particular similarity between the participation dimensions of exchange of information and the activity dimension of communication activities. There is also similarity between participation in social relationships and interpersonal behaviors activities. The difference is delineated, however, using an example of a person's inability to initiate social contact (an activity) and that person's participation in friendships (participation). If other people are not able to accommodate this inability and spend extra time in befriending the person, an effect on participation will occur. However, facilitators such as self-help associations and counsellors could successfully raise the level of participation in this area. Madden and Hogan (1997) make the point that the purposes of measuring participation are mostly orientated toward social policies and services.

Other points to note in the Beta draft of the ICIDH-2 is that the term "disease" has been substituted by the term "health condition" such that disablement associated with ageing, for example, can now be included in the classification scheme. In addition, the term "disablement" as well as the term "functioning" has continued to be used as overarching terms to describe the impairments, activity limitations, and participation restrictions that occur as a result of a health condition.

In summary, there are some inconsistencies between the terms used in the ICIDH-2 detailed classification scheme and the speech pathology literature (e.g., "understanding the description of a single object" as a communicative activity in the activity dimension). The clarification of some of the terms, however, has been helpful. There is still some way to go in the operationalization of the model through refinement of the classification scheme. WHO (1997) notes that future directions for the ICIDH-2 include the development of assessment instrument and the matching of treatments or interventions.

## Conclusion

The benefits of adopting the WHO model and contributing to its future development include (1) gaining international consensus and (2) maintaining consistent terminology with other professions involved in rehabilitation. There is certainly a need for this in the area of functional communication.

The major contribution of the ICIDH-2 has been the statement that functioning refers to all levels of impairments, disabilities, and handicaps. This is consistent with Wilkerson's model cited by Ramsberger (1994) of micro-, middle-, and macro-level functioning. It is also consistent with the speech-language pathology literature to the extent that functioning has been associated with each of the dimensions. The functional approach could therefore be considered an overarching concept to describe the process of disablement that results from a health condition. However, it is argued that the concept of functional communication as used by speech-language pathologists does not extend into the impairment realm and should therefore be reserved for describing the dimensions of activities and participation.

The ongoing debate in the literature about the nature of functional communication appears to be more about which of the approaches described are most functional. Consider the statement of Kagan and Gailey (1993) that functional is not enough. This is relative to the disability level of functional communication measures. Pragmatic assessments and conversational or discourse analyses are more "functional" than acontextual tests. Worrall (1992, 1995) and Parr's (1996a) contention that the client also needs to be involved in establishing what items should be assessed is considered to be more "functional" because the items are then relevant to the individual. Hence, functional communication becomes more "functional" as context increases along the ICIDH continuum.

The conceptual framework of the ICIDH also reinforces the proposal that there cannot be one dimension, assessment, treatment, or service that is functional. There is a need for a diverse range of levels at which speech-language pathologists operate, an argument for a portfolio of assessment instruments available for clinicians, and a demand for a range of treatments and services from which clinicians and clients can choose. Hence, the conceptual framework of the ICIDH could be used by speech-language pathologists to diversify their role.

Currently, however, there is greater need at the participation end of the continuum. There is a demand for more community-based centers such as the Aphasia Center in Ontario and more research is required on how the social model can be adopted by speech-language pathologists. Measuring instruments that capture the participation level of clients are also urgently required.

The development of more tools that measure everyday communicative activities is also a necessity. As WHO (1997) notes, the range of potential activities that could be included in the activities dimension is huge. Ethnographic research needs to identify the simple and complex communicative activities that occur in the everyday life of our clients in the first instance. Then the issues of individual variation, cultural variation, and contextual variation, can be discussed.

Consistency of terminology is imperative for all professions. Speech-language pathologists require more sophisticated terms than "functional communication" to describe the process of disablement resulting from acquired neurogenic communication disorders. As far as possible the terms used should reflect those in the ICIDH-2. Hence, at the impairment level, the terms speech, language, and swallowing impairment should be used. In the activity dimension, the term activity limitation in communication or interpersonal behavior should be used. In the participation dimension, the term participation restriction in social relationships or exchange of information should occur. Madden and Hogan (1997) note that there is a view in developing countries that a change of terminology will be confusing to countries that are only beginning to understand the original concepts. This may also be true for professions such as speech-language pathology. Hence, the terms disability and handicap may continue to be used for some time.

The shift from using the term functional communication to more specific terms may not be a popular change, however, if rehabilitation is to embrace the social model as well as the medical model, a change in terminology may be the catalyst for the process of change.

Speech-language pathologists also need to look to the detail of the classification scheme and extract what is useful and contribute to attempts to make the scheme more operational. The authors of this book have been encouraged to use the ICIDH-2 as a conceptual framework for their discussions. They have also been encouraged to use the terminology of the ICIDH-2 wherever possible. This may ultimately lead us a step closer to describing the true nature of the functional approach to neurogenic disorders. Understanding the nature of disablement will ultimately mean that speech-language pathologists can make a real difference to the real lives of their clients.

## References

American Speech-Language-Hearing Association (1990). *Functional communication measures project: Advisory report.* Rockville, MD: ASHA.

Baker, R. (1995). Communicative needs and bilingualism in elderly Australian of six ethnic backgrounds. *Australian Journal on Ageing, 14,* 81–88.

Beukelman, D. R., Yorkston, K. M., & Lossing, C. A. (1984). Functional communication assessment of adults with neurogenic disorders. In A. S. Halpern and M. J. Fuhrer (eds): *Functional assessment in rehabilitation* (pp. 101–115). Baltimore, MD: Paul H Brooks.

Blomert, L., Kean, M. L., Koster, C., & Schokker, J. (1994). Amsterdam–Nijmegan Everyday Language Test: Construction, reliability, and validity. *Aphasiology, 8,* 381–407.

Carey, R. (1990). Advances in rehabilitation program evaluation. In M. R. Eisenberg and R. C. Grzesiak (eds): *Advances in clinical rehabilitation* (Vol. 3, pp. 217–250). New York: Springer.

Chamie, M. (1990). The status and use of the international classification of impairments, disabilities and handicaps (ICIDH). *World Health Statistics Quarterly, 43,* 273–280.

Chapey, R. (1992). Functional communication assessment and intervention: Some thoughts on the state of the art. *Aphasiology, 6,* 85–94.

Davis, G. A., & Wilcox, M. J. (1985). *Adult aphasia rehabilitation: Applied pragmatics.* San Diego: College Hill.

Dickson, H. G. (1996). Problems with the ICIDH definition of impairment. Clinical commentary. *Disability and Rehabilitation, 18,* 52–54.

Elman, R., & Bernstein-Ellis, E. (1995). What is functional? *American Journal of Speech-Language Pathology, 4,* 115–117.

Enderby, P (1997). *Therapy outcome measures: Speech-Language pathology technical manual.* Singular publishing Group, London.

Ferguson, A. (1994). The influence of aphasia, familiarity and activity on conversational repair. *Aphasiology, 8,* 143–157.

Fairclough, N. (1989). *Language and power.* London: Longman.

Frattali, C. M. (1992a). Functional assessment of communication: merging public policy with clinical views. *Aphasiology, 6*, 63–83.

Frattali, C. M. (1992b). Beyond barriers: A reply to Chapey, Sacchett and Marshall, Scherzer, and Worrall. *Aphasiology, 6*, 111–116.

Frattali, C. M. (1993). Perspectives on functional assessment: Its use for policy making. *Disability and Rehabilitation, 15*, 1–9.

Frattali, C. (1994). Functional assessment. In R. Lubinski and C. Frattali (eds): *Professional issues in speech-language pathology and audiology* (pp. 306–320). San Diego, CA: Singular Publishing Group.

Frattali, C. M., Thompson, C. M., Holland, A. L., Wohl, C. B., & Ferketic, M. M. (1995a). ASHA FACS—A functional outcome measure for adults. *ASHA*, April, 1995, 41–46.

Frattali, C. M., Thompson, C. M., Holland, A. L., Wohl, C. B., & Ferketic, M. M. (1995b). *ASHA functional assessment of communication skills (FACS)*. Rockville, MD: American Speech-Language-Hearing Association.

Gurland, G. B., Chwat, S. E., & Wollner, S. G. (1982). Establishing a communication profile in adult aphasia: Analysis of communicative acts and conversational sequences. In R. H. Brookshire (ed): *Clinical aphasiology: Conference proceedings* (pp. 18–27). Minneapolis, MN: BRK Publishers.

Hartley, L. L. (1992). Assessment of functional communication. *Seminars in Speech and Language, 13*, 264–279.

Holland, A. L. (1980). *Communicative abilities in daily living*. Baltimore, MD: University Park Press.

Holland, A. L. (1982). Observing functional communication of aphasic adults. *Journal of Speech and Hearing Disorders, 47*, 50–56.

Holland, A. L. (1994). A look into a cloudy crystal ball for specialists in neurogenic language disorders. *American Journal of Speech-Language Pathology*, September, 34–6.

Holland, A., Frattali, C., & Fromm, D. (1998). *Communicative activities of daily living—Second edition (CADL-2)*. Austin, TX: ProEd.

Jette, A. M. (1984). Concepts of health and methodological issues in functional assessment. In C. V. Granger and G. E. Gresham (ed): *Functional assessment in rehabilitation medicine* (pp. 46–64). Baltimore, MD: Williams and Wilkins.

Johnston, M. (1996). Models of disability. *The Psychologist*, May, 205–210.

Kagan, A., & Gailey, G. F. (1993). Functional is not enough: Training conversation partners for aphasic adults. In A. L. Holland & M. M. Forbes (eds): *Aphasia treatment: World perspectives* (pp. 199–225). San Diego: Singular Publishing Group Inc.

Lomas, J., Pickard, L., Bester, S., Elbard, H., Finlayson, A., & Zoghaib, C. (1989). The communicative effectiveness index: Development and psychometric evaluation of a functional communication measure for adult aphasia. *Journal of Speech and Hearing Disorders, 54*, 113–124.

Lyon, J. (1998). Treating real-life functionality in a couple coping with severe aphasia. In N. Helm-Estabrooks and A. L. Holland (eds): *Approaches to the treatment of aphasia* (pp. 203–239). San Diego, CA: Singular Publishing Group.

Madden, R., & Hogan, T. (1997). *The definition of disability in Australia: Moving towards national consistency*. AIHW cat.No. DIS 5. Canberra: Australian Institute of Health and Welfare.

Manochiopinig, S., Sheard, C., & Reed, V. A. (1992). Pragmatic assessment in adult aphasia: A clinical review. *Aphasiology, 6*, 519–533.

Marks, D. (1997). Models of disability. *Disability and Rehabilitation, 19*, 85–91.

Nagi, S. Z. (1965). Some conceptual issues in disability and rehabilitation. In M. B. Sussman (ed): *Sociology and Rehabilitation*. Washington, DC: American Sociological Association.

Parr, S. (1996a). Everyday literacy in aphasia: Radical approaches to functional assessment and therapy. *Aphasiology, 10*, 469–479.

Parr, S. (1996b). The road more travelled: Whose right of way? *Aphasiology, 10*, 496–503.

Payne, J. (1994). *Communication profile: A functional skills survey*. Tucson, AZ: Communication Skill Builders.

Penn, C. (1985). The profile of communicative appropriateness: A clinical tool for the assessment of pragmatics. *The South African Journal of Communication Disorders, 32*, 18–23.

Pierce, R. S. (1996). Read and write what you want to: What's so radical? *Aphasiology, 10*, 480–483.

Prutting, C. A., & Kirchner, D. M. (1987). A clinical appraisal of the pragmatic aspects of language. *Journal of Speech and Hearing Disorders, 52*, 105–119.

Ramsberger, G. (1994). Functional perspective for assessment and rehabilitation of persons with severe aphasia. *Seminars in Speech and Language, 15*, 1–16.

Sarno, M. T. (1969). *The functional communication profile: Manual of directions*. New York: Institute of Rehabilitation Medicine.

Sarno, M. T. (1983). The functional assessment of verbal impairment. In G. Grimby (ed): *Recent advances in rehabilitation medicine* Stockholm: Almquist &Wiksell, Int.

Simmons-Mackie, N. N., & Damico, J. S. (1995). Communicative competence in aphasia: Evidence from compensatory strategies. *Clinical Aphasiology Conference Proceedings, 23,* 95–105.

Skinner, C., Wirz, S., Thompson, I., & Davidson, J. (1984). Edinburgh Functional Communication Profile. (Winslow, Buckingham: Winslow Press.

Smith, L. E. (1985). Communicative activities of dysphasic adults: A survey. *British Journal of Disorders of Communication, 20,* 31–44.

Thuriaux, M. C. (1995). The ICIDH: Evolution, status, and prospects. *Disability and Rehabilitation, 17 (3/4),* 112–118.

Ulatowska, H. K. Allard, L., Reyes, B. A. Ford, J., & Chapman, S. (1992). Conversational discourse in aphasia. *Aphasiology, 6,* 325–331.

Ustan, T. B., Cooper, J. E., Van Duuren-Kristen, S., Kennedy, C., Hendershot, G., & Sartorius, N. in collaboration with WHO/MNH Disability Working Group (1995). Revision of the ICIDH: mental health aspects. *Disability and Rehabilitation, 17,* 202–209.

Verbrugge, L. M., & Jette, A. M. (1994). The disablement process. *Social Science and Medicine, 38,* 1–14.

WCC (June,1989). *The ICIDH. A study of how it is used and evaluated.* Nationale Raad voor de Volsgezondheid, WCC, Dutch Classification and Terminology Committee for Health, P.O. Box 7100, 2701 AC Zoetermeer, The Netherlands.

WCC (May, 1989). *Draft WCC-standard. Terms for classifications and definitions.* Nationale Raad voor de Volsgezondheid, WCC, Dutch Classification and Terminology Committee for Health, P.O. Box 7100, 2701 AC Zoetermeer, The Netherlands.

WCC (1994). *A Survey of Criticism About the Classification of Impairments and the Classification of Disabilities of the International Classification of Impairments, Disabilities, and Handicaps (ICIDH).* Nationale Raad voor de Volsgezondheid, WCC, Dutch Classification and Terminology Committee for Health, P.O. Box 7100, 2701 AC Zoetermeer, The Netherlands.

Wilson, I. B., & Cleary, P. D. (1995). Linking clinical variables with health-related quality of life. *Journal of American Medical Association, 273,* 59–68.

Wood, P. H. N. (1980). The language of disablement—A glossary relating to disease and its consequences. *International Rehabilitation Medicine, 2,* 86–92.

World Health Organization (WHO) (1980). *International Classification of Impairments, Disabilities, and Handicaps.* Geneva: World Health Organization.

World Health Organization (WHO) (1997). ICIDH-2 International Classification of Impairments, Activities, and Participation [http://www.who.ch/programmes/mnh/mnh/ems/icidh/icidh.htm].

Worrall, L. (1992). Functional communication assessment: An Australian perspective. *Aphasiology, 6,* 105–110.

Worrall, L. (1995). The functional communication perspective. In D. Muller and C. Code (eds): *Treatment of aphasia.* London: Whurr Publishers.

Wyller, T. B. (1997). Disability models in geriatrics. *Disability & Rehabilitation, 19,* 480–483.

# 2

# *The Assessment of Activity Limitation in Functional Communication: Challenges and Choices*

## Bronwyn J. Davidson
## Linda E. Worrall

Many existing functional communication assessments attempt to measure communicative activity limitation (disability). This chapter explores the concept of activity limitation in the ICIDH-2 in more detail and describes some Australian research that characterizes communication at the Activity level. It then describes several parameters that vary within functional communication assessments at the Activity level. It is suggested that these parameters may be useful for clinicians who are needing to select appropriate functional communication assessments.

## Introduction

The role of the speech-language pathologist is expanding. Not only is there a need to be skilled in assessment of the nature and severity of a communication or swallowing impairment, but increasingly, speech-language pathologists are involved in defining the impact of acquired neurogenic disorders of communication and swallowing on people's everyday lives. Thus, there is a growing demand for functional communication and swallowing measures.

This chapter discusses issues related to the measurement of communication and swallowing at the disability or activity limitation level. It is recognized that "disability" is an overused term; a term often defined differently by those with disabilities, clinicians, policy makers, people in the "disability movement" and by medical and social scientists. In this chapter, the term is used in the context of the World Health Organization's (WHO) International Classification of Impairments, Disabilities and Handicaps (ICIDH) framework (WHO, 1980) as described in Chapter 1. The term "disability" is used interchangeably with "activity limitation" in line with the revised version of the ICIDH (WHO, 1997). Both these frameworks are described in Chapter 1.

The aims of this chapter are threefold. The first aim is to explore the concept of disability in some detail within the ICIDH-2. In addition, a model is proposed that describes the relationship between the Activity dimension and the other aspects of the ICIDH-2. The second aim is to describe some ethnographic research that details the communicative activities that occur in everyday life. The final aim is to identify some parameters that differentiate communicative disability measures so that clinicians and researchers are aware of the many different types of assessments of everyday communicative activity that are required in clinical practice. This chapter draws heavily on examples from the field of aphasiology. It also seeks, however, to be inclusive of measures at the level of disability for the range of acquired neurogenic disorders of communication and swallowing.

## What is a Disability or Activity Limitation?

To briefly summarize some definitions from Chapter 1, in the original ICIDH framework (WHO, 1980), disability is defined as a restriction or lack of ability to perform an everyday activity. The emphasis is clearly on the impact of a particular impairment on that person's ability to engage in his or her usual daily activities. In the proposed revised version, the broad term of disability is replaced by the neutral term Activity, with the negative term being Activity limitation. Upper case is used to distinguish the dimension of Activities in the ICIDH-2 from the everyday use of the term "activities." An Activity is the "nature and extent of functioning at the level of the person. Activities may be limited in nature, duration and quality" (WHO, 1997, p. 13).

While the ICIDH is most noted for its model of disablement, there is also a highly detailed classification scheme creating taxonomies of various Impairments, Activities, and Participation. In the Activity dimension, the classification scheme of the ICIDH-2 lists many Activities ranging from simple actions such as seeing and hearing to complex Activities such as performing a job. A key feature of the Activity code is objectification, that is, the actual limitation or performance as measured in everyday life. It is assessed against a norm. Activities may also be carried out using an aid or with the help of another person. The classification scheme divides the Activity dimension into 10 "chapters" or sections: (1) seeing, hearing, and recognizing; (2) learning, applying knowledge, and performing tasks; (3) communication activities; (4) movement activities; (5) moving around; (6) daily life activities; (7) care of necessities and domestic activities; (8) interpersonal behaviors; (9) responding to and dealing with particular situations; and (10) use of assistive devices, technical aids, and other related activities.

WHO notes that the potential range of Activities that could be included is wide. However, despite its complexity, the ICIDH-2 classification scheme has the potential to inform speech-language pathologists seeking to assess the consequences of a hearing, voice, speech, language, or swallowing impairment on the everyday activities of an individual. Activities that require communication skills are spread throughout the entire Activity dimension although the two chapters on communication activities (3) and interpersonal behaviors (8) deal with Activities specifically affected by a speech or language impairment. The advantages of the ICIDH-2 classification scheme are that it is an international consensus document that aims to be appropriate to all countries and all cultures. It and its successors, therefore, may prove to be a useful scaffold for developing universal measures of functional communication at the disability or activity limitation level.

Consistent with the ICIDH-2 framework, two criteria emerge for defining measures at the disability (activity) level: (1) measurement is focussed at the level of the person and (2) measurement records performance in everyday life activities (i.e., in naturalistic contexts).

These two criteria are illustrated within the WHO model of disablement and it is important to develop an understanding of this model to appreciate the concept of functional communication at the Disability or Activity level. In the next section, a further model is proposed to illustrate the concepts of the ICIDH-2 to speech-language pathologists.

## A Model of Disablement for Speech-Language Pathologists

Figure 2–1 reproduces the model of the ICIDH-2. This illustrates how a health condition impacts on Impairment, Activity, and Participation. The influence is multidirectional. It also suggests that context (environmental and personal) affects Impairments, Activities, and Participation. It does not, however, illustrate

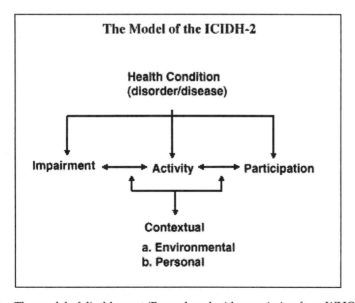

**Figure 2–1.**   The model of disablement (Reproduced with permission from WHO, 1997, p. 7).

particularly well the important relationship between context and the dimensions of Impairments, Activities, and Participation. The relationship between context and the dimensions of the ICIDH-2 is an important concept for speech-language pathologists to understand. Once this relationship is clear, the place of Activity between Impairments and Participation is also clarified.

Figure 2–2 illustrates how the dimensions of Impairments, Activities, and Participation exist in relation to context. The primary feature of this model is the relationship between the amount of context and each of the ICIDH-2 dimensions. In the model, as within rehabilitation, context can be either restricted when assessing impairment (as it is at the base of the cone) or it can be unrestricted when assessing overall participation in life (as it is at the top of the cone). Starting at the base of the cone, context is deliberately restricted when assessing impairment. For example, aphasia test items such as those in the Western Aphasia Battery (Kertesz, 1982), are decontextualized so that clues provided by context do not mask the specific impairment. The base of the cone (the impairments) defines the structural components and provides scaffolding for the other dimensions. Hence, impairment level functions and structures are the basic components that underpin the effect that a disorder may have on a person's communication or swallowing activities and participation in society. Hence, this is why impairment

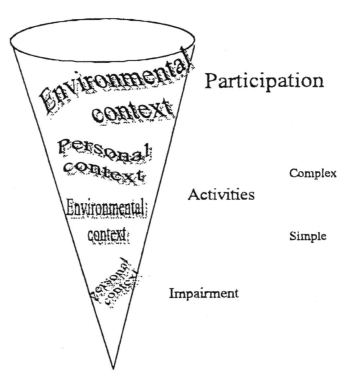

**Figure 2–2.** Model of the relationship between Impairments, Activities, Participation, and Context.

measures are said to be at the body level (i.e., structure and function of parts of the body) rather than Activity measures, which are performed by the person as a whole. Tests that measure at the Activity level such as the Communicative Abilities in Daily Living (Holland, 1980) and its second edition, the Communication Activities of Daily Living (Holland et al., 1998), deliberately include context to determine how well a person performs within the usual cues that are available in everyday settings. At the Participation level, incorporating societal factors (cultural and societal influences) broadens context even further. The increasing role of context within the ICIDH-2 is encapsulated within the definitions that place Impairments at the level of the body, Activities at the level of the person, and Participation at the level of society. Context is divided into personal and environmental context in the ICIDH-2 model. Hence, the Activity dimension focuses on the inclusion of personal and environmental context at the level of the person, rather than at the level of the body or society.

The second feature of this model is that there are no borders between Impairments, Activities, or Participation. For speech-language pathologists, this is an important concept because many assessments and interventions do not fit easily into one dimension or another. Rather, some assessments fit between dimensions or incorporate several dimensions. Hence, it could be argued that Impairments, Activities, and Participation are not separate entities but merely points along a continuum. The boundary between Activity and Participation within a communication context becomes particularly blurred because communication is essentially a participatory activity. The distinction is that while a communicative activity may be performed well by a person with a communication disorder, there may still be barriers to the person's participation in society (e.g., discriminatory policies, lack of understanding of communication disorder by the general public). Both concepts of Activity and Participation are encapsulated within the term functional communication.

The ICIDH-2 separates the Activity dimension into simple and complex activities. Many of the simple activities could be described as speech acts (Searle et al., 1980). These have been used in functional communication assessments such as the Edinburgh Functional Communication Profile—EFCP (Skinner et al., 1984). More complex communicative activities such as "Responds in an emergency (e.g., calls 911)" are contained in assessments such as the ASHA Functional Assessment of Communication Skills for Adults—ASHA FACS (Frattali et al., 1995). Even more complex and integrated activities like phoning to arrange complex travel bookings or phoning to inquire about health-care insurance options are not often contained in functional communication assessments.

## Describing Communication Activities

The model described in the previous section has served to describe some of the features of the Impairments, Activities, and Participation dimensions so that speech-language pathologists can identify Activity level measures of communication and swallowing. The next section focuses on the Activity level in more detail and sets out to describe the nature of everyday communicative activities in particular. First, it describes two issues in Activity level measurement that have a profound influence on the description of communicative activities. The next section explores how communicative activities are described within the ICIDH-2. It then describes an example of ethnographic research that examines the adequacy and complexity of any description of communicative activity.

### Issues in Defining Communicative Activities in Speech-Language Pathology

In the field of speech-language pathology, there has been a tendency to focus on the simple communication activities rather than the more complex. Within interdisciplinary rehabilitation teams, functional assessments need to be transparent to other disciplines, hence the attractiveness of the activity-based descriptions of performance that have gained prominence within the rehabilitation sector.

Another issue in describing communication activities relates to the conceptualization of the function of communication in everyday life. Traditionally, in speech-language pathology, the emphasis in assessments has been on information exchange or "getting the message across." Simmons-Mackie and Damico (1996) provide a timely reminder of the dual role of communicative acts in message transfer (transactional communication activity) and in social affiliation (interactional communication).

### How Does the ICIDH-2 Describe Communication Activities?

Models of disablement such as the ICIDH-2 are beginning to provide the theoretical foundations for the development of Activity based measures. The ICIDH-2 for example has progressed to a level of detail in which a definition of communication activities has been offered. The ICIDH-2 states that

> Communication activities involve at least two active participants, both of whom send and receive messages. They include the ability to formulate messages and interpret and understand messages received. Non-verbal means of communication such as facial expression and gestures are also included. (WHO, 1997, p. 139)

This definition encompasses transactional communication but does not include interactional communication. This is covered to some degree in the ICIDH-2 chapter on interpersonal behaviors that "constitute a person's engagement in social situations. Such situations may range from the familiar to the unfamiliar, may involve few or many people and may be predictable or unpredictable" (WHO, 1997, p. 172). In summary, while the ICIDH-2 classification scheme provides a useful starting point, there is a clear need for speech-language pathologists to examine and modify the classification scheme in this area.

### The Contribution of Ethnographic Research

As speech-language pathologists seek to develop measures that assess Activity limitation, it is of note that there are calls for research which use ethnographic methodology to capture the dynamics of authentic communication and naturalistic interaction (Parr, 1996; Simmons, 1993). Holland (1982) reported on the richness of data collected from systematic observations of 40 people with aphasia. Kagan (1998), Kagan and Gailey (1993), Lyon (1992), Lyon et al. (1997), Parr (1996), and Simmons-Mackie and Damico (1996) are among the clinicians and researchers who have taken up the challenge to undertake detailed and rigorous ethnographic studies of people with acquired neurogenic disorders of communication.

Davidson et al. (1998) have used ethnographic methodologies to document the communicative activities of healthy older people and people with aphasia following stroke in Australia. In this study, a total 240 hours of observation have been coded and the everyday communication activities of 30 older Australians detailed (15 with aphasia compared with 15 healthy older people). The researcher, in the role of participant observer during the person's usual daily activities, took field notes on the communication of each subject for a total of 8 hours over three visits. Diary entries by participants and carers served as a check on the representativeness of the observational period. Integral to the process of coding communication activities was the description/inclusion of contextual features. These included place and time (where and when the communication occurred), the participants in the communication, the mode of communication (written, spoken, gesture, listening, reading, facial expression), and the duration and topic of communication.

A multitude of communication activities was observed. Conversations with family and friends were the foremost communication activities. There was also strong evidence that communication was not only for the exchange of information but also for social affiliation. Greetings, exchanges about the weather, talking to pets, brief comments and asides, expressions of affection, and an affirming touch on the arm were examples of interactional activities. Asking specific questions, requesting shopping items, writing checks, making a speech, doing crossword puzzles, discussing photos, making phone calls, placing bets, listening to directions and television, and reading pamphlets were coded as transactional activities. Conversational activities and telling stories and jokes served the dual roles of interaction and transaction.

While a comparison of the observed communication activities of the group of aphasics and healthy older people suggested that there were no major differences in the types of activities coded, the differences were that the healthy older people communicated more frequently, more elaborately, and for a longer duration. Thus, the Activity limitation is described in quantitative and qualitative terms. Analysis of the types of communication partners also pointed to differences in the nature of communication activities. For example, during the observation period, the aphasic people communicated with more health professionals while the healthy older people were observed communicating with more shop assistants and trades people. Family members, friends, and neighbors were important communication partners for both groups.

This study illuminated important factors in identifying a communication activity. The spontaneity and subtleties of naturalistic communication demanded that a number of interacting factors be recognized. Activities were described in terms of complexity; for example, an episode of communication may have been a simple greeting or a lengthy telephone call involving complex arrangements, discussion of politics, and reminiscences of family gatherings. Contextual variables meant that a communication activity may have occurred in isolation or as part of concurrent activities. Also, the communication activity was detailed in terms of seven variables—place, time, communication partner, topic, duration, interactional/transactional components, and mode of communication (listening, speaking, gesture, writing, reading, and facial expressions).

This study highlighted factors crucial to an understanding of measurement at the level of Activity (disability). Detailed observations of both groups revealed the importance of describing a communication activity in relation to the context in which it took place. In particular, the observational study served to emphasize the clinical importance of finding out who the person's communication partners are. Communication activities are inextricably bound by the nature of the person's relationships (e.g., spouse, daughter, shop keeper, friend, acquaintance, therapist), and the communication environment (e.g., home, shopping center, workplace, club, nursing home, hospital). Any measure of communication disability needs to try to capture an authentic sample of everyday communication activities identified as relevant for the person with a communication impairment. The challenge is to retain a description of the complex, unique, and dynamic features of communication for that person within a clinically feasible assessment. A further challenge is to use observations of real-life communication as a basis for the description of communicative activities in classification schemes such as the ICIDH-2 or as a basis for the selection of items in assessments of communicative activity.

This study has demonstrated the richness of data generated from observations of communication in natural settings. Speech-language pathologists have much to gain from social research including interviewing, observation, and documentation. Qualitative research methods provide tools especially sensitive to the social context in which data are produced (Mason, 1996). The challenge is to translate these techniques into tools that clinicians can use reliably, validly, and efficiently.

In summary, the description of everyday communicative activities is in its infancy. Consensus needs to be sought on some fundamental issues relating to the area. Speech-language pathologists need to contribute to the development of the communication aspects of the classification scheme of the ICIDH-2. Finally, ethnographic research is a particularly powerful method for describing authentic everyday communication and it shows great potential for informing speech-language pathologists about the nature of communicative activities.

## Measuring Communication Activity Limitation: A Matter of Choice

The aim of the following section is to provide clinicians with a framework whereby they can choose a functional communication assessment that suits their needs. In particular, the next section is aimed at describing the distinguishing features of existing measures of communicative activity limitation. Several parameters are described that serve to make the decision-making task in choosing a functional communication assessment easier for clinicians and researchers alike. The decision-making process would typically begin with the clinician or researcher considering a broad range of functional communication assessments, whether or not they focus on the Activity dimension.

Currently there exists a range of measures of functional communication. Each measure has a different emphasis or purpose and it is likely that the range of functional communication assessments will expand in the future in response to demands from clinicians. It is also becoming increasingly evident that no one assessment will suit all purposes. Frattali (1993) cites Carey (1990) as stating that it is unlikely that someone will invent a car that has the luxury of a big car and the fuel efficiency of a small car or the flexibility of a truck used for hauling different farm machinery. It is also unlikely that one functional communication measure will be designed that will suit all individuals, all impairments, and all cultures in all settings.

The parameters that might guide a clinician's choice of functional communication assessment are: (1) the ICIDH-2 dimension upon which the assessment focuses; (2) the purpose of the assessment; (3) the setting for which the assessment was designed; (4) the type of communication disorder for which the measure was designed; (5) the extent of item sampling; (6) the method of data collection; and (7) the method of scoring.

## ICIDH-2 Dimension Focus

The first parameter is whether the assessment focuses on the Activity dimension of the ICIDH-2 or whether it is a measure of Participation. In addition, some measures may have elements of each dimension of the ICIDH-2. While clinicians may not be concerned with whether the assessment neatly fits into one of those categories, it is suggested that clinicians need to have a general sense of the conceptual basis of the assessment.

In a policy climate that encourages the measurement of outcome, clinicians also need to know that they have assessed each dimension. Both Frattali (1998) and Enderby and John (1997) suggest that WHO's ICIDH is a useful framework for measuring outcome. Measuring performance at each level therefore becomes important and clinicians need to be aware of how each assessment is classified using the ICIDH framework. The reader is referred to various chapters within Frattali (1998) for excellent reviews of measures in each of the communication or swallowing disorders. For example, Holland and Thompson (1998) review outcome measures in aphasia and categorize each measure according to whether it assesses impairment, disability, or handicap. Measures of disability, for example, include the ASHA FACS (Frattali et al., 1995) and the Communicative Effectiveness Index—CETI (Lomas et al., 1989). Similarly, the reader is referred to chapters in Frattali (1998), which review measures of impairment, disability, and handicap in cognitive communication disorders (traumatic brain injury, right hemisphere brain damage, dementia), dysphagia, motor speech disorders, and voice disorders.

## Purpose

The second consideration should be the purpose of the assessment. Impairment level assessments are used for screening, diagnostic assessment, assessment for counseling and rehabilitation, and progressive evaluation or change in performance (Spreen & Risser, 1991). Functional communication assessments can also be used for these purposes. With the current emphasis on outcome measurement, many functional assessments are being developed to suit this purpose (see Frattali, 1998). Well-known functional communication assessments such as the ASHA FACS (Frattali et al., 1995), and the Communicative Abilities in Daily Living—CADL (Holland, 1980) were developed to enhance treatment planning, client/family counseling, and documentation of progress. The CETI (Lomas et al., 1989) was developed specifically as a measure of change. Although there are limited assessments designed for screening purposes or discharge purposes, demand for such assessments will grow as services that target functional communication develop.

## Setting

The third parameter is the setting for which the assessment was designed. There is a commonly held perception that functional communication assessment is only relevant to the later phases of a client's management. McCooey et al. (Chapter 17) argue that there is a need to examine the everyday communicative difficulties of clients while they are hospital in-patients. Pye et al. (Chapter 18) state that assessments designed for the hospital setting do not transfer readily to the extended care facility and therefore suggest that there is a need for functional communication assessments specifically designed for that setting. Hence, the third parameter specifies for which clinical setting the assessment was designed.

## Type of Communication Disorder

The fourth consideration is the population or type of communication disorder for which the assessment was designed. While many functional communication assessments have been primarily designed for people with aphasia, several authors in this book (Larkins, Chapter 12; Lubinski and Orange, Chapter 13; Enderby, Chapter 14; and Cherney and Halper, Chapter 16) have described how different disorders affect functional communication. As noted earlier, reviews of measures of impairment, disability, and handicap for each type of voice, fluency, speech, language, and swallowing disorder is contained in Frattali (1998). Functional communication assessments such as the ASHA FACS (Frattali et al., 1995) have been trialed on both people with aphasia following stroke, and cognitive communication disorder following traumatic brain injury. It is therefore suggested that some functional communication assessments will be more suitable for some communication disorders than others.

## Extent of Item Sampling

A further consideration is whether the assessment contains only a basic or core set of everyday communicative activities that are suitable for all clients or whether individual needs are addressed in an extended list of everyday communication items. Several authors (Elman & Bernstein-Ellis, 1995; Frattali, 1992;

Parr, 1996; Pierce, 1996; Sarno, 1983; Smith, 1985; Worrall, 1995) have noted that individual aphasic people have differing needs. Illustrating opposite ends of the spectrum, Worrall (1995) describes a patient who virtually lived the life of a recluse and had few communicative needs, while Elman and Bernstein-Ellis (1995) described a dentist who had many communicative needs. Their communicative needs may be dictated by their present social situation, premorbid communicative activities, the roles that they wish to return to or develop, their personality, their motivation, their existing level of impairment, social network, and the personal support that they receive. This makes it difficult to design a measure that will be applicable to all individuals. For example, in selecting activities for the ASHA FACS, consideration was given to whether the majority of people with aphasia carried out the activity. Hence, only a set of core activities was included in the ASHA FACS. Communicative activities such as reading knitting patterns or chairing meetings were not included because they are highly individualistic.

Another approach is to only assess the performance of the patient on activities identified as important and relevant by that person. This is an approach advocated by Beukelman et al. (1984) and Worrall (1995). Parr (1996) goes further and suggests that the power of the therapeutic relationship must be handed over to the aphasic individual. Parr states that qualitative research methods must determine the needs of the patient rather than the use of a preset menu of possibilities.

Parr (1996) and Sacchett and Marshall (1992) contend that another issue to address in functional communication assessments is whether the assessment is sensitive to important sociolinguistic and cultural differences. For example, Smith and Parr (1986) found that a disadvantage of the CADL (Holland, 1980) for British speech therapists was the North American culture bias. There are two approaches to this problem. One is that functional communication assessments should use activities culturally appropriate to the specific population with whom the assessment will be used. For example, the inclusion of items such as placing bets on horses may be relevant for an Australian and Hong Kong assessment where punting is a popular pastime, but it may be inappropriate in other countries where it is not. The other approach is to only include items that do not have cultural bias. That is, it should be a universal measure. This would lead to a more restricted set of items. This was the approach taken in the ASHA FACS that used field testing and national and international panels to rule out cultural bias. Ideally, clinicians should have access to both types of instruments: the universal and the culturally specific. Clinicians should be able to access those assessments that are designed to assess a broad range of culturally appropriate items for their client base. They should also be able to access instruments that allow them to assess clients without cultural bias that allows them to compare their scores to data obtained elsewhere in the world.

### Method of Data Collection

Another consideration is whether the assessment is based on observation, simulation, or report. One of the issues raised by researchers and clinicians interested in the assessment of everyday communication relates to the method of assessment of functional performance. Three main methods are identified: direct observation, simulation, and reported assessment.

## DIRECT OBSERVATION

Holland (1982) argues the case for real-life observation being the gold standard of evaluation of everyday communication. Four hours of systematic observation was used to validate the CADL (Holland, 1980). Like many gold standards, performance evaluation in the clinical situation that is based exclusively on extensive real-life observation, is impractical. It is time consuming to observe a patient in the wide variety of activities that are demanded when the examiner is attempting to gain a representative sample of everyday communicative activities. It may also not be cost efficient for the hospital-based speech-language pathologist to shadow the patient at home and in the community. Despite these practical constraints, the face validity of direct observation of communication in a natural environment is very high. It is often for these reasons that performance on simulated tasks or reported performance in real-life situations is frequently used as the clinical tool of functional communication assessment.

## SIMULATION

Simulated activities are often criticized for not sampling natural communication. Natural behavior can, however, be elicited in a simulated situation. Eliciting natural behavior is particularly advantageous when rarely occurring behaviors such as "getting help in an emergency" are to be observed or when repeated samples are required (Scherer & Ekman, 1982). The setting does not have to be real-life to sample natural behavior. The chances of obtaining natural behavior increase, however, when the elicitation procedure is as close to real-life as possible. There are also degrees of simulation. On one hand, the examiner can role play a situation that is unfamiliar to the patient using props that are also alien. On the other hand, situations can be created which mimic the real-life of the patient. For example, a patient may wish to be able to place horse-racing bets over the telephone. This is a familiar activity to the patient and the carer was asked for a description of how it was done. In the clinic, that situation is recreated using the day's racing guide in the newspaper, having the number stored in the phone's memory as it is at home, using the same type of phone, and knowing what information the telephone operator requests. Hence, simulated tasks can be quite real.

It is important, however, to verify if communication strategies that are encouraged and practiced in the clinic, are actually used in the dynamic and varied interchanges of social life. Simmons (1993) points out that since speakers' and listeners' goals are not simply transactional, but are also to achieve a socially acceptable and satisfying interaction, unconventional strategies might not be perceived as appropriate.

## REPORTED

There has always been debate about whether carers or speech-language pathologists are better and more accurate observers of everyday communication. Lomas et al. (1989) have used the significant others of people with aphasia to rate communicative effectiveness on the CETI because of the concern that clinicians have limited opportunity to observe functional communication. Clinicians may also be more inclined to rate competence (the potential to do the task) rather than performance (actually doing the task) when opportunities to observe performance are limited. In addition, Lomas et al. cited the study by Shewan and Cameron (1984), which showed that significant others showed a good level of agreement with aphasic patients on the presence or absence of particular communication problems. Helmick et al. (1976) compared spouses' and clinicians' judgment on the performance of aphasic individuals and found that spouses overestimate performance or perhaps clinicians underestimate performance. Holland (1982) found a high correlation between the interview in which significant others were asked to rate the performance of tasks that had an equivalent item in the CADL and the score on the CADL items. Her conclusion was that significant others judge aphasic performance more adequately than the limited amount of literature would predict.

It seems incredible that few studies or assessments report on the communication activities that aphasic people themselves have identified as important for them. How often is measurement of activity limitation driven by the person with the communication or swallowing disorder? What is the role of self-assessment in rating activity limitation? Worrall (1999) stresses the importance of involving the person with the communication disorder in describing the activities that are relevant to his or her everyday life; for establishing baseline measurements and in setting of therapy goals. Parr et al. (1997) record the experiences of people living with aphasia revealed through in-depth interviews. This qualitative research methodology is a powerful tool for unraveling the personal yet common issues surrounding communication activity limitation.

Some questions still need to be asked. Are there differences between ratings based on simulated communication activities, direct observation in a natural context, or reports of communicative behavior? Can the various methods be used interchangeably as in the ASHA FACS (i.e., observation or reports) or are they measuring different aspects of function? Which method is best for measuring performance in everyday communicative activities or are there advantages and disadvantages to each method? Further research is necessary in this pivotal area of functional communication assessment.

## Method of Scoring

The final consideration is how the assessment measures the performance of an activity, that is, how the assessment is rated or scored. Existing measures rate communicative performance differently. Most measures use an ordinal scale but vary on the type of scale used. Scales include a visual analogue scale, a unidimensional rating scale (i.e., one dimension rated on one scale) or multidimensional rating scale (i.e., multiple dimensions rated on one scale). Measures also vary on the anchors of the scale. The anchors or extreme points on the scale may be in absolute terms such as "does" or "does not" or may be relative terms that relate their current abilities to premorbid abilities. The parameters of the scale (e.g., dependency, effectiveness, appropriateness, efficiency) also vary across measures. The advantages and disadvantages of each type of scale are now discussed.

The advantage of the visual analogue scale such as that used by Lomas et al. (1989) in the CETI is that it is easily interpretable by nonprofessional raters. Because the CETI was specifically designed so that non-professionals could rate the communicative effectiveness of the person with aphasia, the visual analogue seems ideal for this measure. In contrast, other measures such as the Functional Communication Profile—FCP (Sarno, 1969) and the CADL (Holland, 1980) use a unidimensional ordinal rating scale. The ASHA FACS (Frattali et al., 1995) uses a unidimensional rating scale for communication independence and also rates qualitative dimensions on separate scales. The FCP and the CETI use a relative scale in which the person's performance is compared to his or her ability before the stroke. The CADL and the ASHA FACS, on the other hand, use an absolute scale with the ASHA FACS asking the examiner to judge whether the person does or does not do it on a seven point scale of communicative independence while the CADL uses a simple three point scale of communicative adequacy.

There is an issue of whether dependency or communicative burden should be seen to negatively affect overall functional communicative ability. The ability to communicate independently is emphasized in the ASHA definition of functional communication and is a primary parameter in the ordinal scales of the Functional Independence Measure (State University of New York at Buffalo, 1990). The ASHA FACS also includes the qualitative dimension of degree of communicative sharing. However, there is a body of literature that describes communication sharing (Kagan, 1998; Lyon, 1992; Parr, 1996) as a positive strategy in living with aphasia, rather than a problem of the person with a communication disability. Autonomy is a state that is sought by many people with aphasia and may well require a greater degree of interdependence in that some communicative "burden" is accepted by the carer (Parr, 1996).

In summary, clinicians and researchers need to become more sophisticated in the choices that are made. First, no one assessment will suit all needs. Parameters such as the conceptual focus of the assessment, purpose of the assessment, the setting and the type of communication disorder for which it was designed, the extent of item sampling, and method of data collection used, need to be carefully considered. The choice of an assessment can then be made with full knowledge of how the assessment differs from others.

## Conclusion

There are many challenges ahead in the development of functional communication measures that assess Activity Limitation. Challenges include the integration of theoretical constructs such as the ICIDH-2 into functional communication assessment within a clinical context. Another challenge is to transfer well-established research methodologies such as ethnographic methodology into the clinical setting. There are challenges to embrace socially driven models of communication and for speech-language pathologists to facilitate the person's identification of those communication activities pertinent to his or her lifestyle, relationships, and needs. A final challenge is to develop a diverse set of Activity-level functional communication assessments that cater to all needs so that clinicians can choose an assessment to meet their particular need. This chapter has sought to provide some groundwork for future efforts aimed at meeting these challenges.

## References

Beukelman, D. R., Yorkston, K. M., & Lossing, C. A. (1984). Functional communication assessment of adults with neurogenic disorders. In A. S. Halpern and M. J. Fuhrer (eds): *Functional assessment in rehabilitation* (pp. 101–115). Baltimore, MD: Paul H Brooks.

Carey, R. (1990). Advances in rehabilitation program evaluation. In M. R. Eisenberg and R. C. Grzesiak (eds): *Advances in clinical rehabilitation* (Vol. 3) New York: Springer.

Davidson, B., Worrall, L., & Hickson, L. (1998). Observed communication activities of people with aphasia and healthy older people. Paper presented at the *8th International Aphasia Rehabilitation Conference*, Kwa Maritane, South Africa.

Elman, R., & Bernstein-Ellis, E. (1995). What is functional? *American Journal of Speech-Language Pathology, 4*, 115–117.

Enderby, P., & John, A. (1997). *Therapy outcome measures: Speech-language pathology technical manual.* London: Singular Publishing Group.

Frattali, C. M. (1992). Functional assessment of communication: Merging public policy with clinical views. *Aphasiology, 6*, 63–83.

Frattali, C. M. (1993). Perspectives on functional assessment: Its use for policy making. *Disability and Rehabilitation, 15*, 1–9.

Frattali, C. M. (Ed) (1998). *Measuring outcomes in speech-language pathology.* New York: Thieme.

Frattali, C. M., Thompson, C. M., Holland, A. L., Wohl, C. B., & Ferketic, M. M. (1995). *ASHA Functional Assessment of Communication Skills for Adults (FACS).* Rockville, MD: American Speech-Language-Hearing Association.

Helmick, J. W., Watamori, T. S., & Palmer, J. M. (1976). Spouse's understanding of communication disabilities of aphasic patients. *Journal of Speech and Hearing Disorders, 41*, 138–143.

Holland, A. L. (1980). *Communicative abilities in daily living* Baltimore, MD: University Park Press.

Holland, A. L. (1982). Observing functional communication of aphasic adults. *Journal of Speech and Hearing Disorders, 47*, 50–56.

Holland, A. L., Frattali, C., & Fromm, D. (1998). *Communication activities of daily living,* 2nd Ed. Austin, TX: Pro Ed.

Holland, A. L., & Thompson, C. K. (1998). Outcome measurement in aphasia. In C. M. Frattali (ed): *Measuring outcomes in speech-language pathology* (pp. 245–266). New York: Thieme.

Kagan, A. (1998). Supported conversation for adults with aphasia: Methods and resources for training communication partners. *Aphasiology, 12*, 816–830.

Kagan, A., & Gailey, G. F. (1993). Functional is not enough: Training conversation partners for aphasic adults. In A. L. Holland and M. M. Forbes (eds): *Aphasia treatment: World perspectives* (pp. 199–225). San Diego: Singular Publishing Group Inc.

Kertesz, A. (1982). *Western Aphasia Battery.* New York: Grune and Stratton.

Lomas, J., Pickard, L., Bester, S., Elbard, H., Finlayson, A., & Zoghaib, C. (1989). The communicative effectiveness index: Development and psychometric evaluation of a functional communication measure for adult aphasia. *Journal of Speech and Hearing Disorders, 54*, 113–124.

Lyon, J. (1992). Communication use and participation in life for adults with aphasia in natural settings: The scope of the problem. *American Journal of Speech and Language Pathology, 1*, 7–14.

Lyon, J., Cariski, D., Keisier, L., Rosenbeck, J., Levine, R., Kumpala, J., Ryff, C., Coyne, S., & Levine, J. (1997). Communication partners: Enhancing participation in life and communication for adults with aphasia in natural settings. *Aphasiology, 11*, 693–503.

Mason, J. (1996). *Qualitative researching.* London: Sage.

Parr, S. (1996). Everyday literacy in aphasia: Radical approaches to functional assessment and therapy. *Aphasiology, 10*, 469–479.

Parr, S., Byng, S., & Gilpin, S., with Ireland, C. (1997). *Talking about aphasia: Living with loss of language after stroke.* Milton Keynes: Open University Press.

Pierce, R. S. (1996). Read and write what you want to: What's so radical? *Aphasiology, 10*, 480–483.

Sacchett, C., & Marshall, J. (1992). Functional assessment of communication: implications for the rehabilitation of aphasic people: reply to Carol Frattali. *Aphasiology, 6*, 95–100.

Sarno, M. T. (1969). *The functional communication profile: Manual of directions.* New York: Institute of Rehabilitation Medicine.

Sarno, M. T. (1983). The functional assessment of verbal impairment. In G. Grimby (ed): *Recent advances in rehabilitation medicine*. Stockholm: Almquist &Wiksell, Int.

Scherer, K. R., & Ekman, P. (1982). Methodological issues in studying nonverbal behaviour. In K. R. Scherer and P. Ekman (eds): *Handbook of methods in nonverbal behaviour research*. Cambridge: Cambridge University Press.

Searle, J. R., Ferenc, K., & Bierwisch, M. (Eds) (1980). *Speech act theory and pragmatics*. Boston: Kluwer.

Shewan, C. M., & Cameron, H. (1984). Communication and related problems as perceived by aphasic individuals and their spouses. *Journal of Communication Disorders, 17*, 175–187.

Simmons, N. N. (1993). *An ethnographic investigation of compensatory strategies in aphasia*. Ann Arbor, MI: University Microfilms International.

Simmons-Mackie, N., & Damico, J. (1996). Accounting for handicaps in aphasia: Communicative assessment from an authentic social perspective. *Disability and Rehabilitation, 18*, 540–549.

Skinner, C., Wirz, S., Thompson, I., & Davidson, J. (1984). *Edinburgh functional communication profile*. Winslow, Buckingham: Winslow Press.

Smith, L. E. (1985). Communicative activities of dysphasic adults: A survey. *British Journal of Disorders of Communication, 20*, 31–44.

Smith, L., & Parr, S. (1986). Therapists' assessment of functional communication in aphasia. *Bulletin of the College of Speech Therapists, 409*, 10–11.

Spreen, O., & Risser, A. (1991). Assessment of aphasia. In M. T. Sarno (ed): *Acquired aphasia* (pp. 73–150). New York: Academic Press.

State University of New York at Buffalo (1990). *Guide for the use of the uniform data set for medical rehabilitation*. Buffalo, NY: Research Foundation, State University of New York.

World Health Organization (1980). *International Classification of Impairments, Disabilities, and Handicaps*. Geneva: World Health Organisation.

World Health Organization (1997). ICIDH-2 International Classification of Impairments, Activities, and Participation. A Manual of Dimensions of Disablement and Functioning. Beta-1 draft for field trials. Geneva: World Health Organization. [http://www.who.ch/programmes/mnh/mnh/ems/icidh/icidh.htm]

Worrall, L. (1992). Functional communication assessment: An Australian perspective. *Aphasiology, 6*, 105–110.

Worrall, L. (1995). The functional communication perspective. In D. Muller and C. Code (eds): *Treatment of aphasia* (pp. 47–69). London: Whurr Publishers.

Worrall, L. (1999). *Functional communication therapy planner*. Oxon, UK: Winslow Press.

# 3

# *Beyond Activity: Measuring Participation in Society and Quality of Life*

## FABIANE M. HIRSCH
## AUDREY L. HOLLAND

**There has been a recent trend towards incorporating the participation (handicap) dimension and quality of life into functional communication assessment. This chapter describes the concepts and some of the issues surrounding participation and quality of life. A number of measures that might be used in speech-language pathology are critically reviewed. This chapter leads the way forward in focusing the attention of the profession on measurement of participation and quality of life issues.**

## Introduction

The end of the twentieth century brings the end of an era in which the scope of a speech-language pathology evaluation was limited largely to an assessment of impairment. With demands for documenting functional outcomes becoming more and more pervasive in research and clinical practice, we find it increasingly necessary to couple assessment and treatment more directly with daily functioning. That necessity, in turn, has spawned renewed interest in measures that evaluate limitations on the activities that comprise daily life. Many such measures are discussed elsewhere in this book. The goal of this chapter is to go beyond assessment of activity limitations to discuss measurement of the impact of acquired communication disorders on individuals' participation in society and their quality of life (QoL).

## Defining Participation and Quality of Life

In the 20 years since the inception of the World Health Organization's (WHO, 1980) model of disablement, speech–language pathologists, and indeed professionals in almost every dimension of health care, have been schooled in the WHO definition of *handicap*; the extent to which an individual is limited in continuing his or her culturally and age-appropriate roles in life. Although speech–language pathology has traditionally focused its clinical methods on impairments, it is difficult to imagine a clinician who fails to consider the handicapping influences of an acquired language disorder. With the release of the 1997 draft of the International Classification of Impairment, Activities, and Participation (ICIDH-2) (WHO, 1997) comes a transition in WHO terminology from handicap to *participation*. Participation is defined as "the nature and extent of a person's *involvement in life situations* (our emphasis) in relation to Impairments, Activities, Health Conditions, and Contextual Factors." The focus is on a person's participation in society and society's response in facilitating or hindering that participation. The ways in which participation might be *restricted* represent the discord between what might be expected of an individual who does not have a health problem and the circumstances of an individual with a given health condition.

The move to a neutral rather than negative term refreshingly diverts the focus away from weaknesses. It also may make it easier to relate the new term in the context of our own lives, allowing us to define this term more insightfully for persons with communication disorders. Consider your experiences over the past several days. Maybe you played racquetball with a friend, had coffee with a colleague, or played bridge with your neighbors. You may have gone to work or school, attended a meeting or conference, or volunteered in your community. Could individuals with acquired communication disorders have been involved in similar situations, if they so desired? Or would their participation have been restricted by their communication deficits?

Few measures of outcome in speech–language pathology specifically address participation in society. Other disciplines, such as pharmaco-economics, physical therapy, occupational therapy, and psychology have recognized the value of such measures and have focused energy on devising appropriate assessment tools. Although difficult to administer to individuals with acquired communication disorders, these tools shed light on how to assess participation restrictions. Thus, they can help guide speech-language pathologists toward the types of questions to ask to understand restricted participation resulting from communication disorders.

But, in our quest to understand acquired communication disorders and their impact on the lives of our patients, we would be quitting prematurely if we limited our assessment to measures of impairment, activity, and participation without considering two other components of the WHO model of disablement: health conditions and contextual factors. A complete picture can be achieved by considering the interactions of *all* components of the model and by appraising an individual's internal or affective response to these components. By evaluating the relevant components and personal responses, we believe that we can characterize an individual's *QoL*.

Historically, QoL has been tied tightly to economics, with the belief that greater material affluence is highly correlated with improved QoL. The end of World War II, however, signaled a new era focusing on the fulfillment of needs that cannot be expressed monetarily (Campbell, 1981). The psychologist Edward Chace Tolman predicted such a shift from what he labeled "economic man" to "psychological man" [as cited in Campbell (1981)]. Tolman believed that as financial security increased, decreased fears of economic disaster and higher levels of education would allow individuals to broaden their horizons and pursue their humanistic interests.

Initially, the use of QoL as a dependent variable was resisted by economists and psychologists. However, in 1969 Norman Bradburn developed his comprehensive survey of life quality and proposed a psychological well-being model based on positive and negative affect, or feeling states (Bradburn, 1969). Following Bradburn's seminal contribution, recognition of the value of studying QoL pervaded many domains, notably that of health care. The WHO confirms the significance of QoL in its definition of health as "a state of complete physical, mental and social well-being and not merely the absence of disease or infirmity" (WHO, 1969) and in its efforts to develop a QoL measure, the WHOQoL (Szabo, 1996). Today, both popular and scientific literature refer frequently to QoL.

Although the concept is intuitively appealing, precise definition of QoL has been elusive (Campbell, 1981; Fries & Singh, 1996; Spilker, 1996). Spilker (1996) has proposed an illuminating model in an attempt to define QoL. He suggests that QoL can be envisioned as a three-tiered pyramid in which an overall sense of well-being is at the apex, broad domains of well-being constitute the middle tier, and components of each domain comprise the base. The sense of well-being at the apex is considered synonymous with an individual's overall satisfaction with life. The five major domains in the middle tier include physical status and functional abilities, psychological status and well-being, social interactions, economic and/or vocational status and factors, and religious and/or spiritual status. Each domain contains a number of specific components; for example, the psychological status domain includes anxiety, cognition, and depression.

Building on Spilker's model, we define the quality of an individual's life not only as an aggregate of broad domains but as the product of personally weighted life domains filtered through the individual's own perspective (see Fig. 3–1). In our model, life domains, such as those proposed by Spilker, each have varying relevance to a particular individual's life, a concept depicted by varying sizes of domain parcels in Figure 3–1. For one person, spirituality may be the most important domain, and would be represented by the largest parcel. For this same individual, economic status may be relatively unimportant, and denoted by the smallest division. For another person, these representations may be reversed. The personal filter allows the domains to be colored by each person's own perspective. For example, for two individuals who hold finances in high regard, a $50,000 annual salary may seem lavish to one yet meager to another. A thorough understanding of QoL, at the point of our model and of life more generally, requires assessment not only of relevant life domains, but also of the personally defined filter.

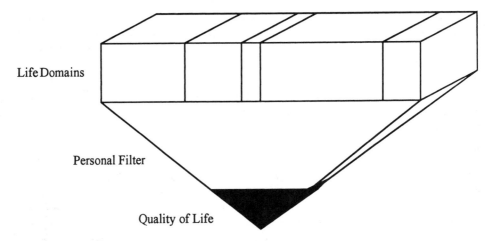

**Figure 3–1.** Model depicting how QoL may be derived.

## Measuring Participation and QoL

In Spilker's definition and our model, QoL is closely associated with facets of participation in society. It is not surprising, then, to find that many assessments aimed at measuring QoL seek information similar to that of participation measures. Thus, the boundary between tools for assessing these two variables is somewhat superficial and is used here only to help organize our discussion. Before discussing individual measures for assessing participation and QoL, however, it is worth addressing general issues of how these variables can be assessed, and, perhaps more critically, examining the difficulties inherent in assessing participation and QoL in individuals with acquired communication disorders.

### How Can Participation and QoL Be Assessed?

Assessing an individual's participation in daily life is relatively straightforward. If questions address involvement in situations appropriate for a given individual, an accurate summary of participation restrictions can be determined. For example, if one wants to find out to what extent someone is working, then direct questioning or direct observation should provide valid and reliable information about that individual's participation in his work environment. Most measures of participation take this approach.

Assessing an individual's QoL, however, is not as simple as evaluating objective circumstances such as salary or health status. Many measures have been developed in efforts to assess QoL; unfortunately, there is little consensus on which measures to use, or even which domains should be tapped. Many investigators interested in QoL develop their own measures because of discontent with available instruments or a need to explore specific issues deemed critical to a population of interest. Most available measures can be classified into one of three categories: generic scales, disease-specific scales, and scale batteries (de Haan et al., 1993). Generic scales are suitable for a variety of patient populations, allowing comparison of QoL information across different groups. However, they are often so broad as to miss the problems critical to a specific patient population. Disease-specific scales are typically more sensitive to these problems, but do not allow cross-disease comparisons. Scale batteries are compilations of assessments aimed at measuring several domains of interest. Although each domain may be studied in depth using this approach, inability to compare findings across studies and the difficulty patients have in completing such extensive batteries may discourage their use. Given these considerations, the general consensus for measuring QoL in patient populations appears to be the use of generic scales supplemented with disease-specific measures (McSweeney, 1990; Spilker, 1996).

### Who Can Assess Participation and QoL?

The reliability of life participation and QoL assessment derives directly from the source of the information. Significant others may be able to accurately report on an individual's involvement in various daily activities (Sander et al., 1997; Tepper et al., 1996; Whiteneck et al., 1992), but judging QoL is likely to be a different matter. In medical settings, rehabilitation specialists, nurses, physicians, social workers, and other health-care professionals may attempt to characterize a patient's QoL as an important outcome indicator. Medical practitioners, however, are probably not the best sources for information about their patients' life quality. Slevin et al. (1988) found low correlations between the reports of doctors and nurses and the reports of patients on a number of assessments of life quality, and concluded that reliable and consistent measurement of QoL must come from the patients themselves. This finding supports Campbell's statement that "the only source of information from which we can learn something directly about the feeling of life is the individual person; the man or woman who is living the life is the only one who can tell us how it feels" (Campbell, 1981, p. 16).

### Limitations of Self-Assessment in Individuals with Acquired Communication Disorders

If the patients themselves are the best reporters of their life quality, gathering information on the QoL of patients who have communication deficits may be difficult. Comprehension deficits, when present, can be significant obstacles, especially given the complex language used in most available measures. To complete these assessment tools, patients must be able to understand not only the instructions but each test item and response choice. Difficulties in expression, such as inconsistency in signaling "yes" and "no," also may affect assessment. Open-ended questions requiring detailed responses may be difficult, if not impossible, to answer effectively. Cognitive deficits, such as difficulty maintaining attention, problems with switching mental set, and perseverative behaviors, may pose additional concerns, as may lack of self-awareness. Visual deficits and neglect may prove problematic when assessment incorporates written material or visual stimuli, and hearing impairments may affect comprehension of auditorily presented material.

Because of these obstacles, communicatively impaired individuals are often excluded from outcome studies that incorporate QoL measures, with resultant neglect of an important patient population in such research (de Haan et al., 1993; Gordon et al., 1991; Hinckley, 1998). But with adaptations, many of the assessment challenges mentioned above can be minimized. Table 3–1 outlines possible compensations. For example, comprehension and speaking difficulties may be minimized if a multimodal approach is implemented in which speech, writing, gesture, and drawing are incorporated into instructions, stimulus items, and response choices. Use of visual scales such as those in the Visual Analogue Mood Scales (VAMS) (Stern et al., 1997) and the Dartmouth COOP Functional Assessment Charts (Nelson et al., 1987) might compensate for comprehension difficulties. Shortening or simplifying questions also might improve an individual's ability to comprehend and respond accurately. Providing a small closed set of response choices is preferable to requiring open-ended description. To avoid potential patient confusion and frustration, formats can be adjusted so that there are few places where switching mental set might be necessary, and memory demands can be minimized. Large print and vertical arrangement of response choices may help to compensate for visual deficits and neglect.

Some measures have implemented strategies such as those listed above. Gordon et al. (1991), for example, reported simplifying their measure, the Structured Assessment of Depression in Brain-Damaged Individuals (SADBD), to require only "yes/no" responses by the patient. Gordon et al. also used a standardized set of visual cues to assist in assessment. For example, the authors describe showing patients an index card with the word "sleep" printed on it. A series of cards with simple phrases linking potential sleep problems is then presented so pa-

Table 3–1. Strategies to Compensate for Deficits When Assessing Individuals with Acquired Communication Disorders

| *Deficit* | *Compensatory Strategies* |
|---|---|
| Comprehension (Auditory and reading) | Multimodality presentation |
| | Visual analogue scales |
| | Simplified language |
| Expression (Speech and writing) | Multimodality responding |
| | Small set of response choices (e.g., yes/no) |
| Cognition | Simplified language |
| | Small set of response choices (e.g., yes/no) |
| | Consistent response set throughout assessment |
| | Careful ordering of items (e.g., all communication items together) |
| | Limited memory demands (e.g., instructions on each page) |
| | Reduced assessment length |
| Vision | Vertical scales (for visual field cuts and neglect) |
| | Large print |

tients can choose the appropriate response. Such adjustments are critical for reliable evaluation of life quality of individuals with communication disorders.

## A Review of Measures

We direct our attention now to specific measures available for assessing participation in society and QoL. Table 3–2 lists the measures reviewed here. We have attempted to assemble a relatively comprehensive inventory, but this list is far from exhaustive.

### MEASURES OF PARTICIPATION

All professionals in rehabilitative medicine should be concerned about the extent to which their patients can resume their participation in society. Unfortunately, the focus of reintegration into society is often restricted to adapting the physical environment. For an individual with a communication disorder, it is typically the social milieu that acts as the greatest stumbling block to successful participation in the community, far more than the physical environment. Kagan discusses these notions more fully by pointing out that although most rehabilitation programs prepare for community reentry by minimizing physical barriers through the use of building modifications, wheelchairs and ramps, quad canes and the like, there is no similar effort made for communicative reentry; there are no communication ramps (Kagan, 1995). The communicatively impaired individual, in effect, may be able to get into the building to attend the party or the meeting, but without communication support, may not be able to participate socially in the event.

Table 3–2. Measures Reviewed in this Chapter

Measures of Participation
  Craig Handicap Assessment and Reporting Technique (CHART)
  Community Integration Questionnaire (CIQ)
  Functional Life Scale (FLS)
Measures of Quality of Life
  Standardized Measures
    Sickness Impact Profile (SIP)
    SF-36
    Dartmouth COOP Functional Assessment Charts
    Affect Balance Scale (ABS)
    Satisfaction With Life Scale (SWLS)
    Ryff Scales of Psychological Well-Being
  Nonstandardized Measures
    Psychosocial Well-Being Index (PWI)
    Behavior, Emotion, Attitude, Communication (BEAC) Questionnaires
    Quality of Life Survey
  Other Assessment Methods
    Single Questions
    Semistructured Interviews
    Direct Observation

Restricted societal interaction is a profound consequence for most individuals following stroke or TBI, and for their families. Consider friends who no longer visit because of their discomfort in conversing with a person who has aphasia, the receptionist who hurries an individual with right hemisphere damage through completion of a form, or the answering service that hangs up because the individual with a head injury responds too slowly. Assessment that fails to address such circumstances is not adequate for truly evaluating an individual's daily participation in life.

A number of assessment tools have been developed to examine physical and social participation of rehabilitation patients. The Craig Handicap Assessment and Reporting Technique (CHART) (Whiteneck et al., 1992) was designed to quantify handicap as a measure of rehabilitation outcomes for people with physical disabilities. Whiteneck et al. chose questions to measure the domains of handicap from the original WHO definition. These domains include physical independence, mobility, occupation, social integration, and economic self-sufficiency. The CHART has recently been revised to include a section on supervision for cognitive problems. Initially applied to a population with spinal cord injuries, the CHART's application to other rehabilitation populations, including head-injured patients, has been demonstrated, and it is recommended by the National Institutes of Health/National Institute of Neurological Disorders and Stroke (NIH/NINDS) Head Injury Centers as part of a research battery for following head-injured patients (Hannay et al., 1996). The Community Integration Questionnaire (CIQ) (Willer et al., 1993) was similarly intended to measure rehabilitation outcomes, but was designed specifically to assess the handicaps of traumatically brain injured individuals. Although it overlaps somewhat with the CHART, it does not address physical independence, mobility, and economic self-sufficiency (Hannay et al., 1996). It has, however, been successful in demonstrating improved outcomes from rehabilitative services (Willer et al., 1993). Finally, the Functional Life Scale (FLS) (Sarno et al., 1973), developed by J. E. Sarno et al. in 1973 to measure overall disability, appears to fit well with the present ICIDH-2 definition of participation. The FLS consists of 44 items grouped into five categories: cognition, activities of daily living (ADL), activities in the home, outside activities, and social interaction. For each item, four qualities (self-initiation, frequency, speed, and overall efficiency) are rated along a five-point functional continuum, where appropriate. Recently, M. T. Sarno reported findings from aphasic individuals participating in a comprehensive rehabilitation program who were evaluated with the FLS at 3-month intervals up to 1 year post-stroke (Sarno, 1997). The fluent aphasia group showed significant improvement on cognition, outside activities, and social interaction subscores, as well as significant change on all four qualities—speed, frequency, self-initiation, and efficiency; the nonfluent group demonstrated significant improvement on home and outside activities subscores; and the global aphasia group showed significant improvement only on the self-initiation quality.

The three measures just discussed look strictly at what an individual does, with no regard for how he or she feels. Many measures, often in addition to looking at what the individual does, also consider the personal attitudes, feelings, and beliefs of the individual. As such, these measures extend beyond a stringent assessment of participation and attempt to reveal a more comprehensive picture of the individual, a picture of his or her QoL.

MEASURES OF QUALITY OF LIFE

Although QoL is vaguely defined, most people agree that life situation alone does not determine an individual's life quality. If QoL was highly predictable from one's objective life circumstances, we could use easily measured indicators like incidence of illness, number of hospital stays, degree of impairment, and so forth, to determine life quality, and there would be no need to develop direct measures of well-being. But life quality appears to result from an interplay between objective facts about one's life situations and such things as the resilience one brings to them and one's values and hopes.

### Standardized Measures

Several available QoL measures include subsets of questions aimed at evaluating objective life situations, but supplement them with questions that address the perception of, and personal response to, these situations.

### Sickness Impact Profile

Prompted by the observation that standard clinical measures were often insensitive to patients' reports of progress, an interdisciplinary team at the University of Washington developed the Sickness Impact Profile (SIP) (Bergner et al., 1981; Damiano, 1996a, 1996b), one of the first measures of overall health. The SIP is a measure of perceived health status designed to be sensitive enough to detect differences in health status between diagnostic groups and over time. It consists of 136 items describing activities of daily life that fall into 12 categories: sleep and rest, emotional behavior, body care and movement, home management, mobility, social interaction, ambulation, alertness behavior, communication, work, recreation and pastimes, and eating. Subjects check those SIP items that are related to their health and that apply to them on the day they are tested. The questionnaire may be administered as an interview or self-administered, taking 20–30 minutes to complete. Scoring is based on the number and type of items marked, each item having a scale value. Three resultant scores can be calculated: dysfunction in each of the 12 categories, dysfunction in psychosocial and physical aggregate domains, and overall dysfunction. In field trials, the SIP was found to have good internal consistency, good ability to discriminate patient groups, good test–retest reliability, and good criterion validity (Bergner et al., 1981; Damiano, 1996a, 1996b; de Haan et al., 1993). The SIP has been used extensively in clinical trials, epidemiological studies, and program evaluations. Published scores are now available for a variety of diseases and conditions to allow comparative analyses [see (Damiano 1996b) for references].

Damiano (1996a, 1996b) has noted that certain patient populations, such as those with lower extremity fractures, hyperthyroidism, cataracts, or chronic lung disease, demonstrate discrepancies between SIP category scores. The same may prove true for individuals with acquired communication disorders. It may be possible to demonstrate efficacy of speech-language services using the SIP by showing that improvement in overall scores is related to improvement in relevant categories, such as communication and social interaction, while others, such as ambulation, remain constant. Although more burdensome to administer than shorter measures, the SIP may provide a sensitive measure of change. It is, however, primarily a behavioral measure, and supplementing it with questions on feelings of well-being and life satisfaction is recommended (de Haan et al., 1993).

### SF-36

The Medical Outcomes Study (MOS) 36-Item Short-Form Health Status Survey (SF-36) also was designed to describe population health in comprehensive terms and to compare the relative burden of diseases and the relative benefits of alternative treatments (Ware, 1996; Ware & Sherbourne, 1992). The SF-36 was intended as a short, practical measure. Its 36 items can be categorized into eight scales: physical functioning, role activities—physical, bodily pain, general health, vitality, social functioning, role activities—emotional, and mental health. Items in these scales can be further aggregated into summary measures of physical health and mental health. Both standard (4-week) and acute (1-week) recall versions have been published. The survey can be given by a trained interviewer, self-administered, or computer-administered, and takes approximately 5 to 10 minutes to complete. Internal consistency and test–retest data have revealed good reliability. Good content, concurrent, criterion, and construct validity also have been reported. In addition, predictive validity for utilization of health-care services, the clinical course of depression, loss of job within 1 year, and 5-year survival has been demonstrated (Ware, 1996). Communication and cognitive functioning scales are not included in the SF-36, a serious limitation on its applicability for individuals who have communication disorders; however, the diversity of scales included in the measure may make it a good indicator of well-being that can be supplemented with other measures of communication and cognition. Ware suggests just this approach, using the SF-36 as a "generic core" and supplementing it with other more specific measures (Ware, 1996). An appealing feature of the SF-36 is that, having achieved widespread usage, norms are available for general and specific populations. Recently, an even more abbreviated version, the SF-12 has been made available (Ware et al. 1996). Both the SF-36 and the SF-12 can be examined further on-line at http://www.sf-36.com.

### Dartmouth COOP Functional Assessment Charts

Another brief measure used to study many of the previously discussed domains is the Dartmouth COOP Functional Assessment Charts (Nelson et al., 1987, 1996). These Charts were developed by the Dartmouth Primary Care Cooperative ("COOP") Information Project, a network of community medical practices cooperating on research activities concerned with primary medical care. They were designed to measure the functional status of patients in busy medical office practices.

Nine charts constitute the complete assessment, each chart focusing on a different aspect of functional status: physical fitness, feelings, daily activities, social activities, pain, change in health, overall health, social support, and QoL. Each chart contains a single question. Responses are on a five-point ordinal scale and are arranged vertically below each question. Each written response option is also depicted by a drawing indicating a level of well-being or functioning. Patients are asked to read the question and choose the response that best describes them during the past 2 weeks, or the past month, depending on the version used. Administration time is 2 to 3 minutes. The COOP Charts are reported to have good test–retest reliability, good convergent and discriminant construct validity (de Haan et al., 1993; Nelson et al., 1996), and moderate indications of interobserver reliability (de Haan et al., 1993).

The COOP Charts are potentially useful for individuals with reading and auditory comprehension deficits, as the illustrations may facilitate comprehension of both the questions and the response options. For example, for social activities, rather than just progressing from a happy to a sad face, the illustrations depict a range from an individual interacting with a group of people to an individual isolated from the group. The illustrations are appealing and appropriate for adult use. Unfortunately, some of the questions as written are long and complex and the correspondence between the written information and the pictorial information is not precise. However, it does provide a valuable model of illustration use for assessing life-quality domains.

One concern expressed by de Haan et al. (1993) is the utility of the COOP Charts for research purposes. Because only one item is used to measure each domain, de Haan et al. suggest that the Charts' value may be limited in stroke outcome studies. Clinically, however, they have proven very valuable. Not only do they provide baseline measures of functional abilities, they reportedly make it easier for patients and clinicians to discuss functional problems and assist in helping clinicians understand the patient's view of the impact of a health problem on the patient's daily life (Nelson et al., 1987).

*Affect Balance Scale*

In contrast to the COOP Chart that asks an individual to rate his or her QoL outright (Chart #9: QoL), other measures attempt to determine a person's perception of life quality less directly. Some of these measures tap subjective appraisal of a person's life circumstances to the exclusion of objective measures of the components affecting QoL.

Perhaps the best known of such measures is the Affect Balance Scale (ABS) (Bradburn, 1969). A small section of a comprehensive assessment distributed as one of the first national surveys of well-being in America, the ABS consists of a set of 10 questions designed to look at positive and negative affect. Administration is estimated to take 2 to 3 minutes. The format of the ABS incorporates a carrier phrase defining time span ("During the past few weeks did you ever feel . . .") followed by five completions concerned with positive feeling-state (e.g., "Pleased about having accomplished something?"), and five completions concerned with negative feeling-state (e.g., "Bored?"), with a yes/no response format. In pilot work, Bradburn (1969) found that scores on the positive-item set or negative-item set alone did not correlate well with self-reports of happiness; however, the difference between scores on the positive and negative sets was related to happiness self-reports. Hence, a score calculated from the difference between these two sets is used to define an individual's well-being status. Test–retest reliability over an average of 3 days was high, suggesting that response stability is adequate for identification of meaningful change. To test validity, Bradburn compared ABS scores with responses on three general indicators of happiness and life satisfaction included in the general survey and found good convergent construct validity.

However, the construct validity of the ABS has been challenged because of its weak theoretical underpinnings. Ryff (1989) questioned Bradburn's demonstration of independence of positive and negative affect, suggesting that it appeared to be a "serendipitous finding of a study conceived for other purposes" (p. 1070), those purposes focusing on social change rather than on defining the structure of well-being. Other criticisms have also been noted. For example, Diener suggested that the positive affect items reflect arousal content more strongly than the negative affect items; that the items contain much specific nonaffective content; that occurrence of feelings, rather than intensity or frequency of feelings, is assessed; and that the scale may be affected by acquiescence-response bias and ceiling and floor effects (Diener, 1984).

Despite criticism, the ABS has been used in a number of studies of language-impaired individuals. Lyon et al. (1997), for example, used the ABS as an outcome measure for their Communication Partners treatment program. Differences between pre- and post-treatment ABS scores were not significant. Records et al. (1992) found no differences in ABS scores between adults with histories of specific language impairment and age-matched comparison subjects.

*Satisfaction With Life Scale*

The Satisfaction With Life Scale (SWLS), a five-item instrument developed by Diener et al. (1985), was designed to measure global life satisfaction as a judgment process to the exclusion of related concepts such as positive and negative affect. Items revealed by factor analysis to relate to affect were specifically eliminated in the final scale. The SWLS items are reproduced here.

- In most ways my life is close to my ideal.
- The conditions of my life are excellent.
- I am satisfied with my life.
- So far I have gotten the important things I want in life.
- If I could live my life over, I would change almost nothing.

Each item is scored on a seven-point scale, from strongly disagree (1) to strongly agree (7), with a resultant possible range from 5 (low satisfaction with life) to 35 (high satisfaction with life). Administration time is estimated to be 2 to 3 minutes. Test–retest correlations over a 2-month period were high, and item-total correlations revealed good internal consistency. Correlations with other scales of positive functioning have been found to range from moderate to high for college student and geriatric samples (Diener et al., 1985; Pavot et al., 1991). Normative data are available for diverse populations, including abused women, elderly caregivers, religious women, prison inmates, and doctoral students (Pavot & Diener,

1993). Although the questions do not appear applicable for pre- and post-treatment assessment, significant changes on the SWLS have been reported following psychotherapy (Pavot & Diener, 1993).

It is not clear, at least for the purpose of evaluating QoL in individuals with acquired communication disorders, if it is valuable to exclude affect, as Diener did in developing the SWLS. If satisfaction with life and affect are two components of well-being, as Ryff (1989) suggests, neither the SWLS nor the ABS alone is adequate for our purpose here, and we must look at either using both of these measures or turning to a more comprehensive measure that includes both components.

### Ryff Scales of Psychological Well-Being

Lamenting the general neglect of theory in the development of early QoL measures, Ryff et al. (1989; 1995) developed scales based on theoretical frameworks of alternative domains of positive psychological functioning, namely developmental (life-span) psychology, clinical psychology, and mental health. Feeling that positive affect, negative affect, and life satisfaction failed to fully define QoL, Ryff reviewed relevant psychological theories and found many similar features that she incorporated into six dimensions: self-acceptance, positive relations with others, autonomy, environmental mastery, purpose in life, and personal growth. The original scales included 20 items for each dimension, but the newer short form contains 14 items per dimension for a total of 84 items. Items from the six scales are mixed to form a single continuous assessment tool. Responses are on a six-point format from strongly disagree (1) to strongly agree (6), with responses to negative items reversed during scoring so that high scores indicate high self-ratings. Administrative time is estimated to be 15–30 minutes for individuals with intact language skills.

Correlations of the original scales with prior measures of positive and negative functioning revealed good convergent and discriminant validity. The dimensions correlated with each other, as well, but loaded onto different factors of well-being, indicating that they measure different constructs (Ryff, 1989). Test–retest reliability coefficients were high. For the short form, internal consistency was high for each dimension as was correlation with the 20-item parent scales. Ryff (1989) noted that although some of her theory-based dimensions were strongly associated with prior indices of well-being, others were not. This suggested that previous measures neglected valuable information, specifically in the dimensions of positive relations with others, autonomy, purpose in life, and personal growth.

Hoen et al. (1997), in evaluating the effectiveness of the community-based aphasia program of the York-Durham Aphasia Center (YDAC), administered the short form of the Ryff Scales (14 questions per dimension) to family members of aphasic participants. Hoen et al. administered an even more condensed form of the Ryff Scales to the aphasic participants. This condensed form was developed by selecting questions that were easier for aphasic individuals to understand, and has only four questions per dimension. Between test sessions separated by 6 months, family members showed significant positive change on five of the six dimensions, with only environmental mastery remaining unchanged. Aphasic participants also demonstrated significant positive change on five of the six dimensions; positive relations with others did not change significantly for this group. Because the Scales were altered in the condensed form, new psychometric testing is needed. But this adaptation of the Ryff Scales shows promise for measuring outcomes of aphasia therapy.

### Nonstandardized Measures

*Psychosocial Well-Being Index*

There are several measures that have not yet been rigorously evaluated but have initial encouraging results with language-impaired patients. One example is the Psychosocial Well-Being Index (PWI) developed by Lyon et al. (1997) as an outcome measure for their Communication Partners aphasia treatment program. The PWI consists of 11 open-ended questions that sample purpose or direction in life, contentment, active participation in life, feelings toward self and others, and comfort levels alone and with others. Lyon et al. had aphasic adults, their caregivers, and adult volunteers from the community (the communication partners) complete the PWI, as well as other measures. The responses were videotaped and scored in two ways: estimates of existing levels of function were marked on a 100-mm vertical line, and estimates of magnitude of change were indicated on a ± 7-point continuum after watching their own earlier videotaped responses. Lyon et al. found significant improvement on PWI scores for all three members of each triad tested, regardless of the scoring method. They also found significant improvement on their Communication Readiness and Use Index (CRUI), another nonstandardized measure, but failed to find significant changes on the *Boston Diagnostic Aphasia Examination* (BDAE) (Goodglass & Kaplan, 1983), *Communicative Abilities in Daily Living* (CADL) (Holland, 1980), or *ABS* (Bradburn, 1969). The authors urge caution in interpreting their findings for two reasons: aphasic adults for whom treatment was deferred for 2 months improved on the PWI and CRUI during this 2-month period, and clinician judgments did not correlate highly with score changes on these two nonstandardized measures. Hence, the PWI and CRUI, although intended to provide more sensitive measures of outcome than the standardized tests, may have overestimated treatment effects. Further research is needed to determine the value of the PWI in aphasia treatment research.

*Behaviour, Emotion, Attitude, Communication Questionnaires*

Another nonstandardized measure was used to evaluate program effectiveness at the York-Durham Aphasia Center. In addition to the modified Ryff Scales discussed earlier, Hoen et al. administered their Behaviour, Emotion, Attitude, Communication (BEAC) questionnaires to aphasic participants and their caregivers to assess change in social function and psychosocial well-being over a 6-month period of participation in the YDAC program (Hoen et al., 1997; Thelander et al., 1994). The BEAC comprises four questionnaires, two that are completed by the aphasic participant and are titled *How I See Myself* and *How I See My Spouse or Family Member* and two that are completed by the caregiver, *How I See Myself* and *How I See My Aphasic Spouse/Family Member*. The questionnaires for rating the aphasic participant (by the aphasic patient and caregiver) contain 31 items. The questionnaires for rating the caregiver are shorter, 16 and 19 questions to be completed by the aphasic patient and the caregiver, respectively. All four questionnaires have a six-point response format, from *strongly no* to *strongly yes*. Thelander et al. (1994) did not find significant change over a 6-month period using these questionnaires, despite the significant changes noted on the condensed Ryff Scales. One possible explanation proffered by the investigators is that because the scoring system had not yet been developed, analysis was completed on an item-by-item basis, which may have been less sensitive to changes. As with the PWI, this measure seems promising, but further development is needed before it can gain widespread use.

### Quality of Life Survey

A more comprehensive assessment of the QoL of aphasic patients is currently being undertaken by N. L. Records (personal communication, June 17, 1997). Similar to the measure used to assess the life quality of young adults with specific language impairment histories (Records et al., 1992), the current measure is a compilation of several QoL assessment tools, plus questions for gathering demographic information. It is currently being field-tested.

### OTHER ASSESSMENT METHODS

To this point, we have primarily considered QoL measurement using questionnaires, but other formats have also been utilized. Some examples are discussed here.

### Single Questions

Several measures reviewed in previous sections use a corpus of questions to gather information about the affective responses of aphasic individuals to their life situations. In contrast, some researchers have used a single question to try to ascertain their subjects' perspective of their life quality. The Dartmouth COOP Charts discussed previously use such an approach; following eight charts that probe various aspects of life functioning, the final chart asks patients to rate the quality of their lives. Similarly, in a questionnaire designed to gather information on lifestyle satisfaction in adults with chronic aphasia, Hinckley (1998) used the single question "Overall, how would you rate your current lifestyle?," with a four-point response scale that included very happy, content, dissatisfied, and discouraged. Other information was also collected, such as self-ratings of general health, continued therapy services, occupation, daily activities, and social contact. Because of the small number of respondents ($N = 32$), lifestyle satisfaction ratings were collapsed into two categories: positive lifestyle rating (very happy or content) and negative lifestyle rating (dissatisfied or discouraged). Logistic regression revealed that only time post onset had a significant impact on the likelihood of positive life satisfaction, and this relationship was negative, with the probability of achieving a good life satisfaction rating decreasing as time post-onset increased. Hinckley warns of a number of factors that could have influenced the results: the questionnaires were sent to subjects' homes for completion, the language was somewhat complex, and there was a poor response rate

(21%). This suggests that subjects with more impoverished language skills and limited support at home were likely underrepresented. Indeed, the respondents were typically young (average age of 50 years, range of 23 to 69 years), healthy, and employed. Hinckley suggests that replication with an improved research design is needed to better determine the predictors of lifestyle satisfaction for aphasic individuals. With respect to the use of a single question for measuring QoL, although something simple is desirable for ease of administration, sensitivity is typically compromised (Fries, 1996).

### Semistructured Interviews

Most investigators of QoL depend on structured assessment tools for gathering life quality information; however, several researchers have relied on semistructured interviews to obtain this information (e.g., Le Dorze & Brassard, 1995; Wahrburg et al., 1997). The PWI discussed previously uses such a format (Lyon et al., 1997). Another example is provided by Le Dorze and Brassard (1995) who used a qualitative research interview that included themes and some focused questions to look at the disabilities, handicaps, and coping strategies of aphasic individuals and their relatives and friends. The interviews were tape-recorded and transcribed. Analysis included identifying statements containing consequences of aphasia, labeling these statements with descriptors, and grouping the descriptors as a disability, handicap, or coping behavior. These investigators were thus able to characterize these variables in the words of the people actually experiencing the consequences of aphasia rather than in the words of researchers. Of note is that some of their findings differed from those of previous investigations. For example, many of the handicaps and coping behaviors reported by participants referred specifically to communication situations rather than the psychological responses of earlier studies, and there was no evidence of unrealistic attitudes of spouses reported by other investigators. Le Dorze and Brassard (1995) suggest that when researchers attempt to design questionnaires, they have a different perspective from that of the individuals affected, that is, "researcher-defined problems may not be very real for the aphasic persons and spouses" (p. 252). If a questionnaire is to be truly reflective of the perspectives of communicatively impaired persons and their families, then it is imperative to begin by listening to what these individuals have to say. However, Le Dorze and Brassard's format, which required verbal responses, restricted its use to aphasic individuals with good verbal skills. In addition, their participants lived in the community and belonged to a self-help group, introducing once again a sampling bias plaguing studies of the QoL of communicatively impaired individuals. They conclude that a more systematic understanding of the handicaps of individuals with a wider range of aphasic symptoms and living environments is critical for establishing a theoretical basis for the design of new therapeutic interventions.

### Direct Observation

Finally, we consider perhaps the most naturalistic of the methods available for collecting information on individuals with acquired communication impairments—direct observation in natural communication situations. The Communicative Profiling System (CPS) (Simmons-Mackie & Damico, 1996) is an assessment procedure designed to profile the communicative handicap of individuals with aphasia. Its goal is to collect information from the perspective of those involved by interviewing speaking partners, similar to Le Dorze and Brassard (1995). But the CPS goes a step further, incorporating actual observation of aphasic individuals in their natural communicative environments. Although focused more on participation in communicative situations than on QoL, the CPS is included here because it is a more holistic assessment approach that fits with the other measures recently designed for use with individuals with acquired communication impairments, and it has the potential to add a new dimension to QoL assessment. The CPS involves four phases of data collection and analysis: (a) interviews of individuals familiar with the aphasic individual; (b) observation of aphasic individuals and collection of anecdotal information; (c) videotaping of natural communicative events; and (d) interpretive analysis by the examiner. The resulting profiles provide information on an aphasic individual's communicative behaviors and strategies, the effects of the environmental context on the individual's performance, and the individual's network of communication partners, which can then be used in planning intervention. Simmons-Mackie and Damico (1996) illustrate this process by demonstrating how the CPS provided a comprehensive summary of the communicative handicap of an individual with severe nonfluent aphasia and mild apraxia of speech, and how the information collected was subsequently used to guide intervention.

## Assessing Caregivers

Throughout this chapter, we have emphasized the problems of individuals with communicative impairments, with only tangential regard for their caregivers. However, we are also aware of the compromises on QoL, or at least potential restrictions on participation in society, that befall those who live with, or care for, the person with the impairment. Along with Satir (1985), we believe that in any family network, the person with the problem is simply "the identified patient." All family members are affected, although to varying degrees. Social life for families can be curtailed; hobbies and interests neglected due to caregiving responsibilities; work outside the home undertaken for the first time in many years to avoid financial disaster, or alternatively, work responsibilities relinquished to care for the impaired individual, and so on. For such reasons, we urge involved clinicians to study caregiver QoL and to be prepared to provide family guidance.

Almost any of the measures we have described can be used with significant others. In fact, using the same measures for patients and family members may provide a more cohesive picture of quality of family life than can be achieved by using different measures. To complete the picture, measures focused on caregiver burden can be utilized. Two examples are the Caregiver Burden Scale, developed by Zarit et al. (1988), and Relatives' Stress Scale, used by Pearson et al. (1988). Neither of these measures was specifically designed for caregivers of communicatively impaired individuals, but their applicability is clear.

## A Comment on Depression

Depression may play a significant role in the QoL of individuals with acquired communication impairments. Gordon et al., for example, found that 56% of their poststroke subjects with left brain damage and 68% of their poststroke subjects with right brain damage were depressed (Gordon et al., 1991). Reportedly, depression is the most studied of all psychological variables of aphasia (Wahrborg, 1991). Depression may affect individuals by diminishing their desire to interact with family and friends, causing reticence toward resuming work functions or retirement activities, and influencing many other domains of daily life. Many measures are available for assessing depression. These include, but are not limited to, the Structured Assessment of Depression in Brain-damaged Individuals (SADBD) (Gordon et al., 1991), the Geriatric Depression Scale (GDS) (Yesavage et al., 1983), the Beck Depression Inventory (BDI) (Beck et al., 1996), and the Hamilton Rating Scale for Depression (HRS) (Hamilton, 1960). In-depth discussion of depression is beyond the scope of this chapter. Interested readers are referred to review articles by Swindell and Hammons (1991) and Sapir and Aronson (1990) and Wahrborg's book (1991).

## Conclusion

There are many approaches to measuring participation in society and QoL of individuals who have acquired communication disorders. However, few have been adequately field-tested with this population, and in only a limited number of cases have measures been modified for use with communicatively impaired individuals. As a result, we have much speculation about QoL and restricted ability to participate in society, but little data to support or refute our speculations. As interest in these issues grows, and as speech–language pathologists become more comfortable with the knowledge acquired by other disciplines, this picture should become more clear. When it does, we should be better able to understand the social restrictions experienced by communicatively impaired individuals and their families. We should also be better able to identify successful coping strategies and key characteristics of individuals who rise to the challenge of their impairments. Ultimately, we should be able to incorporate this new information into intervention strategies targeting successful reintegration into society and improved life quality.

## Acknowledgment

This work was supported, in part, by the National Multipurpose Research and Training Center Grant DC-01409 from the National Institute on Deafness and Other Communication Disorders.

## References

Beck, A. T., Ward, C. H., Mandelson, M., et al. (1961). An inventory for measuring depression. *Archives of General Medicine, 4*, 53–63.

Bergner, M., Bobbitt, R. A., Carter, W. B., et al. (1981). The Sickness Impact Profile: Development and final revision of a health status measure. *Medical Care 19*, 787–805.

Bradburn, N. M. (1969). *The structure of psychological well-being.* Chicago: Aldine Publishing Company.

Campbell, A. (1981). *The sense of well-being in America: Recent patterns and trends.* New York: McGraw-Hill Book Company.

Damiano, A. M. (1996a). The Sickness Impact Profile. In B. Spilker (ed): *Quality of life and pharmacoeconomics in clinical trials,* 2nd ed. (pp. 347–354). Philadelphia: Lippincott-Raven.

Damiano, A. M. (1996b). Sickness Impact Profile: User's manual and interpretation guide. Baltimore, MD: Johns Hopkins University.

de Haan, R. Aaronson, N., Limburg, M., et al. (1993). Measuring quality of life in stroke. *Stroke, 24,* 320–327.

Diener, E. (1984). Subjective well-being. *Psychology Bulletin 95,* 542–575.

Diener, E., Emmons, R. A., Larsen, R. J., et al. (1985). The Satisfaction With Life Scale. *Journal of Personality Assessment, 49,* 71–75.

Fries, J. F., & Singh, G. (1996). The hierarchy of patient outcomes. In B. Spilker (ed): *Quality of life and pharmacoeconomics in clinical trials,* 2nd ed., (pp. 33–40). Philadelphia: Lippincott-Raven.

Goodglass, H., & Kaplan, E. (1983). The Assessment of Aphasia and Related Disorders. Philadelphia, PA: Lea & Febiger.

Gordon, W. A., Hibbard, M. R., Egelko, S., et al. (1991). Issues in the diagnosis of post-stroke depression. *Rehabilitation Psychology 36,* 71–87.

Hamilton, M. (1960). A rating scale for depression. *Journal of Neurology and Neurosurgery Psychiatry 23,* 56–62.

Hannay, H. J., Ezrachi, O., Contant, C. F., et al. (1996). Outcome measures for patients with head injuries: Report of the outcomes measures subcommittee. *Journal of Head Trauma Rehabilitation, 11,* 41–50.

Hinckley, J. J. (1998). Investigating the predictors of lifestyle satisfaction among younger adults with chronic aphasia. *Aphasiology 12,* 509–518.

Hoen, B., Thelander, M., & Worsley, J. (1997). Improvement in psychological well-being of people with aphasia and their families: Evaluation of a community-based programme. *Aphasiology, 11,* 681–691.

Holland, A. L. (1980). Communicative abilities in daily living. Baltimore, MD: University Park Press.

Kagan, A. (1995). Revealing the competence of aphasic adults through conversation: A challenge to health professionals. *Topics in Stroke Rehabilitation, 2,* 15–29.

Le Dorze, G., & Brassard, C. (1995). A description of the consequences of aphasia on aphasic persons and their relatives and friends, based on the WHO model of chronic diseases. *Aphasiology, 9,* 239–255.

Lyon, J. G., Cariski, D., Keisler, L., et al. (1997). Communication Partners: Enhancing participation in life and communication for adults with aphasia in natural settings. *Aphasiology 11,* 693–708.

McSweeney, A. J. (1990). Quality-of-life assessment in neuropsychology. In D. E. Tupper and K. D. Cicerone (eds): *The neuropsychology of everyday life: Assessment and basic competencies* (pp. 185–217). Boston: Kluwer Academic Publishers.

Nelson, E. C., Wasson, J. H., Johnson, D. J., et al. (1996). Dartmouth COOP functional health assessment charts: Brief measures for clinical practice. In B. Spilker (ed): *Quality of Life and Pharmacoeconomics in Clinical Trials,* 2nd ed. (pp. 161–177). Philadelphia: Lippincott-Raven.

Nelson, E., Wasson, J., Kirk, J., et al. (1987). Assessment of function in routine clinical practice: Description of the COOP Chart method and preliminary findings. *Journal of Chronic Diseases, 40,* 55S–63S.

Pavot, W., & Diener, E. (1993). Review of the Satisfaction With Life Scale. *Psychological Assessment 5,* 164–171.

Pavot, W., Diener, E., Colvin, C. R., et al. (1991). Further validation of the Satisfaction With Life Scale: Evidence for the cross-method convergence of well-being measures. *Journal of Personal Assessment 57,* 149–161.

Pearson, J., Verma, S., & Nellett, C. (1988). Elderly psychiatric patient status and caregiver perceptions as predictors of caregiver burden. *Gerontologist, 28,* 79–83.

Records, N. L., Tomblin, J. B., & Freese, P. R. (1992). The quality of life of young adults with histories of specific language impairment. *American Journal of Speech-Language Pathology, January,* 44–53.

Ryff, C. D. (1989). Happiness is everything, or is it? Explorations on the meaning of psychological well-being. *Journal of Personality and Social Psychology 57,* 1069–1081.

Ryff, C. D., & Keyes, C. L. M. (1995). The structure of psychological well-being revisited. *Journal of Personality and Social Psychology 69,* 719–727.

Sander, A. M., Seel, R. T., Kreutzer, J. S., et al. (1997). Agreement between persons with traumatic brain injury and their relatives regarding psychosocial outcome using the Community Integration Questionnaire. *Archives of Physical and Medical Rehabilitation 78*, 353–357.

Sapir, S., & Aronson, A. E. (1990). The relationship between psychopathology and speech and language disorders in neurologic patients. *Journal of Speech and Hearing Disorders, 55*, 503–509.

Sarno, M. T. (1997). Quality of life in aphasia in the first post-stroke year. *Aphasiology, 11*, 655–679.

Sarno, J. E., Sarno, M. T., & Levita, E. (1973). The functional life scale. *Archives of Physical and Medical Rehabilitation, 54*, 214–220.

Satir, V. (1985). *Conjoint family therapy*, 3rd ed. Palo Alto, CA: Science and Behavior Books.

Simmons-Mackie, N. N., & Damico, J. S. (1996). Accounting for handicaps in aphasia: Communicative assessment from an authentic social perspective. *Disability Rehabilitation 18*, 540–549.

Slevin, M. L., Plant, H., Lynch, D., et al. (1988). Who should measure quality of life, the doctor or the patient? *British Journal of Cancer 57*, 109–112.

Spilker, B. (1996). Introduction. In B. Spilker (ed): *Quality of Life and Pharmacoeconomics in Clinical Trials, 2nd ed.* (pp. 1–10). Philadelphia: Lippincott-Raven.

Stern, R. A., Arruda, J. E., Hooper, C. R., et al. (1997). Visual analogue mood scales to measure internal mood state in neurologically impaired patients: description and initial validity evidence. *Aphasiology, 11*, 59–71.

Swindell, C. S., & Hammons, J. A. (1991). Poststroke depression: Neurologic, physiologic, diagnostic, and treatment implications. *Journal of Speech and Hearing Research 34*, 325–333.

Szabo, S. (1996). The World Health Organization Quality of Life (WHOQOL) assessment instrument. In B. Spilker (ed): *Quality of life and pharmacoeconomics in clinical trials*, 2nd ed. (pp. 355–362). Philadelphia: Lippincott-Raven Publishers.

Tepper, S., Beatty, P., DeJong, G. (1996). Outcomes in traumatic brain injury: Self-report versus report of significant others. *Brain Injury 10*, 575–581.

Thelander, M. J., Hoen, B., & Worsley, J. (1994). York-Durham Aphasia Center: Report on the Evaluation of Effectiveness of a Community Program for Aphasic Adults. Toronto.

Wahrborg, P. (1991). *Assessment and management of emotional and psychological reactions to brain damage and aphasia.* San Diego, CA: Singular Publishing.

Wahrborg, P., Borenstein, P., Linell, S., et al. (1997). Ten-year follow-up of young aphasic participants in a 34-week course at a Folk High School. *Aphasiology 11*, 709–715.

Ware, J. E., Jr. (1996). The SF-36 Health Survey. In B. Spilker (ed): *Quality of life and pharmacoeconomics in clinical trials*, 2nd ed. (pp. 337–345). Philadelphia: Lippincott-Raven.

Ware, J. E. J., & Sherbourne, C. D. (1992). The MOS 36-item short-form health survey (SF-36): I. Conceptual framework and item selection. *Medical Care 30*, 473–483.

Ware, J. J., Kosinski, M., & Keller, S. D. (1996). A 12-Item Short-Form Health Survey: Construction of scales and preliminary tests of reliability and validity. *Medical Care 34*, 220–223.

Whiteneck, G. G., Charlifue, S. W., Gerhart, K. A., et al. (1992). Quantifying handicap: A new measure of long-term rehabilitation outcomes. *Archives of Physical and Medical Rehabilitation, 73*, 519–526.

Willer, B., Rosenthal, M., Kreutzer, J. S., et al. (1993). Assessment of community integration following rehabilitation for traumatic brain injury. *Journal of Head Trauma Rehabilitation, 8*, 75–87.

World Health Organization (1980). *International Classification of Impairments, Disabilities, and Handicaps: A manual of classification relating to the consequences of diseases.* Geneva: Author.

World Health Organization. (1989). *Constitution of the World Health Organization.* Geneva: Author.

World Health Organization (1997). *ICIDH-2: International Classification of Impairments, Activities, and Participation. A manual of dimensions of disablement and functioning, beta-1 draft for field trials.* Geneva: Author.

Yesavage, J. A., Brink, T. L., Rose, T. L., et al. (1983). Development and validation of a geriatric depression screening scale: A preliminary report. *Journal of Psychiatric Research 17*, 37–49.

Zarit, S., Reever, K., & Bach-Peterson, T. (1988). Relatives of the impaired elderly: Correlates of feelings of burden. *Gerontologist, 20*, 649–655.

# 4

# Perspectives and Priorities: Accessing User Views in Functional Communication Assessment

## SUSAN P. PARR
## SALLY C. BYNG

**This chapter highlights the central role of the service user or consumer perspective in rehabilitation. It suggests that current functional communication assessments do not capture the essence of social and cultural experiences of the person with a communication disability. Drawing on a study comprising in-depth interviews with people with aphasia, the potential contribution of qualitative methodology to functional assessment is explored, together with the nature of the disabling barriers faced by people with communication impairment. This chapter reports on the developments in qualitative assessment that have been occurring at the centre for people with aphasia in London's City University.**

## Introduction

Functional communication [defined by the American Speech-Language-Hearing Association (ASHA) in 1990 as "the ability to receive or convey a message, regardless of mode, to communicate effectively and independently in a given environment"] seems a relatively straightforward concept. But layers of debate and uncertainty, perhaps most memorably represented in the Clinical Forum headed by Frattali (1992) have built up around the topic since its conceptualization some decades ago. These have raised fundamental ontological and epistemological questions regarding functional communication: In what terms can it be defined, and from whose perspective? What are its features and parameters? How can it be assessed? How can clinicians best promote functional recovery? What evidence can be gathered to show whether they have or have not achieved this? Clearly, the concept is by no means as unproblematic as it first seems.

In this chapter, we consider these issues with reference to changing priorities within general health care, discuss the developing role of the service user, and describe how user priorities and concerns might be ascertained. Finally, we discuss the implications of different theoretical models of disability for the principles and process of functional assessment.

## Dilemmas in Functional Assessment: The Health-care Context

Functional assessment can be conceptualized and addressed in different ways. Those working with people who have acquired neurogenic impairments may bring various clinical constructs to the task of assessment, depending upon their purpose. They may wish to explore the complex consequences of neurological conditions; to investigate the relationship between impairment, disability, and quality of life; to gauge the outcomes and benefits of treatment; to explore the nuances of interaction; to demonstrate the efficacy of their interventions; to give an account of functional losses to insurers and other stakeholders; to make a clear and unequivocal case for service provision to purchasers.

No one assessment tool can cover this range of purpose, as Worrall comments in the opening chapter to this book. The multifaceted nature of the functional endeavor strengthens the imperative to establish some kind of underlying conceptual coherence, to attach the billowing concept of functional assessment to a sturdy theoretical framework. The 1980 World Health Organization (WHO) classification of Impairment, Disability and Handicap (revised in 1997 to Impairment, Activities, and Participation) constitutes one useful and useable taxonomy, which has had considerable influence in the rehabilitation culture. However, there continues to be a lack of consensus about the meanings of these different terms and how they relate to functional assessment.

The uncertain nature of functional assessment may seem somewhat disconcerting, especially given the urgent need to respond appropriately to the demands of purchasers of health-care services. But the struggle to reach conceptual clarity is being played out simultaneously in a number of different disciplines concerned with rehabilitation, against a common background of demographic change and developments in health-care policy. The debates concerning functional assessment mirror conceptual struggles on a much larger scale.

The backdrop is one of a changing health profile, at least for the world's "developed" nations. Improved living conditions, advances in medical treatment, and increasingly ageing populations mean that chronic illnesses have replaced infectious diseases as major causes of mortality and morbidity. This has led to a focus on managing the long-term disabling consequences of chronic conditions within the community, a concern with maintaining quality of life and an emphasis on health promotion through the process of lifestyle change. Health-care policy now has a social dimension, highlighted by the advent of diseases such as AIDS and concern about the impact of environmental degradation. The growth of scepticism regarding professionalism and expertise has combined with increasing awareness of individual rights and responsibilities. In many systems, people have been reconstituted as "consumers" rather than recipients of health care, within health marketing systems which struggle with finite resources (Popay & Williams, 1994). Patients are starting to share responsibility for decisions regarding their treatment, to demand evidence as a basis for informed choice, to evaluate services (Coulter, 1997), and to participate in research (NHS Executive, 1997).

The debates around functional assessment in acquired neurogenic disorders blend into and reflect this complex and changing background. Clinicians are concerned to address the everyday difficulties that people who have acquired neurogenic disorders face in their own homes and communities. They seek to enhance the quality of life of those who struggle with long-term disabling conditions (Sarno, 1997). The nature of professional relationships with clients is starting to shift as they engage in shared decision-making and goal-planning (Pound, 1998).

## The Role of the Service User in Functional Assessment

The functional status and needs of people with acquired neurogenic disorders have been investigated in numerous ways and for different purposes, according to diverse theoretical conceptualizations of functional communication and the varying severity of the impairment. Different assessments, whether part of more general rehabilitation instruments or specifically dedicated to communication disorders, have been reviewed in detail elsewhere so will only be outlined here. Assessments can variously address the impaired individual's ability to convey basic needs and to act in an emergency (Lomas et al., 1989); to effect basic communicative functions (Skinner et al., 1984); to undertake a range of everyday communicative activities (Holland, 1980); to reflect on quality-of-life issues (Thelander et al., 1994). As a general rule, assessments aspire to meet minimal psychometric standards, although with varying success (Frattali, 1992). In particular, those used as outcome measures are required to be valid, reliable, responsive, generalizable, and applicable (Long, 1994). Enderby's (1997) therapy outcome measurement tool meets these basic psychometric requirements, mapping impairment levels, functional limitations, and restricted participation onto the WHO taxonomy.

Despite their diversity, many functional assessments involve the use of rating scales or standardized scoring systems, which vary in complexity. The rating is most often done by the clinician but in some cases a close family member performs this task (Lomas et al., 1989) or is consulted in the rating process (Sarno, 1969). Self-rating by the client is more unusual, but has been undertaken in some cases (Enderby, 1997; Thelander et al., 1994). What is at issue here is not so much the content of the assessment, or the parameters upon which functional performance is judged, but the role of the person who has the impairment. For the most part, participation in functional assessments has involved being rated by others (clinicians and family members) or rating oneself on constructs generated by others. Thus, those whose functional performance is assessed using the Communicative Abilities in Daily Living (CADL) (Holland, 1980) are required to enact activities generated by researchers and validated in consultation with a small group of aphasic people.

A number of problems are posed by measures or evaluation tools that involve rating a performance on parameters generated by others. For example, some measures have been found to be insensitive to change within individuals over the long periods of time spanned by a chronic impairment (Guyatt et al., 1987). They may fail to take into account factors that are of critical importance to the person with the condition, such as the sense of uncertainty, stigma, and lack of control described by people who experience severe and disabling illness (Fitzpatrick et al., 1990; Scambler, 1989). The assumption that functional literacy assessment tasks have a blanket relevance has been criticized (Parr, 1992). Functional assessments may lack sensitivity to the diversity of individual concerns:

> Although health status instruments attempt to assess by different methods the sever-
> ity of different problems, they generally have not addressed the problem that patients
> will differ considerably in the extent to which an aspect of disability or health-related
> quality of life is a concern or considered something for the doctor to address. It has
> been suggested that, if patients selected aspects of health status or quality of life that
> were of particular concern to them, this would be a more appropriate base-line from
> which to evaluate interventions. Such variation between patients within categories of
> health problem can only be addressed by methods that elicit individual concerns and
> expectations. (Fitzpatrick, 1994, p. 194)

## What Are the Priorities for Users?

We recently completed an in-depth qualitative investigation of the long-term consequences and significance of aphasia. In-depth interviews with a purposively selected sample of 50 people confirmed considerable variation in the concerns and priorities of those who have aphasia and in the ways in which they interpret and understand the condition (Parr et al., 1997). Individuals give different accounts of aphasia, fitting it to idiosyncratic health beliefs and adjusting their personal biographies and identities in their own way. For some, aphasia remains a personal tragedy, in which the limitations imposed (including functional losses) are continuously rehearsed. Some take an heroic identity in their own stories and assume the role of inspiring, helping, and advising others. Others come to see aphasia as an opportunity to live differently, to shed themselves of unsatisfactory lifestyles. Yet others become politicized and focus on challenging the ways in which their rights as disabled people are undermined or violated. Some assume total responsibility for improving their own health status, others look to the ministrations of doctors, healers, and therapists to bring about recovery. Such diverse interpretations of illness and health are not limited to people who have aphasia (Stainton-Rogers, 1991). Indeed some writers argue that biomedical models of illness fail to take account of the fact that it is inevitably experienced and interpreted in social and cultural terms:

> Impairment is more than a medical issue. It is both an experience and a discursive con-
> struction. It has phenomenological parameters and it can be analysed as an effect of
> discourse and language. (Hughes & Paterson, 1997)

Personal interpretation of the condition determines the relative importance of functional limitations for each individual. Overcoming functional limitations may indeed be a lasting and predominant focus of concern for one individual, whereas another with similar impairment might be concerned more with regaining employment, using an advocate, seeking appropriate educational support, finding company, maintaining status, or getting access to information. Our study suggests that the need for functional losses and regaining functional skills to be acknowledged and addressed becomes relatively less critical as time passes and the long-term nature of aphasia becomes apparent, bringing with it clear perceptions of other, less tangible, needs.

This point is made, in a different context, by Kleinman (1988) in a damning indictment of existing clinical assessment procedures:

> Symptom scales and survey questionnaires and behavioural checklists quantify functional impairment, rendering quality of life fungible. Yet about suffering they are silent. The thinned-out image of patients and families that perforce must emerge from such research is scientifically replicable but ontologically invalid; it has statistical, not epistemological significance. It is a dangerous distortion. To evaluate suffering requires more than the addition of a few questions to a self-report form or a standardised interview; it can only emerge from an entirely different way of obtaining valid information from illness narratives. Ethnography, biography, history, psychotherapy— these are the appropriate research methods to create knowledge about the personal world of suffering. (Kleinman 1988, p. 28)

## Listening to Users: The Qualitative Approach

The methodologies suggested by Kleinman are essentially qualitative and have their provenance in social science. They are increasingly understood to have considerable potential in the exploration of chronic conditions and their sequelae, and the evaluation of interventions (Hunter, 1994). In ontological and epistemological terms, they differ from quantitative approaches. They are concerned with different aspects of social experience, and are particularly able to capture complexity, change, process, detail, and context.

Biomedical research and experimental designs that correspond to the quantitative tradition in research have perhaps been more in evidence because of the prevailing culture within which health-care professions operate, even in those that are concerned with chronic disability, and because of the type of research questions being asked. Priority has been placed on attempting to "prove" the efficacy of treatments, proof being defined as quantitatively measureable change in performance. For health-care disciplines trying to establish their research credentials in a predominantly medical setting, it has seemed important to conform to prevalent ideologies about the nature of evidence and scientific robustness of methodologies, particularly through the use of randomized controlled trials (Hunter, 1993). There is, however, increasing evidence of interest in and use of qualitative methods across all disciplines involved in health research, medical and nonmedical (Pope & Mays, 1995).

Although the paradigms upon which they are based are unlike those underpinning biomedical research, qualitative methodologies can contribute a different kind of knowledge, but one that is equally valid. These demand a similar rigor and meticulous attention to detail in design and implementation. The strengths and limitations of quantitative and qualitative approaches are becoming better understood and the potentially fruitful relationship between the two clarified (Mason, 1996).

Objections to qualitative methods are numerous, and encompass their lack of clinical viability (Ulatowska & Scott Self, 1996). Certainly, the lack of a clear "score" can make pre- and postintervention status and the performance of various individuals difficult to compare. In-depth interviews and ethnographies can be time-consuming to design and carry out, and they can generate unwieldy amounts of data that need trained and skilled analysis.

But it is possible that reallocation of resources might make them a viable option. For example, one person in a community-based team of speech and language therapists might be trained to design, carry out, and analyze in-depth interviews and could be used as a resource by therapists working with different care-groups to evaluate their interventions. In the long term, such approaches might prove as valuable and as cost-effective as more conventional, larger scale methods:

> In depth qualitative interviews have a higher unit cost per interview, but even a very small sample may provide a wide range of information and highlight key problems more effectively than a similarly priced large-sample survey. (Long, 1994, p. 178)

At City Dysphasic Group, a center for people with aphasia that is attached to City University, London, researchers are starting to explore the use of in-depth interviewing to identify clients' needs and concerns as a basis for planning therapy and as a means of evaluating outcomes. Interviews are used in conjunction with other more conventional methods of evaluation. Although limited, experience so far suggests that interviews have the potential to capture specific changes, identify how these are attributed, and provide a useful basis for the design of therapy that addresses the concerns of the individual. Quantitative methods can also capture change: scales and scores allow baselines to be clearly established, and some kinds of comparisons within individuals and between individuals and groups efficient communication of findings. The critical issue is to match the methodology to the question being addressed; if the purpose of the assessment or evaluation is to determine "how much," then a quantitative type of approach may be most useful. A "what kind" type of question suggests that a qualitiative approach may be more informative. These methodologies are not mutually exclusive, but can be used in combination, depending on the nature of the issue to be investigated.

Another concern arises from the use of phenomenological approaches with people who have marked communication impairments, and who are often excluded from such research in a way that perhaps mirrors their exclusion from society. It has been argued that a restricted imagination on the part of the researcher, rather than the respondent's inability to take part, may be the main reason for such exclusion (Booth, 1996). A potential exists to develop interview techniques and resources that support respondents who have marked impairments. These would allow baseline data to be generated that is relevant to the individual. Bearing in mind the need for efficiency in outcomes measurement, it may be possible to develop individual rating systems and scales on the basis of interview data, as suggested by Mackenzie et al. (1986).

Methods such as in-depth and semistructured interviewing and ethnography represent a change in the relationship between the researcher and the researched, the assessor and the assessed. While undoubtedly remaining the subject of an investigation, the person who takes part in a qualitative study is involved as someone who has expertise which is acknowledged, who knows about the effects of a condition, and who contributes their knowledge in the assessment process. Detailed description, drawn from interview or observation data, can capture the complexities and intricacies that may elude simple rating scales.

Other initiatives suggest how the skills and knowledge of the clinician may be harnessed in qualitative evaluations based on interviewing. The Pragmatic Profile of Everyday Communication Skills in Adults (Dewart & Summers, 1996) involves a semistructured interview with the person who has an impairment (and a separate interview with another person if necessary) in which various parameters of interaction are discussed. These include communicative function, response to communication, interaction and conversation, and contextual variation. The procedure results in a detailed profile of individual skills and difficulties, itemized according to a professional taxonomy, elicited in a collaborative manner, but not rated.

One of the striking features of qualitative methodologies concerns the "suspension" of professional constructs. If in-depth interviewing is properly done, it can fully explore an experience from the perspective and in the terms of the person it is about. Our own foray into interviewing involved intensive training by an experienced qualitative researcher. Learning to listen without judging or controlling, and putting aside professional theoretical constructs proved to be major challenges, especially in familiar clinical terrain.

Ethnographic methods may seem even more unwieldy than interviewing, but have been effectively used to create detailed taxonomies of compensatory strategies used by individuals who have aphasia, illuminating the problem of generalization from treatment to real life (Simmons-Mackie & Damico, 1995). They have also been used to document the intricacies of interactions undertaken by a person who has severe aphasia (Goodwin, 1995). As with interviewing, the relationship between the ethnographic researcher and researched is arguably different.

These latter studies highlight the delicate balance between interaction and transaction and the critical importance of the ways in which others respond to someone who has a language impairment. The emphasis falls upon the partnership between the person who has a communication impairment and their interactant. A neurological event such as aphasia impacts not just upon individuals in isolation, but the social systems and networks of which that person is a part. Effectively, aphasia is "co-constructed" by the person who has aphasia and other people. This insight leads us to question the principles upon which functional assessments have traditionally been based.

### Functional Assessment and Theoretical Models of Disability

In 1993, Kagan and Gailey stated that, in their view, the functional deficits of the aphasic individual did not constitute an adequate focus for assessment or treatment. They outlined a different approach to therapy, one which represents a major theoretical shift from the traditional preoccupations of language rehabilitation. Drawing upon their experience of working with groups of people who attended the aphasia center in North York, Toronto, and the volunteers whose support they enlisted, Kagan and Gailey suggest that the efforts of the therapist should be focused, not upon the inabilities of the individual, but upon training those around to reveal and acknowledge the competence, even of the most severely aphasic person.

This simple shift of focus has had profound implications for therapy and traditional functional preoccupations. It accords, at least in part, with theoretical developments which have been generated within the disability movement in the United Kingdom over the past two decades. At the heart of the new theories of disability lies a refutation of the "medical model" of illness and disability (embodied in the original WHO taxonomy). This is replaced with a new "social model," which is primarily concerned with disabling barriers and issues of identity. Social model thinkers revisited the WHO taxonomy, maintaining the description of impairment, but eradicating the term "handicap," which they found inappropriate and redefining disability. The two definitions of disability form a striking contrast:

> *any restriction or lack (resulting from an impairment) of ability to perform an activity in the manner or within the range considered normal for a human being. (WHO, 1980)*

> *the loss or limitation of opportunities that prevents people who have impairments from taking part in the normal life of the community on an equal level with others due to physical and social barriers. (Finkelstein & French, 1993)*

According to the social model definition, disability is seen not as inevitably resulting from impairment, but arising from the barriers and restrictions that every disabled person faces, and that are constructed by a disabling society. The social model places the source of the problem firmly within society. The new WHO definitions do acknowledge the social dimension, but maintain a focus on the impaired individual. It will be interesting to see how members of the disability movement react to the new WHO definitions over time. It is not yet clear whether, despite the change in terminology, disability is now truly being conceptualized within the social framework propounded by proponents of the disability movement. The previous definitions did much to stimulate debate about concepts of disability: will these new definitions provoke a similar reaction?

Our study of the long-term consequences and significance of aphasia suggested that people who have acquired communication impairments face an extensive range of disabling barriers. These take at least four different forms as extracts from the interviews suggest (Table 4–1).

Table 4–1.   Disabling Barriers Faced by People Who Have Aphasia
(from Parr et al., 1997)

*Structural barriers*
These arise from restricted opportunities and lack of provision in work and education, impacting upon the person's financial status. They also arise from restricted access to support and services.
   *"Obviously for meetings for me to express myself is pretty difficult."*
   *"I think: 'Well why nobody to help me? Why? Why?' "*
   *"Social Service...forget it."*

*Environmental barriers*
These arise when a person who has aphasia encounters a hostile physical environment (for example background noise) or a hostile language environment (for example people talking all at once, too quickly or using complex language).
   *"People talking all at once..the noise.. I can't cope with that."*
   *"I go please, please slow down."*
   *"Simple word, not big word."*

*Attitudinal barriers*
These concern the hostile and discriminatory reactions which people who have a language impairment often encounter.
   *"Some of them actually thought I think you are an imbecile."*
   *"When I go to a restaurant or pub, I get ignored totally."*

*Informational barriers*
These arise when people are not given information relevant to their concerns at the right time and in a form which they can understand. This is complicated by the fact that asking for information in the first place may be difficult.
   *"I could have done with a lot more information. I should have asked but I couldn't. I think it would have helped but I couldn't grasp that."*
   *"The thing is, I don't know what I'm entitled to."*

The average time since onset of the 50 people interviewed in our study was 7.2 years. Most had at least 5 years' experience of aphasia, one respondent talking about 21 years of compromised language. Reflecting on their current situation, our interviewees made it clear that they still continue to encounter major barriers years post onset. They continue to grapple with discrimination, loneliness, compromised income, lack of control, loss of status, and bewilderment about what has happened to them.

Another concept central to the new theories of disability that are emerging concerns the assumption, which underpins many rehabilitation programs and practices, that all disabled people aspire to functional independence. The disability movement argues that this is not necessarily the case especially when it involves excessive effort, discomfort and fatigue:

> Health and welfare professionals usually regard independence as a central aim in the rehabilitation process. Disabled people define independence, not in physical terms, but in terms of control. People who are almost totally dependent upon others, in a physical sense, can still have independence of thought and action, enabling them to take full

*and active charge of their lives. Narrowly defined, independence can give rise to ineffi-
ciency and stress, as well as wasting precious time. (French, 1994, p. 49)*

"Autonomy" may be preferable to independence. In the case of a person with
aphasia, this may mean using an advocate, rather than struggling to make phone
calls, fill in forms, and do everything functional for oneself. The findings from
our study suggest that people who have aphasia are not inevitably concerned
about achieving functional goals independently. Rather, they seem preoccupied
with major life-issues such as negotiating benefits, dealing with family crises,
maintaining social contact, accessing support and information, and dealing with
stigma, prejudice, and major changes in their personal and social identities. Respondents with aphasia in Parr's (1992) study of functional literacy practices suggested that, even premorbidly, many literacy-based activities were not carried
out independently, even by people living alone. Instead people made substantial
use of a variety of social networks to complete many reading and writing tasks,
or "traded" different roles related to literacy.

Assumptions that normalization equates with independence are increasingly
challenged. Learning to listen to aphasic people, and to others with acquired neurological conditions, means letting go of professional rehabilitation constructs
such as "independence" and allowing the priorities and concerns of the disabled
person to emerge in their own terms. Oliver (1996) makes the point that rehabilitation experts may find it difficult to do this:

> *The impact of the social model of disability on professional consciousness, let alone
> practice, has been somewhat limited. Medicine is still locked into the treatment and
> cure of impairments; physiotherapy and occupational therapy remain convinced that
> working in a one-to-one situation with disabled people on their functional limitations
> is the only way to proceed. (Oliver, 1996, p. x1)*

Kagan and Gailey's approach accords well with these social model principles.
They are concerned with creating an enabling language environment, fostering
strong personal and social identities, promoting respect and acknowledgement of
competence, and switching the focus from the functional independence of the impaired individual to promoting the "feel and flow" of natural adult conversation,
mainly through intensive training of conversation partners (Kagan, 1998).

Their work clarifies the need, especially for rehabilitation professionals, to focus on two key issues in delivering health care. The first is to shift the emphasis
away from the priority of independence toward facilitation of autonomy and
choice. The second is to consider interventions that focus not just on changes
and adaptations made by the individual, but also on institutional, societal, and
environmental changes to address the often subtle barriers encountered by people with communication disabilties. This underlines the importance of extending
the active involvement of a wider variety of health-care professions in public
health planning and service provision than has up to now been envisaged.

The work of Kagan and Gailey, and of others such as Simmons-Mackie and
Damico, suggests that the therapeutic community could usefully move beyond
traditional assumptions to enable the concerns of those who have communication impairments to be heard, understood, and addressed. Using the new terms
coined by the WHO, the focus could perhaps fall less on "activities," more on

participation, less on the individual, more on the structures and social systems around the individual that can have either an enabling or a disabling effect.

There is an argument to be made that the functional assessment agenda could be extended. Individual concerns and patterns of interaction may be usefully explored and described, but wider issues may also be relevant to the therapeutic endeavor. Perhaps functional assessment has the potential to document the existence of the disabling barriers facing the individual, to assess levels of discrimination and the existence of opportunities and support for participation and contribution, access to advocacy and relevant information.

A precedent has been set for this in a research project, which set out ambitiously to measure disablement in society by investigating the extent to which institutional, social, and economic structures contribute to the exclusion of disabled people (Zarb, 1997). People who have acquired communication impairments feel that they do not count any more. As one of our respondents put it: "You get shunned, pushed down when you can't talk." It seems that from the perspective of those who feel unheard, diminished or excluded, functional may still not be enough.

## References

American Speech-Language-Hearing Association (1990). *Functional Communication Measures Project: Advisory Report.* Rockville, MD: ASHA.

Booth, T. (1996). Sounds of still voices: Issues in the use of narrative methods with people who have learning difficulties. In L. Barton (ed): *Disability and society: Emerging issues and insights* (pp. 237–255). London: Longman.

Coulter, A. (1997). Partnerships with patients: The pros and cons of shared clinical decision-making. *Journal of Health Services Research Policy, 2,* 112–121.

City Dysphasic Group (1997). *A profile of the work of the city dysphasic group.* London: Department of Clinical Communication Studies, City University.

Dewart, H., & Summers, S. (1996). *The Pragramatic profile of everyday communication skills in adults.* London: NFER-Nelson.

Enderby, P. (1997). *Therapy outcome measures: Speech language pathology.* Technical manual. London: Singular Publishing Group.

Fitzpatrick, R. (1994). Health needs assessment, chronic illness and the social sciences. In J. Popay and G. Williams (eds): *Researching the people's health.* London: Routledge.

Fitzpatrick, R., Newman, S., Lamb, R., & Shipley, M. (1990). Helplessness and control in rheumatoid arthritis. *International Journal of Health Sciences, 1,* 17–24.

Finkelstein, V., & French, S. (1993). Towards a psychology of disability. In J. Swain et al. (eds): *Disabling barriers—Enabling environments* (pp. 47–53). London: Sage.

Frattali, C. (1992). Clinical forum. Functional assessment of communication: Merging public policy with clinical views. *Aphasiology, 6,* 63–85.

French, S. (1994). The disabled role. In S. French (ed): *On equal terms: Working with disabled people.* London: Butterworth Heinemann.

Goodwin, C. (1995). Co-constructing meaning in conversations with an aphasic man. In E. Jacoby and E. Ochs (eds): *Research on language and interaction* (pp. 233–260).

Guyatt, G., Walter, S., & Norman, G. (1987). Measuring change over time: Assessing the usefulness of evaluative instruments. *Journal of Chronic Disease, 40,* 171–178.

Holland, A. (1980). *Communicative abilities in daily living.* Baltimore: University Park Press.

Hughes, B., & Paterson, K. (1997). The social model of disability and the disappearing body: Towards a sociology of impairment. *Disability and Society, 12,* 325–340.

Hunter, D. (1993). Let's hear it for R. and D. *Health Service Journal, 15,* 136–142.

Hunter, D. (1994). Social research and health policy in the aftermath of NHS reforms. In J. Popay and G. Williams (eds): *Researching the people's health* (pp. 15–31). London: Routledge.

Kagan, A. (1998). Clinical forum. Supported conversation for adults with aphasia: *Methods and resources for training conversational partners. Aphasiology, 12,* 816–830.

Kagan, A., & Gailey, G. (1993). Functional is not enough: Training conversation partners for aphasic adults. In A. Holland and M. Forbes (eds): *Aphasia treatment: World perspectives*. San Diego: Singular publishing Group Inc.

Kleinman, A. (1988). *The illness narratives: Suffering, healing and the human condition*. New York: Basic Books.

Lomas, J., Pickard, L., Bester, S., Elbard, H., Finlayson, A., & Zoghaib, C. (1989). The communicative effectiveness index: Development and psychometric evaluation of a functional communication measure for adult aphasia. *Journal of Speech and Hearing Disorders, 54*, 113–124.

Long, A. (1994). Assessing health and social outcomes. In J. Popay and G. Williams (eds): *Researching the people's health*. London: Routledge.

Lyon, J. (in press). Treating real life functionality in a couple coping with severe aphasia. In N. Helm-Estabrooks and A. Holland (eds): *Approaches to the treatment of aphasia*. San Diego: Singular Publishing Group.

Mackenzie, R., Charlson, M., DiGioia, D., & Kelley, K. (1986). A patient-specific measure of change in maximal function. *Archives of International Medicine, 146*, 1325–1329.

Mason, J. (1996). *Qualitative researching*. London: Sage Publications.

NHS Executive (1997). *Research: What's in it for consumers?* First report of the Standing Advisory group on Consumer Involvement in the NHS R and D Programme to the Central Research and Development Committee 1996/1997. London: NHS Executive.

Oliver, M. (1996). Foreword. In L. Jordan and W. Kaiser (eds): *Aphasia: A social approach*. London: Chapman and Hall.

Parr, S. (1992). Everyday reading and writing practices of normal adults: Implications for aphasia assessment. *Aphasiology, 6*, 273–283.

Parr, S., Byng, S., & Gilpin, S. (1997). *Talking about aphasia*. Buckingham: Open University Press.

Popay, J., & Williams, G. (Eds) (1994). *Researching the people's health*. London: Routledge.

Pope, C., & Mays, N. (1995). Reaching the parts other methods cannot reach: An introduction to qualitative methods in health and health services research. *British Medical Journal, 311*, 42–45.

Pound, C. (1998). Therapy for life: Finding new paths across the plateau. *Aphasiology, 12*, 222–227.

Sarno, M. (1969). *The functional communication profile: Manual of directions*. New York: Institute of Rehabilitation Medicine.

Sarno, M. (1997). Quality of life in aphasia in the first post-stroke year. *Aphasiology, 11*, 665–6679.

Scambler, G. (1989). *Epilepsy*. London: Routledge.

Simmons-Mackie, N., & Damico, J. (1995). Communicative competence in aphasia: Evidence from compensatory strategies. *Clinical Aphasiology Conference Proceedings, 23*, 95–105.

Skinner, C., Wirz, S., Thompson, I., & Davidson, J. (1984). *Edinburgh Functional Communication Profile*. Buckingham: Winslow Press.

Stainton-Rogers, W. (1991). *Explaining health and illness: An exploration of diversity*. New York: Harvester Wheatsheaf.

Thelander, M., Hoen, B., & Worsley, J. (1994). *Report on an Evaluation of Effectiveness of a Community Programme for Aphasic Adults*. York: Durham Aphasia Centre.

Ulatowska, H., & Scott Self, J. (1996). Is ethnographic assessment a reality in aphasia? *Aphasiology, 10*, 469–503.

World Health Organization (1997). *ICIDH-2 International Classification of Impairments, Activities and Participation*. {http://www.ch/programmes/mnh/mnh/ems/icidh/icidh.htm}.

World Health Organization (1980). *International Classification of Impairments, Disabilities and Handicaps*. Geneva: World Health Organization.

Zarb, G. (1997). Researching disabling barriers. In C. Barnes and G. Mercer (eds): *Doing disability research*. Leeds: University Press.

# 5

# Health-Care Restructuring and its Focus on Functional Outcomes in the United States

## Carol M. Frattali

In an era of increased accountability in health care systems throughout the world, increasing importance has been given to functional communication assessment. This chapter describes concepts and terms such as managed care, gatekeeper functions, utilization review or management, treatment authorization, discounted fee-for-service and capitation. There is evidence to suggest that the focus on functional outcome measures by speech-language pathologists world-wide reflects a similar change in health care in other countries. This chapter provides some recommendations and examples of a way forward where quality speech-language pathology services are provided in the context of economic constraints.

## Introduction

I recently met with a group of clinical aphasiologists who were preparing case studies for a book on approaches to the treatment of aphasia (Helm-Estabrooks & Holland, 1998). Wearing the payer's hat, I presented an unpopular perspective. This perspective took into account, as a salient factor, the economics of clinical care. Taking their clinical case studies, I subjected them to criteria commonly used by payers or administrators to make decisions about reimbursable care. These criteria included the following:

- an expectation of significant practical improvement;
- establishment of functional goals;
- estimated duration and frequency of treatment;
- comparable pre-/post-treatment measures to document change;

- documentation of progress and relationship to functional goals; and
- retention of gain at follow-up.

In general, the case studies compared well to these criteria. What remained questionable for a few of these cases, from the reimbursement standpoint, were the times post-onset of the communication disorder, and the lengths of treatment provided. As stated in a chapter included in the Helm-Estabrooks and Holland publication (Frattali, 1998)

> It is generally, although erroneously accepted that maximal rehabilitation benefit occurs during the first 3 months post-onset of stroke. Some may extend the period to 6 months. But we have learned here (and elsewhere in the professional literature in both group and single-subject experimental studies) that significant and functional improvements can occur long after the first 3 to 6 months post-stroke, even with only a short period of treatment. (p. 256)

These criteria emphasize *functional outcomes*, or, as a payer might describe them, practical results in the shortest amount of time (Cornett, in press). Sutherland Cornett illustrates the importance of a functional approach by borrowing from a scenario written by Preston Lewis about the outcomes of treatment of an 18-year-old student who had participated in numerous years of individual treatment. Some of his comments are presented:

> He can put 100 pegs in a board in less than 10 minutes while in his seat with 95% accuracy, but he can't put quarters in a vending machine.

> He can sing the alphabet and tell me the names of the letters when presented on a card with 80% accuracy, but he can't tell the men's room from the ladies' room at McDonald's.

> He can sort blocks by color, up to 10 different colors, but he can't sort white from dark clothes for the washing machine.

> He can identify with 100% accuracy 100 different Peabody picture cards by pointing, but he can't order a hamburger by pointing to a picture on a menu or gesturing.

> He can count to 100 by rote memory, but he doesn't know how many dollars to pay the clerk for a $2.59 McDonald's coupon special.

Matters of economic interest that carry functional themes can also be rephrased as questions. Consider these questions from a recent journal article addressing alternatives to conventional aphasia rehabilitation:

> Given that speech therapy may work for some patients . . ., what is the cost-to-benefit ratio of the gains made? Do the gains made as a result of therapy translate into practical use that improves the patient's functional independence or quality of life? How does speech therapy compare in cost benefit with other potential uses of medical resources for these patients, e.g., personal care services, adaptive equipment, etc? (Weinrich, 1997, p. 107)

The purposes of this chapter are to describe some of the prominent features of change in the U.S. health-care delivery system, address the implications of these changes on conventional clinical practice given its focus on functional approaches to assessment and treatment, offer some alternatives that are being tried in clinical care, and make some recommendations for the future.

## Changes to the U.S. Health Care System

What follows is excerpted from an earlier publication (Frattali, 1998). Predictions are that, in the near future, all U.S. health care will be managed in one form or another. The growth of managed care represents the drive for dictating the "where's," "how's," and "how long's" of patient care. Patients are being discharged "quicker and sicker" from acute care hospitals, giving rise to another level of care called "subacute care," to denote its position between acute care and nursing facility care. Short hospital stays have nurtured the growth of industries such as nursing facilities, home health, and outpatient care. Cost cutting has resulted in caps on services and limits on number of sessions, length of treatment, and level of reimbursement. As a result, patient assessment and treatment plans must be modified. Given these constraints, we must decide how to best use the shrinking resources for providing quality care. To make these decisions, it is important that we first have a general understanding of changing health-care systems.

## Managed Care

In the United States, the most sweeping changes in health care have involved managed care in all its hybrid forms. Generally, managed care describes a cost-effective system that integrates both the financing and delivery of health-care services. It is defined by the American Association of Health Plans (American Managed Care and Review Association, 1995), the national trade association representing managed care organizations, as a comprehensive approach to health-care delivery that encompasses planning and coordination of care, patient and provider education, monitoring of care quality, and cost control. Under this model, the financing and delivery of care are managed under one roof or by the same operational entity.

In the 1980s, at the height of the "health-care crisis" in America, managed care was considered an answer to spiraling costs. But the preoccupation with cost was thought to place the quality of care at risk. Cost consciousness, however, is not necessarily bad when it is accompanied by an ethical sense of decision making and honest yardsticks against which to measure the quality of patient care.

### Common Care Management Features

Three features of care management are important to clinicians: *gatekeeper functions, utilization review* or *management*, and *treatment authorization*. A *gatekeeper* is the coordinator of a patient's care. The gatekeeper approach requires the patient to gain access to the entire system of care through a single, experienced primary-care physician. Thus, the gatekeeper decides what care the patient needs and usually at what intensity and scope of service. *Utilization review/management* (UR) (recently being called *resources management*) is a systematic process of reviewing and controlling patients' use of health-care services and providers' use of health-care resources. UR procedures include second opinions, precertifications, treatment authorizations, discharge planning, chart reviews, and so on. Finally, *authorization* is approval for care or services. These features create a system of checks and balances designed to prevent unnecessary, inappropriate, or excessive care and ensure the quality of care. In effect, they lead to compliance with the regulations for rehabilitative services imposed by Congress for federally qualified HMOs. The Federal HMO Act of 1973 states:

> *Federally qualified HMOs must provide or arrange for outpatient service and inpatient hospital services which shall include short-term rehabilitation and physical therapy, the provision of which the HMO determines can be expected to result in the significant improvement of a member's condition within a period of two months. (Code of Federal Regulations, Title 42, Section 110.102[1990])*

The emphasis here is on "short-term." Although 2 months was specified in the regulatory language as a minimum time period of treatment, it often is interpreted by managed-care administrators as a maximum. In all, the language of the federal law carries great significance for clinicians whose usual ways of providing care extend well beyond this time period.

## Common Forms of Payment

The two common forms of payment to practitioners who work in managed-care contexts are *discounted fee-for-service* and *capitation*. *Discounted fee-for-service* is a discount from the provider's usual or customary fee, paid after services are rendered. As a cost-containment strategy, this option has failed. To offset the impact of the discounts, providers have increased usual rates or increased the frequency and types of services. *Capitation* is a fixed amount of money set by contract between a managed-care organization (MCO) and the provider, to be paid on a per-person (per capita) basis regardless of the number of services rendered or costs incurred. Capitation is usually expressed in cost units of "per member per month (PMPM)." Typically, the MCO sets aside a percentage of the payment to safeguard against unexpected costs. At the year's end, any money left in this risk pool is returned to the providers. Capitation is a shared risk arrangement, which provides incentives for physicians (often the gatekeepers of care) to limit special tests, special services (including rehabilitation), and hospitalization for the enrollees. The scope of services in a capitation contract can range from limited primary-care physician services to all health-care services. As providers are expected to share more risk, the primary payment arrangement is shifting to capitation.

*Fee-for-service* gives caregivers little or no financial incentive to be concerned about the cost and use (or overuse) of services. Thus, to earn more money, the incentive is to increase utilization. This payment arrangement rewards piecework; the more services providers render, the more money they make. Conversely, *capitation* fundamentally changes the financial incentives of traditional fee-for-service system because it is a fixed revenue system that pays the same amount each month no matter how many or how few services are actually provided. Effectively, the fewer services provided, the more the providers are rewarded. Under capitation, the provider's primary objective is to maximize quality of care and patient satisfaction and minimize the total cost of care, per person per year. *Value* (good quality at a low cost), then, becomes the primary demand of major purchasers of health care (i.e., employers) and consumers.

**Typical Managed Care Coverage Limitations**

For speech-language pathology and other rehabilitative services, MCOs may impose one or more of the following restrictions by limiting services to:

- 60 days;
- 10 sessions for speech-language pathology services;
- 10 sessions for physical therapy, occupational therapy, and speech-language pathology services combined;
- 2 weeks with authorization for continued treatment;
- care that adheres to the MCOs critical path (interdisciplinary treatment regimes that organize, sequence and time-specify clinical interventions for defined patient groups).

## *Payer and Accrediting Agency Requirements*

Although it is convenient to cite managed care as the reason for change in health care, other economic and regulatory forces have contributed, in substantial ways, to these changes. As summarized in Table 5–1, outcome-oriented standards are common in accreditation agency requirements and payer guidelines. They reflect a trend toward accountable care in terms relevant to everyday life activities. The requirements are not dissimilar from concepts of accountable and relevant clinical care beginning with documentation of baseline performance, establishment of a plan of care based on that performance, development of functional goals of treatment, reassessment of performance using the same baseline measures, and clinical decision making (e.g., continue treatment, modify treatment, end treatment) based on the findings.

In the requirements cited in Table 5–1, the emphasis is on "functional." Regulatory agencies in the United States operate largely with a definition of medical rehabilitation as "those services intended to optimize function." Thus, functional status measures have become instruments of choice in documenting a patient's status or change in status. That said, there is a need to emphasize the danger of using functional measures at the exclusion of other tests or measures that are used for differing but equally important purposes. A functional measure can neither be used for sensitive and differential diagnostic purposes, nor can identify strengths and weaknesses in specific parameters of speech, swallowing, language, and cognition. These purposes are reserved for our conventional standardized behavioral and instrumental tests and procedures that measure at the impairment level. Furthermore, functional measures may not capture aspects of health-related quality of life, which are more adequately addressed by a growing number of psychosocial, wellness, and quality-of-life self-assessments. Payers may likely not appreciate the differences among these classes of measures. There-

Table 5–1.    Some Requirements of Payers and Accrediting Agencies.

| Source | Requirements |
|---|---|
| Joint Commission on Accreditationof Health Care Organizations  (JCAHO) (1997) | PE 1.3.1 All patients referred to rehabilitation services receive a functional assessment. TX 6.3 Rehabilitation restores, improves, or maintains the patient's optimal level of functioning, self-care, self-responsibility, independence, and quality of life. |
| The Rehabilitation Accreditation Commission (CARF) (1997) | 6. A Medical Rehabilitation Program should demonstrate that the persons served are making measurable improvement toward accomplishment of their functional goals. 33. The exit/discharge summary should delineate the person's: a. Present functional status and potential. b. Functional status related to targeted jobs, alternative occupations, or the competitive labor market. |
| ASHA Professional Services Board (PSB) (1992) | b. The plan for ongoing quality improvement periodically addresses all standards, with particular attention to services that are of high volume or that carry added risk, emphasizing <br> • Client evaluation and/or treatment outcomes; these may include, but are not limited to, identification of disorder, acceptance of recommendations, functional change in status, client/family satisfaction... |
| Medicare Intermediary Manual (Guidelines) (1991) (See also Medicare outpatient billing forms 700 and 701) | Section 3905.3: Plan of treatment: The plan of treatment must contain the following: <br> • Functional goals and estimated rehabilitation potential..., estimated duration of treatment <br> A. Functional goals must be written by the SLP to reflect the level of communicative independence the patient is expected to achieve outside of the therapeutic environment. The functional goals reflect the final level the patient is expected to achieve, are realistic, and have a positive effect on the quality of the patient's everyday functions. Examples include: Communicate basic physical needs and emotional status (feelings). Communicate personal self-care needs. Engage in social communicative interactions with family and friends. Carry out communicative interactions in the community. 3905.4 Progress reports. Obtain: The initial functional communication level. The present functional level. The patient's expected rehabilitation potential Changes in the plan of treatment.. [The medical reviewer may approve the claim if there is still a reasonable expectation that significant improvement in the patient's *overall functional ability* will occur] |

fore, clinicians must inform payers of the various purposes of different types of assessment tools, and the importance assigned to each to yield a total picture of the patient, which is necessary for appropriate intervention.

## Health-Care Changes in Other Countries

Byng et al. (1998) detail a thorough account of the health-care changes occurring in the United Kingdom. As well, Hesketh and Sage (in press) document these same changes and discuss the activities related to development and use of outcome measures in the United States, Canada, Australia, and the United Kingdom. From this international perspective, the focus on functional measures is apparent. Byng et al. report, "In the United Kingdom in recent years, as in North America, the attention of health care professionals has been focused ever more sharply on the need to assess and evaluate the impact of intervention" (p. 558). These authors discuss the emergence of a profound change to health-care provision in the United Kingdom since the introduction of its National Health Service. Its government signaled the importance that evaluation of effectiveness would have on the development of health services in its strategy document "Health of the Nation" (1991):

> The development of a better understanding of the effectiveness—and cost effectiveness—of interventions is essential. It is fundamental not only to setting strategic objectives; it is fundamental to all health planning and to each individual decision about how to use resources, from choice of treatment for individual patients to legislation on environmental protection. (p. 43)

Within the U.K. Research and Development Program, a number of initiatives has been established through which the development of outcome measures is promoted.

According to Byng et al. (1998), outcomes measurement is a relatively recent concept in the United Kingdom. Data collection in the United Kingdom has focused on measures such as admissions, discharges, and waiting times, the number of times a client has been in contact with a service, and so forth. Outcomes measurement, therefore, has been limited to information on the pattern of admission and discharges, with little or no systematic collection of information on the pattern of recovery or even the amount of intervention a client with a particular condition might receive. But, in addition to the need for quantitative outcomes data, Byng et al. emphasize the use of qualitative outcomes research methods. In the United Kingdom, there is a growing awareness that the means of investigating the client's perspective must move beyond conventional assessment procedures. They cite Worrall (1992) who suggests that the disabling aspects and functional implications of a communication disorder can only be properly assessed through some form of consultation between patient and professional. This orientation encourages the use of qualitative methods to investigate communication disorders and their effects in terms of everyday life.

Pope and Mays (1995) tell us that the goal of qualitative research is "the development of concepts which help us to understand social phenomena in natural (rather than experimental) settings, giving due emphasis to the meanings, experiences and views of all the participants" (p. 43). Thus, in Byng's et al. words, "It investigates the social world, and perspectives on that world, in terms of the concepts, perceptions, and accounts of the people it is about, a departure and contrast from the process of testing out constructs developed by professional experts" (p. 567).

Hesketh and Sage (1999) begin their discussion centered on the importance of outcome measures by stating that clinicians are likely to look at outcomes that are directly relevant to the management of the individual client. By this, they mean that clinicians tend to choose conventional measures of impairment as preferred outcome measures. They support this position, in part, by the results of a survey (Hesketh & Hopcutt, 1997) about use of outcome measures in the field of aphasiology in the United Kingdom. They found that many respondents were using impairment-based measures such as the Psycholinguistic Assessment of Language Processing in Aphasia (PALPA; Kay et al., 1992) and the Boston Diagnostic Aphasia Examination (BDAE; Goodglass & Kaplan, 1983) to monitor change over time. Similar survey results have been reported in the United States (ASHA, 1996) and Australia (Worrall, 1998).

Hesketh and Sage (1999) acknowledge that incorporating the opinions of service users is increasingly becoming a part of measuring health-care outcomes. They reveal a problem inherent in this approach, however. Speech-language pathologists are challenged by clients with communication disorders who find it difficult or are unable to self-report perceptions of change or aspects of quality of life. They identify several options. Simpler measures can be devised; family members/caregivers can serve as proxies; assessment tools can be adapted by incorporating visual analogue scales with few verbal descriptors or pictures to augment written text. Finally in-depth interviews can be conducted by the skilled clinician to uncover the unique perceptions and opinions of the client.

Perhaps most importantly, Hesketh and Sage (1999) dispel a commonly held belief that "any therapy is better than none." They use Culyer's (1992) argument that ineffective care is unethical, particularly because it denies limited health-care resources to those who can derive benefit. In this context, they propose that outcomes measurement occur at three levels: at the individual client level to inform the direction of treatment; at the service level to allow managers to establish a strong relationship and dialogue with health-care commissioners; and at the community/population level to allow health-care commissioners to obtain information about treatment efficacy and effectiveness and to use the information to set realistic performance targets for the services that they are commissioning.

## A Managed-Care Case Example

Returning to the discussion of health-care changes in the United States and the pressure to find effective alternatives to conventional treatment, I would like to share an example that is borrowed from the same earlier publication (Frattali, 1998). Clinicians must develop effective strategies for working within a system of managed care. To accomplish this, they first must understand differences between managed care and traditional approaches to clinical care. The following case example, summarized from the ASHA publication, *Managing Managed Care* (1994), illustrates how services are being limited:

> The patient (FC) was a 78-year-old male who sustained a left hemisphere stroke with right hemiparesis and mild to moderate aphasia. Prior to the stroke, FC was independent and living at home. He was insured by an HMO that contracted with an individual practice association (IPA) to service Medicare patients for a capitated rate of payment for the full extent of health care.
>
> FC was hospitalized for 6 days in an acute care hospital. During his hospital stay, he received SLP services, after which he was discharged home with home health care. Utilization review (UR) authorized a speech-language pathology evaluation, after which his speech-language pathologist was to send the report to UR for its review. Because UR had authorized only a single-visit evaluation, testing was abbreviated to what could be accomplished within the single session. FC had difficulty formulating both verbal and written language. Evaluation findings were as follows: FC's speech was fluent but characterized by literal paraphasias and neologisms. He could communicate basic needs at sentence level, but, longer, more complex utterances were difficult. Auditory comprehension was reduced to following 66% of three-step directions and understanding 50% of paragraph-level information. Reading was 80% accurate at sentence level, but FC was unable to read anything at paragraph level. Writing was severely impaired. He could write his name, but was unable to formulate written words or phrases. Before his stroke, FC had written letters to family members frequently.
>
> On the SLP's recommendation, treatment was authorized, but for a limit of two sessions. Because basic needs were being communicated verbally and on FC's request, these sessions focused on writing skills. At the end of the two sessions, FC was able to write the alphabet and was beginning to write phrases when given a stimulus word. A home program was developed and his spouse was instructed to complete verbal and written exercises with FC.
>
> On the basis of FC's progress and motivation, the SLP requested authorization for additional treatment. The physician who served as the gatekeeper requested copies of treatment notes and a progress report with justification for continued treatment, then forwarded the documentation to UR. Authorization was received for four more visits. At the end of the four visits, FC was formulating short sentences with 75% accuracy, writing the names of objects with 90% accuracy, and formulating and writing short sentences with 77% accuracy. His spouse was further instructed to use compensatory strategies and to encourage self-correction of errors.
>
> Because FC was continually improving, the SLP requested four more sessions. Two visits were authorized with notification that no further SLP services would be approved. The last two sessions focused on family training. Further progress would depend on good follow-through by the family at home.

As a result of four separate UR authorizations, only one evaluation session and eight treatment sessions constituted the posthospital SLP treatment program for this patient. This treatment program would be considered by many speech-language pathologists to fall far short of the need for this patient, particularly in the presence of continual gains. Another factor that interfered with a smooth course of treatment was the fragmented approach to authorization. In this example, the SLP was only given a few sessions per authorization in which to render service, never knowing whether treatment would be reauthorized. Consequently, a fragmented approach to treatment resulted. This might be an example of "living by systems." It is important to recognize, however, that in these times of change, systems, too, are changeable.

### Suggesting Ways to "Manage" Managed Care

From the above example, some suggestions can be made for what might have been done differently to prevent an unacceptably brief and fragmented course of treatment:

1. *Understand the practices of the restructured health-care system:* Learn what drives decision making and who makes the decisions in the health-care plan. Once key decision makers are identified, effective negotiations can take place. The best time to negotiate a treatment package is before coverage terms are delineated or a contract is signed. Speech-language pathologists, working independently or collectively, can negotiate with decision makers at local HMOs or other managed-care offices to reach consensus on service provisions.

   Practitioners in hospitals could also discuss service policy with the hospital employee who is responsible for managed-care negotiations, usually a vice president for managed care or the chief financial officer (Griffin & Fazen, 1993).

2. *Support treatment claims with data:* Once speech-language pathologists have the attention of decision makers, they need objective data to support claims of acceptable levels of care. If eight sessions are insufficient, SLPs must provide convincing data that demonstrate cost savings in other areas covered by the managed-care plan or improvements in medical status, functional status, independence, consumer satisfaction, and quality of life. Decision makers will respond to these areas because these persons value economics and the areas translate into cost savings (as well as retention of satisfied consumers) for the health plan.

3. *Team with physicians and patients/family members to advocate for needs:* Clinicians can work with referring physicians and family members to ensure that an insurance company has an appropriate perception of a patient's needs. Such initial steps can avoid conflicts down stream, such as denials of treatment authorization requests as noted in the previous example. Consumers often are their own best advocates. Clinicians can inform them of appeals processes and of the right to pursue legal action, if options for rehabilitation are inappropriately restricted. Consumers can also involve their employers. Large employers particularly have clout when they represent a large segment of enrollees in a specific plan. Consumer satisfaction is vital to financial viability for many plans, and they may adjust coverage to retain enrollees.

4. *Develop and foster acceptance of critical paths:* Another clinical tool that decision makers are beginning to accept is critical paths. If clinicians can provide a

"map" that delineates the process of care with associated outcomes along a time line, which ideally is supported by clinical research findings, they may make considerable progress in adjusting overly restrictive terms of rehabilitative care.

5. *Educate patients and their families about managed care restrictions:* In a system of managed care, patient/family education becomes vital. From the outset of intervention, patients and families should be advised of their plan's limitations and their options once benefits are exhausted. These options may include investigation of other sources of funding, self-pay, referral to a lower cost clinic (e.g., university clinic), group treatment, or family or self-training to continue therapy. There should be no surprises that result in a premature end to the treatment program and leave patients unprepared to cope adequately with an impairment. Discharge should be anticipated from the outset.

6. *Explore alternatives to traditional treatment practices:* Once options to extend treatment are exhausted up front, one must make the best use of what has been authorized by the managed-care company. One questions if in the above example, the chosen treatment approach was best given the circumstances. Other innovative methods that are of known or expected treatment effectiveness and efficiency might have been used. These methods might have included a functional approach to treatment, training of family members as clinician volunteers, instruction of self-cueing, computer-assisted treatment, enrollment in a stroke club, or a homework regimen, in any combination that could be grouped into a brief treatment package.

## Toward the Future

What does the future hold? In the United States, reform of prevailing managed-care systems and their myopic focus on economics is a good educated guess. Managed-care reform has become a weighty consumer issue with the U.S. Congress as a result of mounting information of erosion of quality of care. Bills are being introduced that propose benefits, such as offering patients a choice of providers and access to appropriate levels of care, holding managed-care companies accountable for care that is denied or delayed by ensuring plan liability and due process for patients and providers, requiring that managed-care providers state all the reasonable options for care, and prohibiting discrimination against non-physician providers who qualify under state licensing or certification to participate in the health plan (Schmidt, 1998). A member of ASHA's Governmental and Social Policies Board, Becky Sutherland Cornett, states well that health care is about people, not simply profits (Schmidt, 1998).

More recently, a new bill was introduced in the U.S. House of Representatives that would repeal a $1500 Medicare cap that was jointly imposed on speech-language pathologists and physical therapists for their outpatient services to beneficiaries (per patient, per year). The bill, The Rehabilitation Benefit for Seniors Act of 1998, would remove the arbitrary health-care service limit. "Rather than limiting the availability of medically necessary services by imposing an arbitrary annual dollar limitation, the new system would be based on patient need. Payments would be based on patient classification by diagnostic category and would take into account prior use of services in both inpatient and outpatient settings" (Schmidt, 1998).

At the state level, legislation is being passed that increases the accountability of managed health-care plans. For example, the Pennsylvania House of Representatives unanimously passed a bill that would establish the Managed Care Accountability Act. The bill would define certain managed-care terms and require businesses that review HMO decisions to become certified by the Insurance Department every 3 years. The bill would also require that only licensed physicians or psychologists be the ones to deny coverage and would prohibit MCOs from excluding from their physician network doctors who protest managed-care decisions to deny treatment (ASHA, personal communication, 1998).

The above state and federal legislative activity in the United States suggests that perhaps that pendulum is swinging to some point in the middle ground of good care at a reasonable cost. This means that a focus on functional outcomes may remain, but as driven more by the consumer than by the payer or regulator.

A particularly insightful personal account of life after a stroke was documented by Varon (1997), and punctuates the importance of a functional approach to intervention. She describes "watching the unfolding interaction between my somewhat impaired self and the people in my workplace. There is no way that I am fully competent. . . . But people have been willing to make a place for me anyway and to regard my contribution as valuable" (p. 65). This perspective carries a strong message to clinicians interested in measurement of the effects of a language disorder in real-world contexts, and in rehabilitation aimed at reducing psychosocial barriers to optimal functioning in places where it is most meaningful—the natural environments of patients.

## Some Recommendations

The challenge for clinicians is to provide care in the most appropriate setting; at the right time and intensity; coordinated with the best combination of professionals, support staff, and volunteers; at a low cost; and with the best outcomes. The following recommendations acknowledge current limitations of clinical practice and encourage the clinician to discover new opportunities designed to either fit within or modify these limitations to foster care in the best interest of patients:

1. Become knowledgeable about changing health-care systems and discuss the issues with key decision makers to influence change.

2. Develop and test new approaches to clinical intervention that embrace functional approaches to care. Beyond diagnostic and remedial aspects of clinical care, explore interventions that can occur outside the clinic and in a patient's community (e.g., address the need for adaptations in the patient's natural environments and interventions with a patient's family and friends or co-workers to enhance communication and, by extension, quality of life).

3. Intensify clinical research efforts using efficacy and outcomes research methodologies to document key outcomes (including functional communication and health-related quality of life) and disseminate research results in pub-

lic forums, including professional journals, special interest newsletters, study clubs, and local, state, and national conferences.

4. Develop and test cost-effective alternatives to traditional practice including involvement of family members/partners in treatment, use of support personnel, and use of brief treatment packages, group treatments, and co-treatments that have been shown to be efficacious.

5. Develop/use reliable and valid outcome measures in clinical practice and clinical research along the full continuum of the consequences of disease—from differential diagnosis and identification of specific strengths and weaknesses, to the effects of specific speech and language deficits on functional communication, to the effects of communication disabilities on overall wellness and quality of life.

## Conclusion

Robert T. Wertz has been quoted as saying, "It's not a perfect world—people are making up answers to questions based on economics and not efficacy. Our goal is to come to some agreement between the two" (in Frattali, 1998). The dynamics of the U.S. health-care system and its effects on the provision of care teaches us a lesson—listen and respond to the softest voices. These voices, I believe, are the consumers' of speech-language pathology services. They know what is best and what they need in terms of optimal functioning in their natural environments. Our job is to discern how to best meet their needs in a reasonable and cost-responsible way, given the current constraints of the system. When ways become unreasonable, it is the job of the clinician in tandem with appropiate other involved parties, to work toward reform of unworkable systems.

I am encouraged to believe that the next change in U.S. health care will be one of displacement of political power, with the recipients of health care taking the lead. Our goal is to meet their needs by scrutinizing conventional clinical approaches, allowing ourselves to walk away from what simply does not work nor work well in a reasonable period of time, and being flexible enough to try new and innovative interventions—chief among them, functional approaches that address clients in contexts and environments in which they naturally belong.

## References

American Managed Care and Review Association (AMCRA) (now American Association of Health Plans). (1995). *Managed health care fact sheet*. Washington, DC: Author.

American Speech-Language-Hearing Association. Quality Improvement Study Section of ASHA Special Interest Division 11: Administration and Supervision. (1996). Clinical use of outcome measures: Results of a survey. *Special Interest Division 11 Newsletter, 6*, 2–8.

American Speech-Language-Hearing Association, Ad Hoc Committee on Managed Care. (1994). *Managing managed care: A practical guide for audiologists and speech-language pathologists*. Rockville, MD: Author.

American Speech-Language-Hearing Association, Council on Professional Standards. (1992, September). Standards for professional service programs in audiology and speech-language pathology. *ASHA, 34*, 63–70.

Byng, S., van der Gaag, A., & Parr, S. International initiatives in outcomes measurement: A perspective from the United Kingdom. In C. Frattali (ed.): *Measuring outcomes in speech-language pathology*. New York, NY: Thieme Medical Publishers.

(CARF) The Rehabilitation Accreditation Commission. (1997). *Standards manual and interpretive guidelines for medical rehabilitation*. Tucson, AZ: Author.

Culyer, A. (1992). The morality of efficiency in health-care—Some uncomfortable implications. *Health Economics, 1*, 7–18.

Frattali, CM. (1998). Clinical care in a changing health system. In N. Helm-Estabrooks & A. Holland (eds): *Approaches to the treatment of aphasia* (pp. 241–266). San Diego, CA: Singular Publishing Group.

George Washington University, Center for Health Policy Research (1997). Negotiating the new health system: A national study of Medicaid managed care contracts. Washington, DC: Author.

Goodglass, H. & Kaplan, E. (1983). *Assessment of aphasia and related disorders*. Philadelphia: Lea & Febiger.

Griffin, K., & Fazen, M. (1993, winter). A managed care strategy for practitioners. *Quality improvement digest*. Rockville, MD: American Speech-Language-Hearing Association.

Health Care Financing Administration. (1991, June). Medicare intermediary manual, Part 3—Claims Process, section 3905, Medical review Part B, intermediary outpatient speech-language pathology bills. [Transmittal no. 1528]. Washington, DC: U.S. Government Printing Office.

Health of the Nation. A Consultative Document for Health in England. (1991). London: HMSO.

Helm-Estabrooks, N. & Holland, A. (eds). (1998). *Approaches to the treatment of aphasia*. San Diego, CA: Singular Publishing Group.

Hesketh, A. & Hopcott, B. (1997). Outcome measures for aphasia therapy: It's not what you do, it's the way that you measure it. *European Journal of Disorders of Communication, 32* (Special Issue), 198–203.

Hesketh, A. & Sage, K. (1999). For better, for worse: Outcome measurement in speech and language therapy. *Advances in speech-language pathology. 1*, 37–46.

Interstudy. (1996). Projections of HMO growth: 1996–2000. Chicago: Author.

Joint Commission on Accreditation of Healthcare Organizations. (1997). *Accreditation manual for hospitals*. Oakbrook Terrace, IL: Author.

Kander, M. (1996, November). Federal legislation and other federal activities: Impact on rehabilitation service delivery. *ASHA Special Interest Division 11 Newsletter, 6*, 15–16.

Kay, J., Lesser, R., & Coltheart, M. (1992). *Psycholinguistic assessment of language processing in aphasia*. Hove, UK: Lawrence Erlbaum Associates.

Pope, C. & Mays, N. (1995). Reaching the parts other methods cannot reach: An introduction to qualitative methods in health and health services research. *British Medical Journal, 311*, 42–45.

Schmidt, N. (1998). Outcome-oriented rehabilitation: A response to managed care. In E. Dobrzykowski (ed.): *Essential readings in rehabilitation outcome measurement* (pp. 41–45). Gaithersburg, MD: Aspen Publications.

Sutherland Cornett, B. (in press). *Clinical practice management in speech-language pathology: Principles and practicalities*. Gaithersburg, MD: Aspen Publishers.

U.S. General Accounting Office. (1993). Medicaid: States turn to managed care to improve access and control costs. [GAO/T-HRD-93-10]. Washington, DC: Author.

Weinrich, M. (1997). Computer rehabilitation in aphasia. *Clinical Neuroscience. 4*, 103–107.

Worrall, L. (1992). Functional communication assessment: An Australian perspective. *Aphasiology, 6*, 105–111.

Worrall, L. (1998). National survey of speech pathology outcome measures. Paper presented at the Speech Pathology Australia Conference, Freemantle, Western Australia. 11–15 May, 1998.

# 6

## The Assessment of Functional Communication in Culturally and Linguistically Diverse Populations

### ROSEMARY BAKER

**The assessment of functional communicative abilities of people from diverse cultural and linguistic backgrounds presents the speech-language pathologist with many challenges. This chapter explores the notions of cultural and linguistic diversity and examines their influence on communication assessment. The suitability of existing approaches for application to diverse populations is considered. An approach to developing appropriate functional communication assessments for these populations is then discussed.**

### Introduction

This chapter focuses on the challenge of assessing functional communication in settings characterized by cultural and linguistic diversity. First, the nature of this diversity, the ways in which it is manifested in language use and communicative performance, and its implications for assessment in speech–language pathology are outlined. The suitability of existing assessment procedures for use with diverse populations, and on their administration in translated form are commented on. Finally, possible ways of approaching the design of assessment procedures suitable for particular populations are considered and developmental work on an approach for the Australian multilingual setting is described.

This discussion relates primarily to people with acquired neurogenic language impairment, who, premorbidly, used more than one language in their everyday lives, that is, those displaying at least some degree of bilingualism or multilingualism. However, some of the issues raised apply also to people who would normally be regarded as speaking different varieties rather than distinct languages. The term 'variety' is defined by Hudson (1996; p. 22) as "... *a set of linguistic items with similar social distribution,*" and thus encompasses the notions of "language," "dialect" (whether regionally or socially determined) and "register" or "style." Furthermore, some of the points discussed here are relevant to monolingual speakers of nonstandard varieties of the dominant language in their setting, or of varieties not generally spoken by those responsible for assessing their communicative function.

This chapter is thus concerned with situations in which premorbid language use was one of the following:

1. The client made exclusive use of one or more languages or varieties not shared by the assessor;
2. The client could function (to varying degrees) in the language or variety normally used for assessment, but also spoke one or more others.

The use of different codes is not, however, the only issue. Intertwined with this already challenging set of situations are cultural factors that influence all aspects of communicative behavior. Adequate provision for the situations outlined above requires an understanding of the implications of cultural and linguistic diversity for the assessment process at every stage, from determination of appropriate content and format, to the interpretation and use of results.

## Cultural Diversity

### Cultural Background

Pauwels (1995) notes that definitions of culture are almost as numerous as the scholars who write on the topic. A frequently quoted, and comprehensive, definition is that of Samovar, Porter, and Jain (1981):

> *Formally defined, culture is the deposit of knowledge, experiences, beliefs, values, attitudes, meanings, hierarchies, religion, timing, roles, spatial relations, concepts of the universe, and material objects and possessions acquired by a large group of people in the course of generations through individual and group striving. Culture manifests itself in patterns of language and in forms of activity and behavior that act as models for both the common adaptive acts and the styles of communication that enable us to live in a society within a given geographic environment at a given state of technological development at a particular moment in time. (Samovar et al., 1981, p. 24)*

For our present purposes, however, the following less formal definition, given by the same authors, is adequate:

> *... culture is the form or pattern for living. People learn to think, feel, believe and strive for what their culture considers proper. Language habits, friendships, eating habits, communication practices, social acts, economic and political activities, and technology all follow the patterns of culture. (Samovar et al., 1981, p. 23)*

We are taught some of these patterns of culture explicitly, but most are learned unconsciously from the behavior of those around us. Although much of this learning takes place during childhood, people who later migrate to another country usually also take on, to varying degrees, some of the cultural traits of their new setting, a process referred to as acculturation. The next generation, brought up in this setting, will normally be exposed to cultural patterns from their parents' country of origin as well as those of their own country of residence, and will thus learn aspects of both.

Culture does not necessarily correspond with racial or ethnic background. Although members of a particular culture often have a shared background, people of similar background do not always share the same culture. Battle (1993), for example, describes the cultural gulf she observed between African-American visitors to Senegal and the local villagers with whom they shared ancestral links, thus highlighting the differences in cultural identity, personal history and view of the world that can be found among people of similar racial background.

Further, within each broad cultural group there is variation associated with factors such as age and gender roles, region, social and economic status, and educational level. Such factors, as well as other, individual characteristics, can influence aspects of people's lives and behavior in ways that cut across cultural backgrounds.

## Cultural Differences

Cultural differences have been described (from a Western viewpoint at least) on a number of dimensions. The analyses summarized by Pauwels (1995) include the following: world view, beliefs concerning human nature, the perception of self, features of social organization, orientation toward activity or work (i.e., whether the focus is on doing or being), time orientation (the conceptualization and importance of time), space management (the distinction between private and public spheres), toleration of uncertainty, and individualism versus collectivity (i.e., the extent to which priority is given to the individual's own interests as compared with those of the family, social or work group). Individualism is considered to be a strong feature of Western cultures, whereas in many other cultures responsibility to the group is paramount.

Cultural background influences the ways in which people regard illness, disability and rehabilitation. Several authors discuss the cultural characteristics of major groups in the United States, including Kayser (1998), Payne (1997), and contributors to the volume edited by Battle (1993). Kayser (1998) summarizes some differing views of impairment, disability, and handicap found among these groups. These include differences in beliefs concerning the causes of diseases and disabilities, approaches to healing, conditions regarded as handicapping, and degrees of acceptance of disability within the family.

Cultural variables are found to affect access to and utilization of language intervention services in a number of ways. Wallace (1993) notes that when a cultural tradition dictates that a sick person should be taken care of, the notion of rehabilitation may not be acceptable, and in some cases the need to be taught to function independently would be seen as a source of shame to the family. One of Whitworth and Sjardin's (1993) case studies of aphasia in migrants to Australia exemplifies the "sick role" that may be adopted by the patient, and the conflict between this role and rehabilitation objectives. On the other hand, cultural stereotypes may lead health professionals to overestimate the support provided by the person's family network. As Payne (1997) points out, family structures and values can in any case change as a result of acculturation, and so a particular level of involvement by family members cannot be assumed.

Penn (1993) raises some of the problems with access to services in South Africa, where poverty and lack of transport and facilities can make formal assessment inappropriate. Wallace (1993) mentions the lack of awareness of speech–language pathology services among some groups in the United States, and points to the need for "creative service delivery options" (p. 248), which might include home-based treatment, particularly if timeliness or the keeping of appointments is a problem.

One aspect of cultural difference that is not often mentioned is the increased anxiety and fatigue experienced when coping in an unfamiliar culture (Gallois & Callan, 1997; Klopf & Park, 1982). Gallois and Callan attribute this to the greater risk of misunderstanding and social mistakes. Even after long periods of contact or residence in a new setting, people vary in their ability to operate effectively and comfortably in its cultural framework. This difference represents an additional potential burden for those with neurogenic communication disorders.

A lack of understanding of cultural differences can lead to mistrust (Payne, 1997). A major hindrance to the development of trust and respect across cultures is ethnocentrism. This is explained by Samovar et al. (1981) as follows:

> In studying other cultures, and in making cultural comparisons, we do so from the perspective of our own culture. Our observations and our conclusions are colored by the specific orientation of our culture. . . . There also is a danger that we might allow our judgments to take on evaluative interpretations. . . . This inclination to believe that our own group is superior and the only basis for judging other groups (or cultures) is called ethnocentrism. (Samovar et al., 1981, p. 19)

Clearly, if intercultural contact between speech–language pathologists and clients is to proceed successfully, ethnocentrism needs to be recognized and overcome, so that different systems of beliefs and values are understood rather than judged. In gaining a knowledge of other cultures, however, and in applying this in intercultural encounters, it is important to guard against the tendency to view people in terms of stereotypes.

Most authors point to the heterogeneity that exists within any community, and stress that information about cultural characteristics should not be overgeneralized or oversimplified. Among migrant groups, variation among generations and individuals is such that one should not make assumptions about maintenance of the cultural values of the country of origin, or indeed about acculturation to the adoptive country. These issues underscore the value of a detailed individual history in forming a clear picture of the cultural framework in which clients and their family members operate.

### Culture and Communication

It is generally held that culture determines, governs, or, at the very least, strongly influences, the ways in which people communicate. Samovar et al. (1981) offer the following view of the relationship between culture and communication:

*Culture and communication are inseparable because culture not only dictates who talks with whom, about what, and how the communication proceeds, it also helps to determine how people encode messages, the meanings they have for messages, and the conditions under which various messages may or may not be sent, noticed, or interpreted. In fact, our entire repertory of communicative behaviors is dependent largely on the culture in which we have been raised. Culture, consequently, is the foundation of communication. And, when cultures vary, communication practices also vary. (Samovar et al., 1981, p. 24)*

Culturally based variation occurs, for example, in choosing to speak versus remaining silent (in that silence carries different meanings in different cultural settings), speaking simultaneously (which may be regarded as normal or impolite), and making direct eye contact (which may indicate polite interest or seem intrusive). There are also differences in conventions for turn-taking, volume and pitch, body posture (e.g., when greeting or leaving), and for the acceptability or otherwise of physical contact such as touching a person's head (Strevens, 1987).

Gallois and Callan (1997) emphasize that because the culture-specific social rules that govern our communication may not be easily accessible to us, we may become aware of them only when they are broken. In communication between people of different cultural backgrounds, messages are encoded within one person's cultural framework and decoded within that of the other. When the participants' rules do not coincide, the listener may attribute the wrong meaning to the speaker's message, or may understand it only partially or indeed not at all. Equally, the speaker may inadvertently produce a message that to the listener is inappropriate in some way, or, at worst, offensive. Alternatively, the speaker may fail to produce the particular type of utterance that the listener's rules for appropriate and polite interaction would demand in a given situation. Either person may infer a message when none was intended, as a result of differences in paralinguistic and nonverbal aspects of communication.

Payne (1997) mentions some sources of potential misinterpretation in clinical contexts, such as the avoidance of direct gaze among Native Americans, and the head nodding which may be used by Vietnamese people to indicate respect but not necessarily understanding. Kayser (1998) draws out the implications of preferred Native American discourse styles for speech–language pathology, noting in particular the likely avoidance of direct gaze, of familiarity with acquaintances, and of drawing attention to oneself or to others. Silence may indicate not that a person is unable to respond, but that the clinician's questioning is regarded as too personal. Kayser (1998) also raises the issue of potential disagreement between clinicians and clients' families in their views of what constitutes improvement. The family may not perceive progress unless it improves the person's ability to communicate in a specific cultural role.

Assessing the ability to communicate in people of different cultural backgrounds thus requires a knowledge of characteristics of communication that are often different from the speech–language pathologist's own. As Samovar et al. (1981, p. 19) explain, "It is difficult to see and to give meaning to words and movements we are not familiar with. How, for example, do we make sense of someone's silence if we come from a very verbal culture?" Erroneous inferences can be avoided only by being aware of culturally based assumptions that might affect intercultural communication, and by gaining an understanding of our own and of other people's perceptual frames of reference.

## Linguistic Diversity

### Linguistic, Cultural, and Individual Factors

Despite the close link between culture and language, it is helpful for purposes of language assessment to maintain a distinction between cultural and linguistic considerations. Speakers of different languages may share similar cultural frameworks, so that the provision of appropriate assessment materials entails differences in linguistic code but not in substance. Conversely, apparent linguistic similarity can link populations superficially with distinct cultural differences. Assessment materials developed in English in the United States, for example, are largely understandable to speakers of British, Australian, South African and Indian varieties of English, but do not necessarily reflect their usage, their communicative settings, or their social rules of interaction.

Furthermore, considerable linguistic and communicative differences can be found among subpopulations within a particular geographical setting. In the United States, for instance, the broad categories used to designate ethnicity comprise a wide range of national, cultural, and linguistic backgrounds. Yeo (1996) lists at least 13 subgroups subsumed under the Asian/Pacific Islander designation, and notes that even within some of these (e.g., Chinese) several different languages are represented. The designation "Hispanic," too, comprises people of varied national origin and cultural background, including Mexican, Caribbean, Cuban and Puerto Rican, who may carry with them different combinations of African, Indian and European influences (Kayser, 1998).

Materials developed according to the linguistic and cultural framework of a particular dominant group can give rise to erroneous interpretations when administered to members of other groups. The major problem when using test materials with populations other than those for whom they were developed is that of distinguishing differences from deficits, as the volumes edited by Taylor (1986a, 1986b) affirm.

It must also be recognized that our communicative behavior is not determined solely by culture, but also by a range of social, physical and psychological factors (Samovar et al., 1981). In developing assessment procedures, it is important to keep in mind the individual variation that results from these additional factors, and to avoid overestimating the homogeneity of the target population(s).

According to Hudson (1996, p. 29), the clear delineation of speech communities on the basis of linguistic variables has proved impossible. He presents instead a view of individuals as using language ". . . to locate themselves in a multidimensional social space." He emphasizes the importance of social networks in shaping people's linguistic behavior, noting in particular the strong influence of relatively small social groups such as family, friends, neighbors, colleagues, and fellow members of organizations.

Even in members of moderately homogeneous groups, the speech–language pathologist will be aware of differences in premorbid communicative styles. With the addition of linguistic and cultural variables, the range of possibilities becomes even greater, and so additional information on these will be needed for meaningful interpretation of poststroke performance or progress.

## Bilingualism and Multilingualism

Although each person's communicative behavior is in some respects unique, it is nevertheless possible to identify general categories of speech community found throughout the world (see, e.g., Holmes, 1992; Hudson, 1996). This section focuses on communities characterized by multilingualism and bilingualism. An understanding of language use in such communities is important to the assessment of functional communication because of its direct relevance to decisions concerning the language(s) in which a person is to be assessed, and the choice of appropriate content.

Holmes (1992) notes that more than half of the world's population is bilingual, and indeed that many people use several languages for different purposes in their everyday interactions. Some individuals acquire more than one language as a result of their particular personal history, for example, through having parents of different language backgrounds, or through attending schools in different countries. Commonly, however, bilingualism and multilingualism occur at a national or community level.

In some nations (e.g., Canada and Switzerland), the existence of distinct linguistic communities is acknowledged by the recognition of more than one official language. In many countries, including Australia, Canada, New Zealand, South Africa, the United States and European countries, numerous languages are used in addition to the declared or *de facto* national languages. In Australia, for example, it is estimated that 150 aboriginal languages and 75 to 100 "immigrant" languages are spoken (Clyne, 1982, 1991).

In multilingual and bilingual communities, different languages tend to be associated with different communicative purposes. The languages of immigrant communities, for example, are used predominantly in domestic and social settings. In some communities, two languages or varieties are used in a consistent and complementary way for formal versus informal communication, a phenomenon known as "diglossia." In Arabic-speaking countries, for example, everyday communication is conducted in regional colloquial varieties, while classical Arabic is reserved for formal purposes.

The repertoire of languages and varieties acquired by an individual in any setting is determined by social, economic, and geographic factors (Penn, 1993), and by factors such as exposure and attitudes to the different varieties, and the functions and status of each within the community. Language choice in bilingual and multilingual speakers is sometimes described with reference to this linguistic repertoire (Holmes, 1992). Just as monolingual speakers draw from the range of styles and registers available to them those that suit a particular social context, bilingual and multilingual speakers select the appropriate languages or varieties. The situational variables that can influence this choice include domain (e.g., family, religion, employment) factors relating to the interlocutor (e.g., degree of familiarity, linguistic repertoire), and physical setting. Numerous examples of language choice based on such variables can be found in the sociolinguistics literature (see, e.g., Holmes, 1992; Hudson, 1996).

Countries and communities do not fit neatly into categories of multilingualism, bilingualism and diglossia, however, and different forms occur in complex combinations. Within multilingual Switzerland, for example, speakers of German exhibit diglossia in their use of dialects of Swiss German versus standard German. Further, the relative status of varieties can change over time, and as a consequence of social and political changes. In Greece, for example, which was once commonly cited as a clear case of diglossia, the relative prestige of the formal and informal varieties has changed since the end of military rule, with an informal variety finally having been accorded official status (Holmes, 1992). It should be noted also that formal and informal varieties do not have clear-cut boundaries, but are more realistically viewed as forming dialect continua (Hudson, 1996).

The aspects of bilingualism discussed so far have clear implications for assessment. It is known that people's languages can be differentially affected in aphasia [see Paradis (1993) for a description of possible patterns of recovery]. Assessment in more than one language is thus likely to increase diagnostic accuracy, as well as providing a comprehensive picture of residual communication ability for use in planning therapy. Awareness of the range of languages and varieties used premorbidly by a client is thus fundamental to the assessment process. Knowledge of the typical contexts of use of different languages and varieties is also necessary, so that assessment can reflect the real-life communication of bilingual and multilingual speakers.

A further important characteristic of normal bilingual behavior is the use of more than one language or variety within the same conversation or discourse. This can take a number of forms: "Sometimes switching occurs between the turns of different speakers in the conversation, sometimes between utterances within a single turn, and sometimes even within a single utterance" (Milroy & Muysken, 1995, p. 7). Appropriate code-switching forms part of the pragmatic competence of bilingual and multilingual speakers, and as such is relevant to the assessment of functional communication in aphasia.

In normal circumstances, people are often not consciously aware of their code-switching, or that of others; however, inappropriate choices or mixes would seem odd to conversational partners. In a reanalysis of published case studies of bilingual aphasia, Hyltenstam (1995) estimated that in up to 40% of these cases, there were inappropriate choices of language for the situation, with some individuals clearly aware of this problem, and others seemingly not. This aspect of communication in bilingual speakers with aphasia requires further study.

The points emerging from this discussion reinforce the view of Grosjean (1989), that assessment of communication in bilinguals should take account of their characteristic patterns of language use, rather than being based on monolingual norms. A final noteworthy feature of bilingualism, and one that has particular relevance to age-related communication disorder, is its dynamic nature in the individual. Hyltenstam and Obler (1989) offer the following insights:

> In the case of bilingual speakers, the life-span variation in linguistic behavior is, of course, often quite spectacular. A large number of factors surrounding the acquisition and use of each language and the interplay between them at various phases of the individual bilingual's life conspire to determine the individual's linguistic "status" at any given point in time. Of obvious importance in this respect is, for example, whether

*both languages initially developed simultaneously, or whether one was acquired prior to the other, whether both languages were used throughout the life-span, or whether there were periods when there was no need for one of them or no possibility of using it—or its use was socially problematic. Further important factors are whether the second language was learned in a formal classroom setting or acquired in an informal communicative situation, whether one of the languages was eventually lost or retained in modality or domain specific uses. (Hyltenstam & Obler, 1989, p. 3)*

This individual variation highlights the desirability of investigating communication disorder in relation to personal history and communicative repertoire over time.

## Variation in Proficiency Levels

From the point of view of communication assessment, it is important to note that among migrant groups, and in countries with a history of colonization, considerable variation is found in people's levels of proficiency in the major language(s) of the country of residence. This can range from inability to communicate at all in these languages to a native-speaker-like command, depending on opportunity, motivation, and personal history. The status of the mother tongue in such situations, and the extent to which it is maintained by subsequent generations, is a further contributory factor to the variation in degrees of functional bilingualism so frequently observed. First generation migrants from other linguistic backgrounds, and both migrants and indigenous people with limited educational opportunities, are among those for whom communication assessment is most likely to be affected by low proficiency.

Low proficiency in the language of the country of residence can be found in migrants even of many years' standing. Li (1994) and Baker (1995) report this in relation to members of communities in the United Kingdom and Australia, respectively. Milroy and Muysken (1995) cite the work of Klein and Dittmar (1979), in which they observe that among migrant workers in Germany, length of residence is a poorer predictor of proficiency in German than the proportion of social ties contracted with monolingual speakers of German.

The issue of proficiency has obvious implications for the choice of language(s) for the assessment of communication. However, even if it were always possible to assess people in all of their languages, or in those they speak best, there is the additional question of sensitivity to client preference. People may prefer to use their second language for reasons of pride, and so as not to feel that their proficiency is regarded as inadequate. In some cases, the first language has painful associations with the past (Butcher, 1996). Further, assessment needs to take account of the person's communicative needs, which may involve frequent use of the second language. In any event, results must be interpreted in the light of information on premorbid proficiency levels in the languages assessed.

## Dialectal Variation

A further aspect of linguistic diversity that impacts on assessment is that of regional and social dialectal variation, and the variation between contact languages such as creoles and the standard varieties from which they originate. The resemblance, and yet the differences, between related varieties can give rise to inappropriate assessment practices. The assessment of speakers of nonstandard varieties according to standard language norms is discussed by Dronkers, Yamasaki, Ross and White (1995), who describe the consequences of trying to assess speakers of Hawaiian English Creole in standard English.

For assessments that focus on communicative effectiveness rather than solely on linguistic form, one would expect the effects of dialectal variation to be less serious. However, the clinician still needs to be aware of differences in communicative styles among speakers of nonstandard varieties, and of differing levels of comprehension and control of the standard variety. It must be remembered, too, that language varieties are not discrete entities, but shade into one another along a continuous scale, departing in differing degrees from any given standard or dominant variety. Each individual will have control of a certain range of the scale, which may or may not include this standard variety.

Although it may seem reasonable to suggest that people be assessed according to their own linguistic repertoire, the clinician also needs to be sensitive to the possibility that clients may perceive their own nonstandard varieties as being inappropriate for use in the therapeutic setting because they lack the prestige of the standard variety (Payne, 1997). Thus, there is a need not only for awareness of the particular varieties used by clients, but also for an understanding of the status and connotations of the different varieties.

## Use of Existing Assessment Procedures

The aspects of diversity discussed above have important implications not only for intercultural understanding and successful communication between speech–language pathologists and their clients, but also for the suitability of existing assessment procedures for diverse populations, in their original languages and in translated form.

### Suitability for Diverse Populations

Kayser (1998), in a discussion of outcome measures, reports that for the past 30 years, speech–language pathologists in the United States have attempted to assess individuals from culturally and linguistically diverse populations using standardized instruments that were developed for monolingual speakers of English. She points to some of the problems associated with this, including bias, lack of linguistic authenticity, lack of appropriate norms, and failure to reflect cultural background.

Awareness of the need for linguistically and culturally appropriate clinical assessment for diverse populations has become increasingly evident in position statements prepared by professional bodies such as the American Speech–Language–Hearing Association (see Kayser, 1998; Taylor, 1986a, 1986b) and the Australian Association of Speech and Hearing (1994). However, an important obstacle to the changes advocated has been the lack of representation of diverse groups within the profession. In 1994, only 1% of speech–language pathologists in the United States reported themselves to be bilingual (Payne, 1997). Whitworth and Sjardin (1993) remark that speech–language pathology in Australia is a largely monolingual profession in an increasingly multicultural community. Penn (1993), too, reports that the great majority of speech–language pathologists in South Africa are English- and Afrikaans-speaking, and that no properly standardized versions of tests have been developed for aphasic patients in the South African setting.

According to Dronkers et al. (1995), the assessment of bilingual aphasia assumes that both patient and examiner speak the same languages and dialects. In many settings, this is clearly not the case. Indeed, the languages in which assessment is conducted are often not actively selected, but are determined by the availability of suitable personnel, as in the case of the multilingual stroke patient described by Penn (1993). The languages in which he was assessed had been rated as his first, fourth, fifth, and sixth out of ten in order of premorbid proficiency.

As regards the extent to which existing procedures take account of cultural diversity, Payne (1997) reports that of nine listed communication assessment instruments developed in the United States, only three included elders from one or more of the four major ethnocultural groups other than European in their normative data: those of Frattali and colleagues (1995), Holland (1980), and Payne (1994). Although these groupings are broad, their inclusion is at least a first step toward reducing sources of bias in assessment.

The appropriateness of the content of existing measures of functional communication for specific subpopulations does not appear to have been widely examined. Some evidence is reported by Baker (1995), in relation to the communicative needs of Australian elders from Dutch, Latvian, Polish, Croatian, Vietnamese, and Italian backgrounds. In this study, data were gathered from 72 people without communication impairment. Group procedures were used to elicit participants' own accounts of the typical settings in which they needed to use language to communicate. Individual interviews were then conducted, to find out which of 49 communicative activities drawn from existing needs assessment procedures and measures of functional communication were applicable to each person. Overall, the results showed that communication in the family and social domains figured most highly, and that the most widely applicable communication activities in the public domain involved shopping, medical services, and religion.

The content of some existing measures of functional communication focuses on transactional communication outside the home setting, such as at the doctor's office and in shops. Indeed, one such measure, the Amsterdam–Nijmegen Everyday Language Test, explicitly restricts its content to communication in the public domain, on the grounds that ". . . other domains such as family interactions are prone to contain idiosyncratic elements" (Blomert, Kean, Koster, & Schokker, 1994, p. 4). Although test content concerned with shopping and medical purposes would be relevant to most of the participants mentioned above, the omission of the domestic and social setting does not seem to be consistent with their stated communication needs. It is possible that, as Lo Castro (1987) comments, the transfer of information is not the most important function of language, and the use of language to promote and maintain social relations is far more frequent in everyday life. The selection of content for measures of functional communication would therefore benefit from having a stronger empirical basis.

Existing measures of functional communication use a range of formats, including role-play, self-report, report by significant others, direct observation, and elicitation. One might expect these to vary in their suitability for diverse populations; this remains to be investigated, however.

### Translations and Interpreters

For people of low proficiency in the usual language of assessment, or for people who are bilingual or multilingual, it is sometimes assumed that translated versions of an existing measure, or the presence of a professional interpreter during testing sessions, will provide a satisfactory solution. Some possible pitfalls of translation, however, are the lack of direct linguistic and conceptual equivalence between languages, and the fact that readily translatable items can differ in difficulty across versions, or can be inappropriate for cultural reasons (Taussig & Pontón, 1996). An example of this last aspect would be the translation of questions on personal or family matters, or requests for directions, for administration to Native Americans, who would be likely to regard such questioning as unacceptable (Kayser, 1998).

There are additional considerations that apply particularly to the assessment of functional communication in bilingual or multilingual speakers. For example, the administration of translated versions of an assessment procedure assumes that people use their different languages or varieties in the same communicative contexts. As Grosjean (1989) explains, bilinguals have differential needs for their languages, and the languages have different social functions. Merely rendering the same test content in different languages fails to capture these aspects of bilingualism.

Further, the use of separate versions does not take account of code-switching, which often features prominently in bilingual language use. The administration of tests in separate languages treats the client as though he or she were always in "monolingual mode" (Grosjean, 1989) in either one language or the other. Although bilinguals may need to operate separately in their languages when speaking with monolingual speakers of each; this practice does not address the question of how well the person can function in "bilingual mode," when speaking with others who share his or her languages.

A related point concerns the applicability of versions in separate languages to people who, in reality, speak varieties influenced by language contact. Taussig and Pontón (1996), for example, mention the elements of "Spanglish" observed in the speech of older Hispanic people after long periods of residence in the United States. In Australia, too, one hears terms such as "Australitalian" to refer to a blend of Italian and English elements (Clyne, 1991). One would therefore need to be wary of assessing members of migrant populations, particularly those of many years' residence, using procedures developed in their countries of origin. Furthermore, the divergence tends to become even greater in the long term, as the language in the country of origin gradually evolves.

Although the use of a carefully selected interpreter can allow a better match between the language background of the client and the variety used for assessment, there are also limitations associated with this option. For example, it does not allow for the process of back-translation, in which the semantic integrity of a written translation is checked by having the new version translated back into the original language.

The use of interpreters in the assessment of functional communication can also raise issues concerning privacy, and the client's attitudes toward the person chosen to interpret. In one of the cases described by Whitworth and Sjardin (1993), for example, a client was anxious about revealing his condition to another person from the same small migrant community. This case also illustrates the consideration that may need to be given to personal characteristics such as the sex of the interpreter, and to political sensitivities associated with conflict in the country of origin.

Although the use of interpreters takes account of linguistic background, it does not address the question of translatability or cultural appropriateness of content. Indeed, the role of a professional interpreter is to convey meaning as faithfully as possible, not to serve as a cultural arbiter of test content. Equally, it is not part of the interpreter's role to evaluate or assess the client's language, and yet functional assessment typically requires judgments concerning the quality or effectiveness of communication.

It is widely recommended that a professional interpreter be used rather than having a family member interpret in clinical settings, for reasons of accuracy, impartiality, and confidentiality. Although in general this seems desirable, there may be occasions in the context of speech–language pathology when a family member is better able to understand the client than an outsider. If judgments of the client's linguistic and communicative performance are required, it would in any case seem necessary for this to be done not by interpreters, but by trained bilingual and bicultural staff, as indeed Payne (1997) recommends.

## Development of Appropriate Procedures

The inadequacy of current provisions for the needs of diverse populations has been highlighted, but there have been few practical suggestions as to how one might address these needs in the context of functional communication assessment in aphasia. Here the requirements for an approach that would be valid, useful and practicable, taking into account the issues discussed so far, are considered.

### Reconciling Validity and Feasibility

Recent discussions of validity in assessment focus on the accuracy of the inferences drawn from assessment results and on their usefulness for their intended purposes (Bachman, 1990). In the present context, valid assessment would permit the speech–language pathologist to make correct inferences regarding an individual's residual capacity for effective communication, and would provide a basis for planning, conducting, and evaluating the efficacy of therapy. To be feasible, however, it must be done within institutional constraints of time, money and expertise, and within the limitations of current understanding of communication.

These limitations immediately become apparent when one considers the comments of Strevens (1987, p. 171), on the complexity of language in use: "It includes the subtle and only partly comprehensible mechanisms for interpersonal communication which are grouped under the general rubric of discourse. These mechanisms are partly linguistic, partly paralinguistic, and partly non-linguistic; they include the individual's rules for social comportment; they are subject to individual variability." Although assessment in any sphere assumes (if only implicitly) that a definable construct underlies performance, language test development usually has to proceed in the absence of a fully specified or agreed definition of the construct. Functional communication is no exception to this.

The relative merits of different conceptualizations of functional communication are not within the scope of this chapter. However, a major concern is the relative applicability of the resultant approaches across a range of cultural and linguistic contexts. Procedures based on detailed analyses of samples of discourse, for example, require expertise that is not immediately available for application in multiple languages, and thus are not at present a feasible option. Procedures based on a less sophisticated, "checklist" approach, on the other hand, might not rate so highly in authenticity, but would at least be practicable.

The determination of test content on the basis of ethnographic studies of communicative activities and bilingual language use holds great appeal from the point of view of validity, but entails obvious practical difficulties. It might, however, be possible to find a compromise, perhaps in the form of communication diaries completed by clients and their relatives, so that at least some of the relevant information is collected in natural settings.

Any measure of functional communication must reflect realistic communicative activities, and for bilingual and multilingual speakers this includes their uses of their different languages. However, great flexibility is needed in incorporating this, because, according to Auer (1995, p. 118), "Many speech activities are not tied to one particular language, and even among those which have a tendency to be realised more often in one language than in another, the correlation is never strong enough to predict language choice in more than a probabilitistic way."

Other major considerations are the languages in which people are to be assessed, and by whom assessment is to be conducted. In the absence of bilingual and bicultural speech–language pathologists or trained co-workers, assessment procedures will need to be suitable for administration by others, and yet yield information that meets the clinician's requirements, at least to some degree. Family members and caregivers form a valuable resource which is already tapped in some existing measures, such as the Communicative Effectiveness Index, or CETI (Lomas, Pickard, Bester, Elbard, Finlayson, & Zoghaib, 1989). In bilingual and multilingual settings, their contribution could help compensate for the lack of suitable personnel.

The possible choice of formats and styles of assessment may be affected by factors such as attitudes to formal clinical settings, experience of assessment, and willingness or capacity to enter into activities such as role-play. Indeed the notion of formal assessment may be inappropriate altogether. All of these constitute potential threats to validity, and so questions of format must receive careful consideration.

The interpretation of results will need to incorporate an element of comparison with premorbid communicative ability. Although information in absolute terms is needed on clients' current ability to perform communicative tasks, the use of this in planning therapy will depend in part on what they were able to do previously. One needs to know, for example, whether communication difficulty in a particular language is the result of stroke or of low premorbid proficiency. One needs also to know to what extent a person's languages were mixed when operating in bilingual mode (Grosjean, 1989), to judge whether any mixing observed after stroke is normal for that person or not.

Hyltenstam (1995) remarks that most published case studies of bilingual aphasia explicitly mention comments made by family members about changes in the person's linguistic behavior. In view of the impossibility of obtaining information on premorbid bilingual language behavior or levels of language proficiency by any other means, it seems reasonable to try to harness the perceptions of family members in a more systematic way.

It was mentioned earlier that homogeneity of target populations should not be overestimated. At the same time, though, one needs to avoid an ad hoc approach, by seeking out common ground for meaningful assessment. The next section describes an attempt to steer a course between consistency and flexibility, while at the same time addressing the sometimes seemingly irreconcilable considerations of validity and feasibility.

## Towards an Approach for a Multilingual Setting

The work summarized in this section is described in full by Marsh and Baker (1999). It involved the initial development of an approach for assessing functional communication following stroke in Australian residents from a range of language backgrounds other than English. This project sought to combine the requirements of validity and feasibility outlined above, with a view to the eventual production of an assessment procedure that would be culturally acceptable, linguistically appropriate, and clinically useful for at least some of the many subpopulations in Australia.

Selection of content for a trial measure was based on detailed investigation of the pre- and poststroke communicative needs and activities of 10 people with aphasia, from Chinese, Dutch, El Salvadorean, Finnish, Italian, Polish, and Russian backgrounds. The participants comprised five males and five females, ranging in age from 35 to 77 years, with a mean age of 62 years. Three methods of data collection were used to determine the most important and frequent needs:

1. individual interviews, designed to elicit from the participants the most important communicative purposes in their current daily lives;
2. individual oral administration of a checklist containing 57 items drawn from existing measures of functional communication and needs assessment procedures, to determine for each person a set of communicative activities engaged in (a) before the stroke and (b) currently, and which language(s) would normally be used in each case; and
3. communication diaries, completed by participants and/or their significant others, to record all the types of interaction that arose during a period of 5 days, and any communication difficulties experienced.

The diaries were designed as a practicable and nonintrusive substitute for direct observation, and yielded specific instances of communication that reflected each person's daily life. The use of multiple methods of data collection allowed a check on the consistency of responses, as well as compensating for possible omissions. Data collection was carried out in different languages, according to participants' and significant others' preferences and levels of proficiency.

From the data gathered in these ways, communicative activities for inclusion in the trial measure were selected according to the following criteria: (1) broad applicability to participants of different backgrounds and with differing levels of severity of impairment; (2) importance and frequency of the type of interaction; (3) variety in the communicative situations sampled, in terms of domains, topics, interlocutors, and pragmatic functions; (4) coverage of different modalities, including nonverbal, listening, speaking, reading, and writing; and (5) potential to differentiate pre- and poststroke communicative function. The preliminary set of 19 items identified in this way included activities such as showing that you understand what is being said, listening to and understanding medication instructions, answering questions about family, and asking where items are in a shop or supermarket.

A strong theme throughout this chapter has been the need for assessment procedures to reflect the widespread use of different languages and varieties, in different social settings and within the same conversation. However, direct assessment of communicative performance was not a possible option for the proposed new procedure because of the current scarcity of bilingual speech–language pathologists or trained bilingual co-workers in the wide range of languages spoken in Australia. In addition, the role of professional interpreters had to be restricted to that of conveying the meaning of others, and not evaluating communicative function. Given that most speech–language pathologists in Australia would not be able to judge the client's performance in languages other than English, and that any information about this would often be sought informally from relatives, it was decided to incorporate the judgments of significant others formally into the new assessment procedure. Those with regular contact with the client in daily life seemed best placed to observe changes that had occurred in communicative performance, and in many cases would be able to evaluate performance in all of the languages normally used by the person.

The format chosen for this procedure was modelled on that of the CETI (Lomas et al., 1989), which seemed more readily adaptable to the requirements of multilingual administration than most other procedures because of its minimal use of verbal descriptors of performance. Each item was shown with a 10-cm vertical visual analogue scale, with the words "Same as before stroke" at the top and "Cannot" at the bottom, either in English or in other languages. The relative or friend would place a mark on the scale to indicate the client's current ability to perform each item compared with their premorbid ability, in whichever language(s) were normally thought to be used for that activity.

The next phase of the project involved a trial administration of the new measure with the same participants. The content was known to be applicable to all members of this diverse group, all of whom had a stable aphasia, because it had been compiled from data previously provided by them. This enabled us to focus on the feasibility of the approach and to assess the potential reliability of ratings from one occasion to another, without inappropriateness of content or changes in severity as possible confounding factors.

The 10 participants were rated on each of the 19 items by their significant others on two occasions, approximately 2 weeks apart. The marks on the visual analogue scales were converted to numeric scores, and compared for the two administrations. Given that the items and the instructions for raters were in a preliminary form, the total set of 190 pairs of ratings showed a promising level of correspondence across administrations, with a Pearson product moment correlation coefficient of 0.74 ($p < 0.0005$). The less consistent ratings could be traced to four particular items and two particular raters; closer analysis of these patterns may provide the basis for refinements to the items and instructions. However, this approach in general seemed practicable, was acceptable to the participants, and took account of their use of different languages. It also yielded information that would be of value to the speech–language pathologist, but that to date has either not been available, or has been gathered in inconsistent ways. This approach therefore seemed worthy of further investigation, to see whether its applicability could be established for particular subpopulations in the Australian setting.

## Conclusion

This chapter noted the importance of individual variation in ascertaining changes in functional communicative ability in people with acquired neurogenic language disorder, and described the ways in which this is made more complex by the addition of the variables of linguistic and cultural diversity. The additional complexities result not only from linguistic differences, but from culturally determined aspects of communication, as well as attitudes toward illness and rehabilitation.

The quality of any assessment procedure applied in a particular setting depends on the validity of the inferences drawn from the results. Clearly, in the case of speakers of more than one language or variety, we cannot simply generalize from performance in one to the other(s). Quite apart from the possibility of differential impairment, each speaker's premorbid use of his or her languages needs to be taken into account. Similarly, the poststroke communicative performance of a speaker of a nonstandard language variety cannot be interpreted with reference to standard language norms, but must be evaluated in its own terms.

The selection of content for functional communication assessments must sample the real-life communicative uses of the language(s) in question. This means not only that the content of the assessment should reflect important and relevant uses of language, but also that any communicative tasks presented during assessment need to be in the language that the person would previously have used in the domains concerned (in so far as this can be determined in retrospect).

In view of the different possible attitudes and degrees of access to health services, it has been suggested that sensitivity, creativity, and flexibility are needed in determining appropriate approaches to assessment and treatment. Rather than the structures and practices of a predetermined health system being imposed on all clients, appropriate and acceptable styles of service provision need to be arrived at through mutual understanding between service provider and client. On the part of the health system, this requires an appreciation of, and sensitivity to, any additional cultural factors that may be important in each case. On the part of the client it requires an awareness of some of the inevitable constraints under which health professionals work, together with a willingness to contribute to the negotiation of procedures for assessment and therapy that are acceptable and feasible.

In some settings (e.g., the Australian multilingual context described above), the client and his or her usual communication partners are better placed to judge the extent of changes in communicative function than a speech–language pathologist of a different linguistic and/or cultural background. Even where client and assessor share the same linguistic code(s), premorbid data are not normally available as a point of comparison, and direct observation of the client in real communicative settings is not usually feasible. Work in progress by Davidson, Worrall, and Hickson (1998) seeks to establish which of several indirect measures corresponds best with information obtained from direct observation of participation in communicative events in natural settings. For determining the range of communicative situations in which a person can successfully participate, observation in natural contexts (in so far as this is not intrusive) would seem to be the method of choice, and indeed ethnographic methods are increasingly advocated. However, the potential of these for obtaining usable information of sufficient generality, particularly in multilingual and culturally diverse settings, remains to be investigated. In view of the frequency with which the assessor does not share the linguistic code(s) of the client, recourse to the reports of significant others, or of assistants from the relevant linguistic background, seems at present to be the most practicable approach.

Thus, four of the themes highlighted by Worrall in Chapter 1 have been shown here to be of particular relevance to the assessment of communicative function in culturally and linguistically diverse populations: (1) the need for emphasis on the individual's own environment and premorbid communicative activities; (2) the importance of the interactional purposes of communication (e.g., in creating and maintaining personal bonds), and not only the transactional purposes; (3) the need for flexibility and innovation in models of service delivery, with greater possibility for departure from entrenched Western medical models; and (4) the need for measuring instruments that capture the participation level of clients, that is, the extent to which clients can still function in the language(s) of their usual communicative partners, and use these for their premorbid communicative purposes. It is hoped that the present chapter will provide a foundation for the development of approaches that are better tailored to their target populations than has been the case to date.

## References

Auer, P. (1995). The pragmatics of code-switching: A sequential approach. In L. Milroy, P. Muysken (eds): *One speaker, two languages: Cross-disciplinary perspectives on code-switching* (pp. 115–135). Cambridge: Cambridge University Press.

Australian Association of Speech and Hearing (1994). *Speech pathology in a multicultural multilingual society.* Melbourne: AASH.

Bachman, L. F. (1990). *Fundamental considerations in language testing*. Oxford: Oxford University Press.

Baker, R. (1995). Communicative needs and bilingualism in elderly Australians of six ethnic backgrounds. *Australian Journal on Ageing, 14*, 81–88.

Battle, D. E. (1993). Introduction. In D.E. Battle (ed): *Communication disorders in multicultural populations* (pp. xv–xxiv). Boston: Andover Medical Publishers.

Blomert, L., Kean, M-L., Koster, C., & Schokker, J. (1994). Amsterdam–Nijmegen Everyday Language Test: Construction, reliability and validity. *Aphasiology, 8*, 381–407.

Butcher, L. S. (1996). *A descriptive study of the process of aged care assessment with clients of non-English-speaking background*. Brisbane: Ethnic Communities Council of Queensland.

Clyne, M. G. (1982). *Multilingual Australia*. Melbourne: River Seine Publications.

Clyne, M. (1991). Overview of 'immigrant' or community languages. In S. Romaine (ed): *Language in Australia*. Cambridge: Cambridge University Press.

Davidson, B., Worrall, L., & Hickson, L. (1998, August). Observed communication activities of people with aphasia and healthy older people. Paper presented at the 8th International Aphasia Rehabilitation Conference, Kwa Maritane, South Africa.

Dronkers, N., Yamasaki, Y., Ross, G. W., & White, L. (1995). Assessment of binguality in aphasia: Issues and examples from multilcultural Hawaii. In M. Paradis (ed): *Aspects of bilingual aphasia* (pp. 57–65). New York: Pergamon.

Frattali, C. M., Thompson, C. K., Holland, A. L., Wohl, C. B., & Ferketic, M. M. (1995). *Functional assessment of communication skills for adults*. Rockville, MD: American Speech–Language–Hearing Association.

Gallois, C., & Callan, V. (1997). *Communication and culture: A guide for practice*. Chichester: John Wiley.

Grosjean, F. (1989). Neurolinguists, beware! The bilingual is not two monolinguals in one person. *Brain and Language, 36*, 3–15.

Holland, A. L. (1980). *Communicative abilities in daily living*. Baltimore: University Park Press.

Holmes, J. (1992). *An introduction to sociolinguistics*. London: Longman.

Hudson, R. A. (1996). *Sociolinguistics*, 2nd ed. Cambridge: Cambridge University Press.

Hyltenstam, K. (1995). The code-switching behaviour of adults with language disorders—with special reference to aphasia and dementia. In L. Milroy, P. Muysken (eds): *One speaker, two languages: Cross-disciplinary perspectives on code-switching* (pp. 302–343). Cambridge: Cambridge University Press.

Hyltenstam, K., & Obler, L. K. (1989). Bilingualism across the lifespan: An introduction. In K. Hyltenstam, L. K. Obler (eds): *Bilingualism across the lifespan* (pp. 1–12). Cambridge: Cambridge University Press.

Kayser, H. (1998). Outcomes measurement in culturally and linguistically diverse populations. In C. M. Frattali (ed): *Measuring outcomes in speech–language pathology* (pp. 225–244). New York: Thieme.

Klein, W., & Dittmar, N. (1979). *Developing grammars*. Berlin: Springer.

Klopf, D. W., & Park, M. S. (1982). *Cross-cultural communication*. Seoul: Han Shin Publishing.

Li, W. (1994). *Three generations, two languages, one family: Language choice and language shift in a Chinese community in Britain*. Clevedon, Avon: Multilingual Matters.

LoCastro, V. (1987). *Aizuchi*: A Japanese conversational routine. In L. E. Smith (ed): *Discourse across cultures* (pp. 101–113). New York: Prentice Hall.

Lomas, J., Pickard, L., Bester, S., Elbard, H., Finlayson, A., & Zoghaib, C. (1989). The Communicative Effectiveness Index: Development and psychometric evaluation of a functional communication measure for adult aphasia. *Journal of Speech and Hearing Disorders, 54*, 113–124.

Marsh, A., & Baker, R. An approach to the assessment of functional communication in adults with aphasia in a multilingual setting. Manuscript submitted for publication, 1999.

Milroy, L., & Muysken, P. (1995). Introduction: Code-switching and bilingualism research. In L. Milroy & P. Muysken (eds): *One speaker, two languages: Cross-disciplinary perspectives on code-switching* (pp. 1–14). Cambridge: Cambridge University Press.

Paradis, M. (1993). Multilingualism and aphasia. In G. Blanken, J. Dittmann, H. Grimm, J. C. Marshall, & C.-W. Wallesch (eds): *Linguistic disorders and pathologies* (pp. 278–288). Berlin: Walter de Gruyter.

Pauwels, A. (1995). *Cross-cultural communication in the health sciences*. Melbourne: Macmillan Education Australia.

Payne, J. C. (1994). *Communication profile: A functional skills survey*. Tucson, AZ: Communication Skill Builders.

Payne, J. C. (1997). *Adult neurogenic language disorders: Assessment and treatment*. San Diego, CA: Singular Publishing Group.

Penn, C. (1993). Aphasia therapy in South Africa: Some pragmatic and personal perspectives. In A. L. Holland & M. M. Forbes (eds): *Aphasia treatment: World Perspectives* (pp. 25–53). San Diego, CA: Singular Publishing Group.

Samovar, L. A., Porter, R. E., & Jain, N. C. (1981). *Understanding intercultural communication*. Belmont, CA: Wadsworth Publishing Company.

Strevens, P. (1987). Cultural barriers to language learning. In L. E. Smith (ed): *Discourse across cultures* (pp. 169–178). New York: Prentice Hall.

Taussig, I. M., & Pontón, M. (1996). Issues in neuropsychological assessment for Hispanic older adults: Cultural and linguistic factors. In G. Yeo & D. Gallagher-Thompson (eds): *Ethnicity and the dementias* (pp. 47–58). Washington, DC: Taylor & Francis.

Taylor, O. L. (ed). (1986a). *Nature of communication disorders in culturally and linguistically diverse populations*. San Diego, CA: College-Hill Press.

Taylor, O. L. (ed). (1986b). *Treatment of communication disorders in culturally and linguistically diverse populations*. Boston, MA: College-Hill Press.

Wallace, G. L. (1993). Adult neurogenic disorders. In D. E. Battle (ed): *Communication disorders in multicultural populations* (pp. 239–255). Boston: Andover Medical Publishers.

Whitworth, A., & Sjardin, H. (1993). The bilingual person with aphasia—the Australian context. In D. Lafond, R. Di Giovanni, Y. Joanette, J. Ponzio, M. Taylor Sarno (eds): *Living with aphasia: Psychosocial issues*. San Diego, California: Singular Publishing Group.

Yeo, G. (1996). Background. In G. Yeo, D. Gallagher-Thompson (eds): *Ethnicity and the dementias* (pp. 3–7). Washington, DC: Taylor & Francis.

# SECTION 2

# *Functional Communication Therapy Approaches*

# 7

# Functional Communication and the Workplace: A Neglected Domain

## CLAIRE PENN
## DILYS JONES

**Return to work is an important yet neglected area of study for speech-language pathologists. This chapter describes the development of a tool, the Scale of Occupational Functional Communication Demands, that allows the communication demands of the workplace to be matched with the communication skills of the person returning to work. The chapter also summarizes a South African survey of the vocational outcomes for groups of people with head injury and stroke. The survey found a high unemployment rate in both populations. Important information about the variables affecting return to work for people with head injury or stroke is discussed.**

## Introduction

*"Labor omnia vincit"*
*"Work conquers all"*
—Virgil

Over the past two decades there has been increasing emphasis on functional aspects in diagnosis and therapy within the field of speech–language pathology and approaches have been developed that examine the impact of a specific impairment on the individual's daily living and his/her perceived role in society. As this volume demonstrates, the application of such principles to communication and related disorders is widespread, profoundly influencing methods of assessment as well as the goals, contexts, and techniques of rehabilitation.

Despite this burgeoning focus on outcome and functional assessment and therapy, the workplace has been an area that seems to have been relatively neglected by the speech–language pathologist. Ours is a work-oriented society, and the ability to return to work after a disabling event or illness is not only a leading index of recovery, but also a factor proven to link directly to quality of life and self-esteem for the survivor (Crepeau & Scherzer, 1993). In many ways, return to work can be viewed as the functional acid-test of our therapeutic endeavors. This is reflected in the World Health Organization's (WHO, 1997) inclusion of work as an important aspect of the participation level of the new International Classification of Impairment, Disability and Handicap.

Traditionally the workplace has been the domain of the occupational therapist, vocational rehabilitation specialist, or industrial psychologist. However, many of the existing work assessment protocols pay scant attention to the communication dimension. When they do, they fail to differentiate the communication demands of occupations. What remains unclear is when and how communication will affect a patient's ability to return to work. Current functional assessment protocols fail to incorporate the skills required for the workplace. A further point that seems to need acknowledgment and investigation in the literature on rehabilitation outcomes is when and how successful return to work does indeed occur following disability.

The issue of return to work is particularly important for the person with a mild communication disability. For this individual, the goal of return to work may seem a close reality, but may ultimately become an unexpected nightmare. Such a person is least likely to have concomitant physical difficulties such as hemiplegia or incontinence, which have been documented to be linked strongly to failure to return to work (Wade & Heuwer, 1987). In addition, the mild patient is most likely to have the motivation, insight, and often an age advantage for re-employment. Yet, it is precisely those with mild communication disability for whom meaningful return to work becomes particularly difficult. Such a patient may have subtle communication symptoms that may be undetected by others and that may be task-specific (Marshall, 1987; Penn, 1993). This patient, by virtue of this handicap, may also feel more vulnerable, particularly in a context of retrenchment, economic instability, and equal opportunity.

Despite enabling policy and legislation in most countries, employment figures for the disabled population fall far short of the ideal. For example, in South Africa (the context in which this study took place) it is estimated that less than 3% of people with disability of any type are currently employed in the open labor market (Rowland in Lapertosa, 1994). The cost of disability to the economy is high. Snell (1993) indicated that disabling injury and disease has become and will continue to be the United States' number one public health problem. Depending on age of insult and etiology, the loss of earnings is estimated to equal or surpass the total costs contingent upon the actual medical condition (including hospitalization, long-term care, and medical and social services).

Throughout the world, important changes in employment practice have been noted. In South Africa, for example, the White Paper on Integrated National Disability Strategy proposes the promotion and implementation "of policies and programmes which ensure equity in terms of employment benefits, status and condition and the promotion of reasonable and equitable work environments for disabled workers." Specifically, the White Paper has specified the need for "vocational assessment techniques to facilitate the matching of disabled job-seekers with job-related requirements" (Integrated National Disability Strategy, 1997, p. 44). Another factor of importance is the introduction of the Managed Health Care paradigm and the critical issue of type and length of funding for the person involved as well as the nature and role of the case manager. These policy factors in part lead to the rationale for evaluating the workplace in more detail.

Among the mechanisms suggested in legislation is the development of vocational rehabilitation services. The high cost of disability has led to the move by U.S. employers, for example, to consider occupational re-entry a preferable option to paying workers compensation. Companies have become increasingly aware of savings that can be effected by appropriate and early intervention, modified duty, and job accommodation.

This chapter focuses on communication disability and employment variables in stroke and traumatic brain injury (TBI) populations. It includes the results of a return to work survey and the results of a study that investigated the relationship between return to work and various injury and demographic variables. The chapter describes the preliminary development and application of a functional communication tool for the workplace.

## Stroke and Return to Work

Stroke is a leading cause of death and disability throughout the world and the third most frequent cause of all deaths in the developed world (Bonita, 1992). However, despite this high incidence, the reported stroke mortality rates have been declining, particularly in industrialized countries and much current research is geared toward outcome and management of rehabilitation for stroke survivors. More than half of stroke survivors are estimated to have some functional disability at 6 months postonset (Wade & Heuwer, 1987). A number of studies have been conducted on the determinants of outcome after stroke. Communication difficulties are a persistent and significant handicap for the majority of stroke survivors and are reported to affect significantly overall social and vocational readjustment as well as quality of life (Geddes et al., 1996; Smollan & Penn, 1997; Weinberg, 1997).

More than half the cost of stroke in monetary terms has been linked to the inability of the person to return to work (Adelman, 1981). Despite the fact that authors such as Gresham et al. (1979) reported that the most prevalent functional deficit following stroke was decreased vocational function, there is relatively little on return to work following stroke in the literature. One reason for this may be the age of the average stroke patient (the majority of whom are over 60 years old). In addition, the literature often does not differentiate between the outcomes of left-hemisphere stroke and right-hemisphere stroke. Thus, the impact of communication deficits associated with left-hemisphere stroke or aphasia in particular is not singled out.

Joussen and Pascher (1984) interviewed 25 aphasic patients of working age, and their families and found that with few exceptions, patients with chronic aphasia were generally not integrated into the workforce. Hatfield and Zangwill (1975) also pointed out the relatively rare occurrence of occupational resettlement in an aphasic population. Weisbroth et al. (1971) studied a group of patients with hemiplegia and found that 37% of the sample returned to work, but those with poorer communication skills were significantly less likely to return to work than those without communication impairment. Similarly, Matsumoto et al. (1973) found a statistically significant difference on a communication scale between stroke patients who returned to work and those who did not. In their study, only 3% of the stroke patients who had aphasia returned to work. More recently, Hermann and Wallesch (1990) investigated the psychosocial adjustment of patients with chronic aphasia and included details of vocational changes. They found that 80% of their sample were unable to maintain even their premorbid domestic abilities. Thirty-five percent of premorbid close contact with workmates had ceased. In only four cases were the social relations connected to patients' jobs viewed as unimpaired. Neau et al. (1998) examined return to work in a group of 71 consecutive young adults (age 15 to 45) after stroke and found a much higher return to work rate after stroke (73%) than other studies. In contrast, a study conducted in Taiwan (Hsieh & Lee, 1997) with 248 consecutive stroke survivors, found nearly three-quarters not able to resume their usual work roles.

Interestingly, in Hermann and Wallesch's (1990) study, which also examined how different professionals examined the importance of various items on a scale of social adjustment, the ability to return to work received a low rating from most of the professionals. They attributed this to the fact that most of their subjects worked with patients who were 55 and over in a community where people were encouraged to retire at 58 years of age. This pessimistic perspective that stroke patients will not return to work is summed up in a local recent popular magazine article that indicated that "some stroke victims may even return to work" (YOU, 1998).

In a South African study by Weinberg (1997) on outcome 1 year post stroke, not one of the 16 patients interviewed had returned to their premorbid work. The social and economic circumstances in which these patients found themselves, together with lack of access to appropriate rehabilitation facilities, were felt to contribute significantly to poor quality of life for these patients and may well be variables of considerable importance particularly in developing countries in determining return to work.

Le Dorze and Brassard (1995) analyzed the personal accounts of aphasic individuals and their significant others to understand the consequences of aphasia. Among the handicaps identified by this group were reduced employment opportunities and loss of career objectives. Parr (1994) found that loss of work was a reason for deterioration in life satisfaction levels in a group of aphasic patients. In the self-accounts of 50 aphasic people reported by Parr et al. (1997), only one person interviewed returned to the same employment as before on a full-time basis, after the stroke.

## TBI and Return to Work (RTW)

By contrast to the literature on RTW in stroke, a large number of studies have been conducted with head-injured patients and vocational outcome. As the majority of this population falls between the ages of 18 to 25 years, they have a large number of potential work years ahead and may already have an "identity investment in a particular career direction" (Price & Bauman, 1991). A wide range of RTW statistics have been reported in these studies ranging from 12% (Thomsen, 1985) to 100% (Wrightson & Gronwall, 1990). However, direct comparison of RTW statistics is problematic due to variability in sampling methods, heterogeneous subject samples, the use of different indices of severity, and the lack of uniform follow-up over time. Among problems identified for instance is the fact that some studies extend for only several months (e.g., Wrightson & Gronwall, 1990) and others up to 20 years (Thomsen, 1992).

In a carefully controlled study by Ben-Yishay et al. (1987), four comparable groups of 30–50 TBI patients were followed up for 2 years. Although they had undergone traditional vocational rehabilitation and were considered ready for placement, it was found that less than 3% of the sample were able to achieve competitive employment and maintain their positions for 1 year—a pessimistic perspective indeed.

Since the latter half of the 1980s, there seems to have been an improved trend with the funding of intensive multidisciplinary rehabilitation programs. A number of studies, for instance, have shown the positive benefits of such programs in improving participants' ability to readapt to the workplace (Ben-Yishay et al., 1987; Christensen, 1992; Johnson, 1998; Lyons & Morse, 1988; Prigatano et al., 1984; Tollman et al., 1993; Wehman et al., 1995). One issue under discussion, however, has been that many of these programs are time consuming, labor intensive, and costly (see, for example, West et al., 1991) and do not necessarily improve chances of RTW after severe brain injury (Wehman et al., 1995). Some studies have demonstrated no relation between the provision of retraining therapy and RTW, and that the treatment variables of duration and costs are inversely related to outcomes (i.e., patients receiving the longest duration of therapy and accumulating the highest treatment costs displaying the poorest outcome ratings) (Putnam & Adams, 1992). Similarly, Rao et al. (1990) found that a shorter length of stay at an inpatient rehabilitation hospital was a significant predictor of improved vocational outcome, probably a reflection of lesser initial severity.

In a number of these outcome studies, an attempt has been made to identify factors within the client's past as well as injury variables that predict outcome on the vocational domain among other things. The large-scale data base of Dahmer et al. (1993), for example, identifies a number of these variables. Among these are pre-injury demographic variables such as age at accident; gender; first language; prior history of communicative, neurological, or psychiatric problems; education; occupational type; occupational status and time since injury (Brooks et al., 1987; Oddy et al., 1985, etc.). The second set of variables relates to injury, such as injury severity, and the tool used to measure severity and cause of injury. A third category of importance is the type of therapy received. Johnson (1998) and Wehman et al. (1990) argue, for instance, for the effectiveness of good support, gradual RTW, and "in vivo" training.

As with the studies reported on stroke and RTW, communication abilities are strongly correlated with the likelihood and success of RTW in TBI. For example, in a study of RTW 15 years after injury, Dresser (1983) demonstrated that in a closed head injury sample, 80% of those with no speech problems were employed, versus 60% of those with speech problems. Brooks et al. (1987) noted that the ability to understand a conversation and to engage in a conversation was highly predictive in determining RTW for the head-injured sample in their study.

Unfortunately, a number of studies that have considered RTW and its correlates do not specify communication as a variable. Johnson (1998), for example, specifies "other cognitive difficulty" and sensory deficits in addition to memory as being important variables, but the specific nature of these areas remains unspecified.

Perhaps the most logical position to take is that "many factors interact in determining employment outcome after brain injury and outcome cannot be predicted by any one of them" (Dikeman et al. cited in Johnson, 1998, p. 77).

## RTW Survey

We have recently completed a survey on vocational outcome in a group of head-injured patients and a group of aphasic stroke patients. This survey examined the relationship between demographic, neurological, and postmorbid variables and vocational outcome. The survey aimed to:

- examine the relationship between vocational outcome and communicative variables;
- explore the relationship between functional independence [as measured by the American Speech–Language–Hearing Association Functional Assessment of Communication Skills for Adults (ASHA FACS)] (Frattali et al., 1995) and return to work.

The subjects selected for this study were TBI and aphasic patients who were of working age at the time of the assessment (i.e., under 65 years). The clinical records of two groups of subjects were used:

- Sample 1 consisted of 50 TBI subjects who had been evaluated for medico-legal purposes in a private practice. The mean age of this group was 29.1 years.
- Sample 2 consisted of a sample of 91 aphasic patients from a clinical practice and a large University Speech and Hearing Clinic. The mean age of this group was 55.8 years.

These records were perused for the following variables: premorbid educational level, premorbid occupational status, and premorbid occupational type. In addition, findings were correlated with a range of pre-injury and injury variables such as age and severity of disorder.

Using a database comprising 197 variables, a number of demographic pre-injury, and postinjury variables were coded and linked to the RTW variables. The results of this survey have been described in detail elsewhere (Watt et al., 1996), but may be summarized as follows:

## Vocational Outcome

Of the 37 originally competitively employed TBI subjects, nine maintained this level, 10 were downgraded, one retired, and 17 (i.e., 46%) were unemployed. Thus, in effect, only nine subjects (24%) working premorbidly were able to RTW full time in a competitive environment. Although this figure compares favorably to some of the other studies reported, many of which reflect the results of coordinated rehabilitation, it should be borne in mind that this is a highly specific population and that often the occupational status may be affected by the medico-legal status of the patient (who is awaiting potential compensation).

For the aphasic group, the picture is somewhat more bleak, indicating an overall unemployment rate of between 62 and 71% of the sample. The same proportion of individuals in the aphasic stroke sample returned to full-time employment as the closed head injury sample, but a significantly higher number of the group were retired. Neau et al. (1998) found that 26% of their young stroke sample were downgraded in the workplace, while Alfassa et al. (1997) reported relatively high RTW figures (67%) in a younger sample. Both of these studies, however, investigated stroke patients in general and did not isolate the specific influence of aphasia or left-hemisphere stroke.

Interestingly, there was a relatively high proportion of missing data regarding employment status in the clinical records of the aphasia sample, reinforcing the impression that clinicians are often neglectful of these issues (Hermann & Wallesch, 1990). This factor probably relates to the age of the sample under investigation.

## Factors Affecting Vocational Outcome

An analysis of whether premorbid occupational type influenced outcome was undertaken in the TBI group. These findings are illustrated in Table 7–1.

It appears that the more skilled workers (e.g., professionals and managers/executives) had a greater chance of returning to work, albeit sometimes of a different type, than manual or clerical workers, who either carried on in the same capacity or were unemployed. This confirms the findings of Brooks et al. (1987) and can perhaps be attributed to the possibility that professional and managerial workers have a greater resource pool of skills and possibly more flexible work contexts than other grades of worker. Further, white-collar workers are likely to have established work contracts, and access to disability insurance that will ensure some security in the workplace.

Similarly, when an analysis was done on changes in occupational type it appeared that the more skilled workers (e.g., professionals, managers, and execu-

Table 7–1.   Relationship Between Occupation Type and Outcome in the TBI Group

| Pre-Injury Occupation Type | Postinjury Occupation Type |
| --- | --- |
| Manual workers (unskilled, semiskilled, and skilled): $n = 6$ | • 2 (33%) continued in this capacity<br>• 4 (66%) were unemployed |
| Clerical/supportive administrative positions: $n = 7$ | • 2 (29%) were able to continue in this job type<br>• 5 (71%) were unemployed |
| Technical workers: $n = 4$ | • 2 (50%) remained in this job type<br>• 2 (50%) were unemployed |
| Managerial/executive workers: $n = 15$ | • 7 (47%) continued in this capacity<br>• 1 (6%) downgraded to skilled manual work<br>• 2 (13%) downgraded to clerical/supportive administrative positions<br>• 5 (33%) were unemployed |
| Professionals: $n = 5$ | • 2 (40%) continued in their professional capacity<br>• 1 (20%) downgraded to clerical work<br>• 2 (40%) were unemployed |

tives) had a greater chance of returning to the same work than manual or clerical workers who either carried on in the same capacity or were unemployed. This confirms the finding of Brooks et al. (1987) and Hsieh and Lee (1997) who also found the specific employment institution to be a strong predictor of RTW in their study of 248 consecutive stroke survivors. Carreiro et al. (1987) similarly observed: "It is noteworthy that self-employed workers who are motivated and can regulate their work according to their own capacities seem to have an advantage over employees whose poststroke resettlement is strictly regulated by bureaucratic considerations and which do not differentiate between aphasia and other types of handicaps" (p. 672).

## Predictors of RTW

The predictive power of a number of variables was tested statistically in the TBI sample (Watt, 1996). Neither age at onset or time since injury appeared to significantly affect RTW. This is surprising in light of the importance attached to these variables in previous research (e.g., Brooks et al., 1987; Neau et al., 1998; Putnam & Adams, 1992). They were, however, significant in predicting whether the subject might be downgraded.

In terms of age of onset, it was found that those subjects older than 25 years were more likely to be downgraded. This could be attributed to the fact that older workers have a greater support system within their places of work and have developed better rapport with their supervisors and co-workers, which may dispose them to be more flexible regarding the time spent on the job. The younger workers who returned to work generally did so full time in the same capacity as before. However, it must be noted that the two age groups were not of equivalent severity.

In terms of the time since onset, the relationship appears different in those 3 years or longer post onset. This group was significantly more likely to be downgraded once they returned to work. This suggests that with lengthening time since injury, the persistent deficits and work-related shortcomings become increasingly clear. This may also be related to more severe injury.

In the multicultural sample of Watt (1996), first language was found to be a factor that also significantly predicted RTW. Those who spoke European languages, English, or Afrikaans were more likely to RTW than those speaking African languages. The possession of postsecondary school training also significantly improved their chances of returning to work. This confirms the findings of Najenson et al. (1978). In addition, the type of premorbid occupation significantly influenced the chances of RTW in that managerial and professional workers were significantly more likely to RTW than technical or clerical workers.

The three factors of first language, education, and premorbid occupational status are all related in that they reflect the socioeconomic status and type of social and educational advantages enjoyed by the subjects. The legacy of social and racial oppression in South Africa may be seen all too clearly in these findings.

Contrary to previous findings, injury severity alone was not found to be related to RTW. This was surprising, although other authors (Brooks et al., 1987; Ip et al., 1995; Thomsen, 1992) have found similar results. This may indicate that other factors (e.g., socioeconomic status) are more influential in RTW than injury severity or that the indices used for classifying severity may not in fact be particularly useful (see Watt et al., 1996).

Interestingly, there was a statistical relationship between therapy and RTW. The more therapy a subject had, the less likely he/she was to RTW. These results are similar to those of Putnam and Adams (1992) and suggest in the South African context that only severely impaired patients receive therapy—in other words, those least likely to RTW. This has important implications for the role of therapists in informing the medical profession as to whom should be referred to therapy, and for policy makers and payers regarding for whom and how much money should be awarded for therapy (cf. Marshall, 1987), although return to work is obviously not the only intended outcome of therapy.

The following communicative difficulties were closely related to failure to RTW: oral motor abnormalities, high-level receptive difficulties, expressive difficulties, difficulties in reading comprehension and memory tasks, and slowed speed of verbal reasoning. In addition, certain neuropsychological test results were significantly related to failure to RTW. By contrast, only one aspect of physical functioning was related to vocational outcome, that being hemi-paresis or paralysis of arm or leg. A significant relationship was also found between lack of insight and the inability to RTW, correlating well with the findings of Ben Yishay et al. (1987). Of further interest was the fact that those who had returned to work displayed less confidence than those who did not, suggesting the continued failures and frustrations experienced in the workplace. Those who returned to work also reported heightened irritability. In sum, our study highlights the rather pessimistic vocational outcome for TBI subjects and the strong influence of demographic factors on outcome.

In the stroke sample, although less data were available, no significant difference was found between subjects over and under 40 years of age in terms of RTW. A nonsignificant effect was also found for education level in contrast to the findings of Granger et al. (1997). Type of aphasia, on the other hand, yielded a fairly predictable result. The only patients who were able to RTW (either in a full-time or downgraded capacity) were either mild to moderate Broca's or anomic aphasic patients, whereas no severe or Wernicke's aphasic patients were re-employed. This suggests the critical relationship between receptive competence and ability to manage in the workplace. What is particularly disturbing is that about 36% of the sample of working age with symptoms sufficiently mild to enable successful RTW in some capacity, remained unemployed.

The question remains as to whether successful RTW links to the performance on functional measures that are currently available and this remains largely unanswered. To determine whether any of these skills predicted successful RTW, a pilot study of 14 subjects was undertaken as part of a larger study. In a sample of 14 premorbidly employed subjects (nine aphasic and five TBI), there was no correlation between RTW status of the subjects and their performance on the ASHA FACS (Frattali et al., 1995). Although this was at variance with prior research such as the study by Matsumoto et al. (1973), which used Sarno's Functional Communication Profile, it should be acknowledged that the sample size in this study was restricted. However, it did highlight the possibility that even a refined tool such as the FACS does not extend far enough into the communication challenges of the workplace. As Hartley (1995) suggests, an important area of evaluation is an environmental needs assessment, which could take us well beyond the context in which we are used to working (the interpersonal and social domains) and into the workplace for instance. The quality of communicative life supplement to the ASHA FACS, which is currently being developed, will address such work issues, among others.

## The Scale of Occupational Functional Communication Demands (SOFCD)

Work is an area that has been identified as a key issue on the "participation" level of the WHO's (1997) International Classification of Impairment, Activities, and Participation (ICIDH-2) scheme. In this classification, participation is based on an environmental interaction model in which it is viewed as a result of the complex relationship between the type of impairment and disability and the demands and context of the environment. In other words, the degree of restriction of participation is dependent on the mismatch between the requirments of the context and the person's impairment. This notion is central to the philosophy of the SOFCD.

Work contexts are frequently pressurizing and distracting and they make multiple demands on communication processing. Yet Wertz (1983) reminds us that RTW should be a rehabilitation goal as it "provides systematic daily routine—and offers confidence and security" (1983, p. 15).The challenge of successful RTW lies in the matching of the individual to the position, and the role of the therapist in this regard is paramount.

It seems important to have a relevant measure that not only determines accurately the person's capacity to fulfill various jobs, but also the communicative requirements or demands of the job itself. This area is poorly researched: The communicative demands of some positions require a combination of high-level communication skills, whereas many positions do not require even average levels of ability in some communicative dimensions. For example, deaf persons commonly pursue professions such as draughting and architecture. Furthermore, many manual laborers do not require high levels of language skills, particularly in the written modality. It is quite possible to read and write effectively without having to speak or pronounce clearly and it is quite possible to work without needing reading and writing skills.

While not all positions require high levels of competence in all the domains of communication, a number of adaptations can be made in the work environment of an individual to minimize the communicative demands placed on that individual. A person with a hearing loss, for example, may communicate using written modalities or Sign Language, rather than using the spoken mode. A person who has difficulty understanding complex instructions can often be made to understand if the message is short or simple. People with motor speech disorders may function adequately in clerical positions where the need for expression is minimal. Despite such intuition, "there is currently no standardised means of assessing residual language capacities which indicate a possible return to work . . ." (Rolland & Beilin, 1993, p. 225). In an attempt to address this gap, over several years we developed a tool that aimed at describing the communicative demands of the workplace.

More specifically, we aimed to develop a tool that measures reliably the communicative demands of various occupations for the purpose of assisting diagnostic and therapeutic reintegration of patients into the workplace and to document and describe vocational outcome following head injury and stroke. The outcome was the SOFCD. Guidelines for its administration are presented in the Appendix.

The initial version of the SOFCD was based on the important preliminary work of Toffolo and Minns (1993) whose scale of job analysis, the Communication Analysis for Employment (CAFE) had been developed in Australia, after consultation with local industrial psychologists and occupational therapists. The SOFCD was devised with the following principles in mind:

- it should be easy to administer and capable of administration not only by speech–language pathologists, but also other professionals such as occupational therapists and human resource personnel;
- it should be applicable across a wide range of occupational contexts reflecting the diversity that exists in the workplace linguistically and culturally; and
- it should have potential application across a full range of communication disorders.

Eight communication parameters were selected as being critical for the workplace. These were based in part on the literature, on the results of the survey described above (linking outcome to specific communication skills) and to on-site

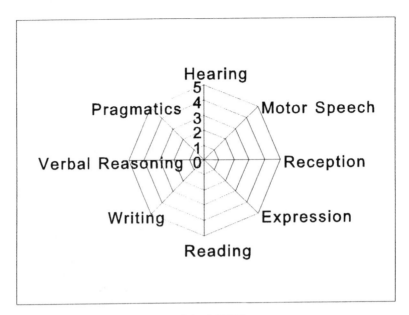

**Figure 7–1.** Schematic representation of the SOFCD.

observations. These were hearing, motor speech abilities, receptive language, expressive language, written skills, verbal reasoning, and pragmatics.

A five-point scale was developed for each parameter, reflecting and exemplifying the different levels of usage, namely low, routine, average, high and intrinsic.

A graphic display of the SOFCD is presented in Figure 7–1. For each communication parameter, these five levels of usage were operationalized into brief descriptions (See Appendix 1). A set of instructions was detailed for raters. The list of instructions and the SOFCD rating guidelines went through several modifications during the course of the study, following validation procedures with a range of judges.

This study explored a number of different occupations graded according to an established scale (the Patterson and Castellion scales of PE Corporate Services Salary Survey, 1995) in several different work contexts (university, factory, offices, and a metropolitan water plant). The communicative demands of 28 different occupations were evaluated using the SOFCD and the tool was refined over this time, using different judges to obtain satisfactory inter-rater reliability (on the weighted Cohen-Kappa scale). This involved interviewing and observation within the workplace. Interviews took place, for example, with the supervisors and the incumbents of the various positions and independent ratings were made by at least two judges in each case. This was then supplemented by a 30-minute observation of the incumbent at work. The communicative profiles of these occupations are summarized in Table 7–2.

Though clearly some expansion of contexts is required, we suggest that the SOFCD has the potential to measure reliably the communicative demands in a number of workplaces, and

Table 7-2. Communication Demands of Different Occupations, as Rated Using the SOFCD

| | Hearing | Motor Speech | Reception | Expression | Reading | Writing | Verbal Reasoning | Pragmatics |
|---|---|---|---|---|---|---|---|---|
| Senior gardener | 1 | 1 | 2 | 2 | 1 | 1 | 1 | 1 |
| Librarian | 3 | 3 | 3 | 3 | 5 | 4 | 3 | 3 |
| Waitress | 5 | 4 | 5 | 4 | 4 | 4 | 4 | 5 |
| Filing clerk | 2 | 2 | 3 | 3 | 4 | 4 | 4 | 2 |
| Teacher | 5 | 4 | 4 | 4 | 5 | 5 | 4 | 5 |
| Driving instructor | 4 | 4 | 3 | 4 | 4 | 3 | 5 | 4 |
| Audiologist | 5 | 5 | 5 | 5 | 5 | 4 | 4 | 5 |
| Security guard | 2 | 2 | 1 | 1 | 1 | 3 | 1 | 1 |
| Electrician | 5 | 2 | 3 | 3 | 3 | 3 | 4 | 3 |
| Electrical apprentice | 5 | 3 | 3 | 3 | 4 | 2 | 3 | 3 |
| Shift supervisor | 4 | 4 | 4 | 4 | 3 | 3 | 4 | 4 |
| B2 End control | 3 | 2 | 3 | 3 | 2 | 1 | 2 | 3 |
| Boiler cleaner | 2 | 1 | 1 | 1 | 1 | 1 | 1 | 1 |
| B3 Fault finder | 1 | 2 | 2 | 2 | 2 | 1 | 3 | 1 |
| Component insertion | 1 | 1 | 2 | 1 | 2 | 1 | 2 | 1 |
| Secretary | 5 | 3 | 4 | 4 | 3 | 4 | 3 | 5 |
| Workshop assistant | 1 | 1 | 2 | 1 | 2 | 2 | 1 | 1 |
| Security guard | 2 | 2 | 1 | 1 | 1 | 3 | 1 | 1 |
| Laboratory assistant | 1 | 3 | 3 | 3 | 3 | 2 | 3 | 3 |
| Kitchen assistant | 1 | 1 | 2 | 2 | 2 | 1 | 2 | 3 |
| Administrative assistant | 3 | 3 | 4 | 4 | 3 | 4 | 4 | 4 |
| Technician | 1 | 2 | 3 | 3 | 3 | 2 | 2 | 2 |
| Kitchen manager/chef | 2 | 1 | 3 | 3 | 3 | 3 | 4 | 4 |
| Assistant registrar | 3 | 3 | 4 | 4 | 4 | 3 | 2 | 4 |
| Security guard/ Access controller | 3 | 3 | 3 | 3 | 2 | 2 | 3 | 3 |
| Supervisor | 4 | 4 | 4 | 4 | 3 | 3 | 4 | 4 |
| Packers | 1 | 1 | 2 | 1 | 1 | 1 | 1 | 2 |
| Quality assurance manager | 4 | 4 | 4 | 4 | 4 | 4 | 4 | 4 |
| Boiler attendant | 5 | 3 | 3 | 3 | 2 | 2 | 3 | 3 |
| Secretary | 3 | 3 | 3 | 3 | 3 | 3 | 3 | 4 |

Key: 1 = low; 2 = routine; 3 = average; 4 = high; and 5 = intrinsic.

- provides an expanded assessment and intervention perspective especially for the person with mild communication problems and may enable a more careful examination of the dimensions of successful RTW in the patient and the environment;
- provides functional parameters that can improve quality of life;
- provides an enabling framework for potential employers of disabled persons; and
- may assist in the implementation of new policy and legislation in the workplace.

In its evaluation of the workplace rather than the client, it provides an environmental-systems based perspective to the client as demonstrated in the work of Lubinski (1994), for example.

## Clinical Application of the SOFCD

To illustrate the potential clinical application of the SOFCD, some detailed interviews were conducted with stroke and TBI patients and a sample of findings from four of these is presented below. The interviews explored factors that appear to be the most important for patients, families, and employers for vocational resettlement. In each of the cases presented, a SOFCD profile of their job (past or current) is provided to illustrate the value of such profiling in the overall consideration of the client. Examples of successful and unsuccessful vocational reintegration are included.

The representations of the communicative demands of the workplaces of each of the four clients are presented in Figure 7–2.

### Case Examples

TWO CASES OF UNSUCCESSFUL RTW

C.H. was 19 years of age when she sustained a closed head injury in a motor vehicle accident, and had just completed high school. The accident took place during the summer vacation, and she had thus not yet commenced working or tertiary education. She received intensive rehabilitation for 6 months and thereafter continued to have speech and occupational therapy for a further 6 months. During this time, she also attended a college which specializes in providing training for disabled people and completed a course in basic computer skills and office management.

Two years post injury she obtained sympathetic employment doing clerical work (this involved filing, typing, and basic bookkeeping), a post that she filled successfully for 3 years. Her supervisor was a family friend who understood the nature of her difficulties and was able to provide a great deal of support and supervision. Nevertheless, she was able to perform this job satisfactorily.

Five years post injury, the company in which C.H. worked was taken over by another company. Her services were retained, but she had a new supervisor and began to experience work failure almost immediately. She was retrenched 3 weeks after the company's take over. At the same time her previously well-

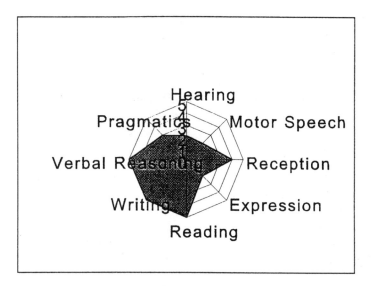

**Figure 7–2.** SOFCD representation of the communication demands of A.A.'s workplace.

controlled epilepsy deteriorated (she had not had a seizure since 1 month after the injury) and to date this has still not been properly controlled.

To explain C.H.'s subsequent failure to reintegrate into the workplace, her cognitive/communicative abilities at that stage will now be summarized. She had mild word-finding difficulties and some difficulty with the comprehension of high-level material (e.g., humor, ambiguity, sarcasm), but coped well in most one-to-one and group social situations. Her memory remained poor and she was reliant on a diary and other external memory aids (notes, reminders, etc). She also tended to be impulsive and this, coupled with some attentional problems, accounted for many of the receptive failures that she experienced—that is, she tended to respond before she had processed information sufficiently. Similarly, she experienced some pragmatic problems mostly related to difficulty in, as she described it as, "thinking before I speak."

On the ASHA FACS seven-point rating scale, she obtained scores of 6 for social communication, 6.7 for basic needs, 7 for reading, writing and number concepts, and 5.8 for daily planning. Her domain mean score for communication independence was 6.57.

C.H. then obtained work in a bank, in a position assisting clients to open checking accounts over the telephone. These interviews were tape-recorded for later verification of client details, and C.H. resigned from this job 1 month later as she had been repeatedly reprimanded for making mistakes in the transcription of the calls (e.g., errors in the sequence of telephone or account numbers). A final attempt at work involved doing dictaphone typing at home. Unsurprisingly, given her attention and receptive language difficulties, this attempt was not successful.

The repeated negative experiences have served to erode C.H.'s confidence and she now believes that she will never be able to work. This case underlines two important points. The first, emphasized by Johnson (1998) is the need for support in the workplace. In C.H.'s case she was successfully employed for a period of 3 years because of the support that her supervisor was able to provide. As soon as this support ceased and she had a supervisor who did not understand her difficulties, she was no longer able to perform appropriately. The second important point is the need to match the person's abilities with the requirements of the job. In both of C.H.'s subsequent attempts to work the jobs placed high demands on attention, listening, and memory skills, without the reinforcement of face-to-face contact. Careful analysis of the job requirements using a tool such as the SOFCD would have helped C.H. to avoid these negative experiences and to re-enter the workplace successfully.

A second example of unsuccessful return to work is L.S., a 40-year-old professional engineer who suffered a stroke resulting in Broca's aphasia. Following rehabilitation, he presented with agrammatic, but expressive and receptive language adequate for most conversational settings. His reading was markedly impaired with no ability to read function words and he was heavily reliant on contextual knowledge to understand what he read. His writing was limited to occasional single words. On the ASHA FACS he scored 5.9 for social communication, 7 for communication of basic needs, 6 for reading, writing, and number concepts, and 7 for daily planning. His domain mean score for communication independence was 6.47.

Despite these difficulties, he returned to work in his premorbid capacity 9 months after his stroke. He experienced severe difficulty, and within a short period he was downgraded into a position as a storeman. As this job required a large amount of reading he found the job difficult. He also experienced a high level of depression in this position, as he felt unsupported and isolated from his former colleagues and friends. He also identified that the job taxed him most in the areas in which he was weakest while not making use of any of his strengths and skills. After a period of 1 month, he resigned from this job, although the company indicated that they had intended to dismiss him, and he was pronounced medically unfit for work.

Two years subsequent to this, L.S. was able to obtain work as a security guard checking invoices in a tile company, a position that he still holds today. This is considered essentially sheltered employment for which he receives a minimal wage, and he considers the work to be menial and boring. However, he comments that "a man must work."

As with C.H., this case highlights the need for careful planning of RTW, analysis of the requirements of the job and liaison between the professional rehabilitation team and the employer. L.S.' employers clearly did not understand the implications of aphasia for his job, and his failure was thus almost inevitable. Furthermore, the social and emotional impact of downgraded employment in the same work context needs to be considered and appropriate support provided.

TWO CASES OF SUCCESSFUL RTW

G.S. was a 20-year-old computer technician employed by the Post Office when she sustained a severe TBI in an assault. She had completed secondary school, but had no formal tertiary education apart from in situ training. She came from a poor socioeconomic background, and had little support, either emotional or financial.

She received a short period of rehabilitation at an acute care hospital and was discharged from treatment when she could walk and had communication skills that were considered to be adequate for daily life. Two years after the accident she referred herself to a university speech clinic as she wished to improve her speech to find work. At that stage, she presented with a marked right hemiparesis mainly affecting the upper limb, memory problems, and some pragmatic difficulties. Her overriding symptoms were agrammatism and deep dyslexia. In addition to individual speech therapy, G.S. joined a support group with other neurologically involved young people, and received counselling from the clinic social worker.

G.S. was highly motivated to re-enter employment and one of the foci of therapy was to assist her to draw up a profile of what types of job she would be able to do and to analyze the likely communicative demands of various jobs that she considered. Numerous job applications were unsuccessful but the support of her new friends in the group, as well as her therapists, enabled her to cope with these disappointments and to incorporate some of the reasons given for her failure as therapy targets. After 18 months, speech therapy was terminated, but G.S. continued to have regular contact with the therapist and with the social worker. She continued in her search for employment and was considered to be capable of making informed and appropriate decisions about the type of job that she would be able to do. She also undertook some voluntary work at her local library—this enabled her to build up her confidence in a sympathetic situation, and in return the librarian assisted her with the writing of letters to prospective employers.

Two years after her initial referral to the clinic she obtained a job doing clerical and administrative work for a children's home. She considers this to be a meaningful and rewarding job where she makes a contribution to society. In a recent telephone call to her former therapist she commented, "now (I am) really better."

Despite her severe communication problem, and the additional disadvantage of lack of training in a community where unemployment is the norm, G.S. is an example of a positive outcome where the need for support was recognized (and initiated by G.S. herself in enlisting the assistance of the librarian) and the communicative demands of the workplace were matched to the individual's communicative strengths.

A second example of successful RTW is A.A., a 50-year-old lecturer at a university where most of the teaching is done by correspondence and small group tutorials. As a result of a left-sided parietal lobe infarct she presented with severe word-finding difficulty, paraphasias, and impaired comprehension, especially for written material. Six months post onset, she scored within the normal range on the Western Aphasia Battery and obtained a communication independence score of 6.9 on the ASHA FACS. However, she still experienced marked difficulty with higher level receptive tasks (e.g., the highest levels of the Token Test) and word finding. She summarized her difficulties as follows: she felt that she needed visual cues and a quiet background to understand what was said and often had to compensate by saying "everyone was talking—I missed that." She felt that she made many mistakes in reading and writing, which required frequent use of a dictionary and other external aids. She also commented on her difficulty with word retrieval and the fact that she often "says what (she) doesn't mean."

Most of A.A.'s therapy made use of work-related material—marked assignments, lecture note preparation, role-played tutorials, etc. A focus of therapy was also identifying the communication demands of her workplace, and completing the SOFCD together with A.A. and a colleague. This had a dual advantage: it allowed client and therapist to identify functional goals specific to the workplace, and it enabled A.A.'s colleagues to understand her potential difficulties and make appropriate modifications to the environment.

Six months after the stroke, A.A. gradually began to RTW. She described this as being "terrifying" and was dependent on the support afforded by therapy. She also commented on the accompanying fatigue, which has been identified by other authors as a major obstacle to RTW (Rolland & Beilin, 1993). This case demonstrates the importance of incorporating work goals into therapy and of gradual, supported return to work.

## Conclusion

The main results of our preliminary work in this area may be summarised as follows:

- RTW for stroke and TBI patients and indeed for the disabled population in general, is a poorly researched area.
- RTW after stroke and TBI is unusual, despite the fact that many individuals have the potential to continue to make a significant contribution to the economy.
- A number of factors may be linked to vocational outcome, including demographic, neurological, cognitive, and communicative predictors.
- RTW seems to be compounded by literacy level, premorbid occupation, difficulties with gaining access to rehabilitation and limited implementation of enabling legislation and undoubtedly by the general context.
- Communication skills required for the workplace are diverse and poorly understood and have an important role in determining effective RTW.
- The SOFCD is a measure that describes the communicative demands of a number of workplaces. It may be used to clarify functional goals for therapy.

As has been shown, the workplace is a neglected domain. This study highlights the importance of extending our assessment and intervention activities into this specific context. While RTW may not be possible for a number of TBI and aphasic patients, as we have seen, it is feasible for a number of individuals, and the role of communication in ensuring successful RTW is important. It therefore seems necessary that some attempt is made to establish the communicative demands of different potential employment contexts for patients. The SOFCD has the potential to do this, encompassing, as it does, a number of the communication behaviors that have been found to be essential for successful return to work.

The results of this study have also suggested the importance of investigating the possible reapportionment of time for therapy. In the context of scarce resources, it is possible that too much energy is allocated on those patients who have little chance of returning to work, although again RTW is clearly not the only goal of treatment. Those with a mild problem, on the other hand, who have the potential of returning to work and contributing to the economy are often neglected. This population should probably receive more therapy and this therapy should be vocationally directed (Johnson, 1998).

We suggest that a tool such as the SOFCD may be an enabling tool that allows for team decisions to be made between the therapist and the workplace for occupational resettlement (Fraser & Baarslag-Benson, 1994). What is important is the modification of the environment and the creation of an awareness on the part of co-workers and employers that sometimes a small change in communication demands of a workplace can make a big difference to the individual concerned. Casey Shannon's self-report (1998) on RTW after a stroke, reflects this aspect. She comments on negative encounters in the workplace and her changing responses to these: "In instances like these, I used to allow myself to be hurt, frustrated and feel less whole . . . It took many encounters with others to realize that this was not my problem. It was *their* problem, caused by lack of knowledge or understanding of disabilities" (p. 163). The results of prior efficacy research on vocational resettlement are encouraging (e.g., Ben Yishay et al., 1987) and lend support to the suggestions that new legislation and monitoring, as well as funding mechanisms should be considered, which incorporate the workplace. The new interest in rehabilitation services in the workplace includes the consideration of "rehabilitation technology" (specialized adapted equipment), case management of individuals, and a recognition among disability insurance carriers of the great savings afforded by satisfactory return to work (see, e.g., Macdonald, 1990).

Many directions for future research have been suggested by our findings, among which include the application of the SOFCD to other categories of disability involving communication such as stuttering and hearing loss; the adaptation of the SOFCD into languages other than English, more systematic and detailed research on the various predictors of RTW, and the adoption and application of the database to a wide range of clinical subjects.

What the study has underlined is the complexities of RTW as a construct, its link to quality of life issues for the patient, and the central role of communication in the workplace.

Nowhere is this point made more clear than in the powerful self-report of one of the informants with aphasia studied by Parr et al. (1997):

> I love work. I love work and it's no good—Eight years ago is on the telephone chat chat chat all day for me. And now is finished—It's a blank—My speech is just tongue-tied. Unbelievable is so awful." (p. 103)

It is certain that such observations and experiences provide compelling motivation to the speech–language pathologist of the future to expand functional assessment and intervention domains into the work arena.

## Acknowledgments

Sincere thanks go to the following persons for their assistance with aspects of this study: Nola Watt whose inspiring research formed the basis for much of the discussion on TBI in this chapter, Odette Vyncke for her tireless support and innovative approach and Lisa Schmaman for her research assistance.

## References

Adelman, S. M. (1981). Economic impact: The national survey of stroke. *Stroke, 12* (Suppl. 1), 69–77.

Alfassa, S., Ronene, R., Ring, H., Dyma, A., Tanir, A., Eldar, R. (1997). Quality of life in younger adults (17–49) after first stroke—a two year follow-up. *Fleischman Unit for Study of Disability, 133,* 249–254.

Ben-Yishay, Y., Silver, S. M., Platesky, E., & Rattock, J. (1987). Relationships between employability and vocational outcome after intensive holistic cognitive rehabilitation. *Journal of Head Trauma Rehabilitation, March,* 35–45.

Bonita, R. (1992). Epidemiology of stroke. *Lancet, 339,* 342–344.

Brooks, D. N., McKinlay, W., Symington, C., Beattie, A., & Campsie, L. (1987). Return to work within the first seven years of severe head injury. *Brain Injury, 1,* 5–19.

Carriero, M. R., Faglia, L., & Vignolo, L. A. (1987). Resumption of gainful employment in aphasics: Preliminary findings. *Cortex, 26,* 667–672.

Christensen, A. L. (1992). Outpatient management and outcome in relation to work in traumatic brain injury patients. *Scandinavian Journal of Rehabilitative Medicine, 26* (Suppl.), 34–42.

Crepeau, F., & Scherzer, P. (1993). Predictors and indicators of work status after traumatic brain injury: A meta analysis. *Neuropsychological Rehabilitation, 3,* 5–35.

Dahmer, O., Skillig, M. A., Hamilton, B. B., Bontke, C. F., Kreutzer, J. S., Ragnarisson, K. T., & Rosenthal, M. (1993). A model systems database of traumatic brain injury. *Journal of Head Trauma Rehabilitation, 8,* 12–25.

Dresser, A., Meirowsky, A., Weiss, G., McNeel, M., Simon, G., & Caveness, W. (1983). Gainful employment following closed head injury. *Archives of Neurology, 29,* 111–116.

Fraser, R. T., & Baarslag-Benson, R. (1994). Cross-disciplinary collaboration in the removal of work barriers after traumatic brain injury. *Topics in Language Disorders, 15,* 55–67.

Frattali, C. M., Thompson, C. M., Holland, A. L., Wohl, C. B., & Ferketic, M. M. (1995). *American Speech–Language–Hearing Association Functional Assessment of Communication Skills for Adults.* Rockville, MD: ASHA.

Geddes, J. M. L., Fear, J., Tennant, A., Pickering, A., Hillman, M., & Chamberlain, M. A. (1996). Prevalence of self-reported stroke in a population in northern England. *Journal of Epidemiology and Community Health, 50,* 140–143.

Granger, C. V., Sherwood, C. C., & Greer, D. S. (1997). Functional status measures in a comprehensive stroke care programme. *Archives of Physical Medicine and Rehabilitation, 58,* 555–560.

Gresham, G., Philips, T., Wolf, P., Kamel, W., & Dawber, T. (1979). Epidemiological profile of long-term stroke disability: The Farmingham study. *Archives of Physical Medicine and Rehabilitation, 60,* 487–491.

Hartley, L. L. (1995). *Cognitive-communicative abilities following brain injury. A functional approach.* San Diego, California: Singular Publishing Group.

Hatfield, F. M., & Zangwill, O. L. (1975). Occupational resettlement in aphasia. *Scandinavian Journal of Rehabilitation Medicine, 7,* 57–60.

Hermann, M., & Wallesch, C. W. (1990). Expectations of psychosocial adjustment in aphasia. A MAUT study with the Code-Muller Scale of Psychosocial Adjustment. *Aphasiology, 4,* 527–538.

Hsieh, C. L., & Lee, M. H. (1997). Factors influencing vocational outcomes following stroke in Taiwan: A medical centre-based study. *Scandinavian Journal of Rehabilitation Medicine, 29,* 113–120.

Integrated National Disability Strategy. (1997). White Paper, Office of the Deputy President.

Ip, R. Y., Dornar, J., & Schentag, C. (1995). Traumatic brain injury: Factors predicting return to work or school. *Brain Injury, 9,* 517–532.

Johnson, R. (1998). How do people get back to work after severe head injury? A 10-year follow-up study. *Neuropsychological Rehabilitation, 8,* 61–79.

Joussen, K., & Pascher, W. (1984). Empirische Untersuchung der sozialen situation von aphasiakern. *Folia Phoniatrica, 36,* 66–73.

Lapertosa, M. (1994). *Employment discrimination and persons with disabilities: Legislative options.* Johannesburg Disability Rights Unit, Lawyers for Human Rights.

LeDorze, G., & Brassard, C. (1995). A description of the consequences of aphasia on aphasic persons and their relatives and friends, based on the WHO model of chronic diseases. *Aphasiology, 9,* 339–255.

Lubinski, R. (1994). Environmental systems approach to intervention strategies in adult aphasia. In R. Chapey (ed): *Language intervention strategies in adult aphasia*, 3rd ed (pp. 269–291). Baltimore: Williams and Wilkins.

Lyons, J. L., & Morse, A. R. (1988). A therapeutic programme for head-injured adults. *The American Journal of Occupational Therapy, 42*, 364–370.

Macdonald, M. (1990). You can control your disability costs. *Business and Health, May*, 21–36.

Marshall, R. C. (1987). Reapportioning time for aphasia rehabilitation: A point of view. *Aphasiology, 1*, 59–73.

Matsumoto, N., Whisnant, J., Kurland, L., & Okazali, H. (1973). Natural history of stroke in Rochester, Minnesota, 1955–1969: An extension of a previous study 1945–1954. *Stroke, 4*, 20–29.

Najenson, T., Sazbon, I., Fizelson, J., Becker, E., & Schechter, I. (1978). Recovery of communicative functions after prolonged traumatic coma. *Scandinavian Journal of Rehabilitation Medicine, 10*, 15–21.

Neau, J. P., Ingrand, P., Moville-Braubet, C., Rosier, M., Condery, C., Alvarez, A., & Gil, R. (1998). Functional recovery and outcome after cerebral infarction in young adults. *Cerebrovascular Disorders, 8*, 296–302.

Oddy, M., Coughlan, T., Tyerman, A., & Jenkins, D. (1985). Social adjustment after closed head injury: A further follow-up seven years after injury. *Journal of Neurology, Neurosurgery, and Psychiatry, 48*, 564–568.

Parr, S. (1994). Coping with aphasia: Conversations with 20 aphasic people. *Aphasiology, 8*, 457–466.

Parr, S., Byng, S., & Gilpin, S. (1997). *Talking about aphasia*. Buckingham: Open University Press.

P.E. Corporate Service General Staff Remuneration Survey in South Africa. April 1995.

Penn, C. (1993). Aphasia rehabilitation in South Africa: Some pragmatic and personal perspectives. In A. Holland, M. Forbes (eds): *Aphasia Treatment: World Perspectives* (pp. 25–54). San Diego: Singular Press.

Price, P. L., & Bauman, W. L. (1991). Working: The key to normalization after brain injury. In D. E. Tupper, K. D. Cicerone (eds): *The neuropsychology of everyday life: Issues in development and rehabilitation* (pp. 125–168). Boston: Kluwer.

Prigatano, G., Fordyce, D. J., Zeiner, H. K., Roueche, J. R., Pepping, M., & Wood, B. C. (1984). Neuropsychological rehabilitation after closed-head injury in young adults. *Journal of Neurology, Neurosurgery and Psychiatry, 47*, 505–513.

Putnam, H. S., & Adams, N. M. (1992). Regression based procedures of long-term outcome following multidisciplinary rehabilitation for traumatic brain injury. *The Clinical Neuropsychologist, 6*, 383–405.

Rao, N., Rosenthal, M., Cronin-Stubbs, D., Lambert, R., Barnes, P., & Swanson, B. (1990). Return to work after rehabilitation following traumatic brain injury. *Brain Injury, 4*, 49–56.

Rolland, J., & Beilin, C. (1993). The person with aphasia and the workforce. In D. Lafond, R. DeGiovani, Y. Joanette, J. Ponzio, M. T. Sarno, (eds): *Living with aphasia. Psychological issues* (pp. 223–242). San Diego: Singular Publishing Group.

Shannon, C. (1998) Aha! There is a reason. In W. Sife (ed): *Life after stroke: Enhancing quality of life*. Binghamton: Haworth Press.

Smollan, T., & Penn, C. (1997). The measurement of emotional reaction and depression in a South African stroke population. *Disability and Rehabilitation, 19*, 56–63.

Snell, R. (1993). Medical Rehabilitation and Public Policy Document drafted for Senate Budget Committee. US senior advisor at the offices of Senator Lawton Chiles.

Thomsen, I. V. (1985). Late outcome in very severe injuries with special reference to psychosocial sequelae. *Ugekr Laeger, 147*, 2689–2694.

Thomsen, I. V. (1992). Late psychosocial outcome of very severe blunt head trauma: A ten to fifteen year follow up. *Journal of Neurology, Neurosurgery and Psychiatry, 47*, 260–268.

Toffolo, D., & Minns, M. (1993). Real life functional assessment. Paper presented at First National Aphasiology Symposium of Australia, Sydney.

Tollman, S., Watts-Runge, A., & Nell, V. (1993). Traumatic head injury to a productive life: An evaluation of a Holistic Neuropsychological Programme. Paper presented at the 5th National Neuropsychology Conference (SACNA). Durban: University of Natal.

Wade, D., & Heuwer, R. (1987). Functional abilities after stroke: Measurement, natural history and prognosis. *Journal of Neurology, Neurosurgery and Psychiatry, 50*, 177–182.

Watson, K. (1998). An investigation of the applicability and efficacy of the ASHA FACS in the South African hospital setting. Unpublished Research Report, University of the Witwatersrand.

Watt, N. (1996). Predictors and indicators of outcome following closed head injury in South Africa. Unpublished Masters Dissertation, University of the Witwatersrand.

Watt, N., Penn, C., & Jones, D. (1996). Speech–language evaluation of closed head injured subjects in South Africa: Cultural applicability and ecological validity. *South African Journal of Communication Disorders, 43*, 85–92.

Wehman, P. H., Kregel, J., West, M., & Cifu, D. (1994). Return to work for patients with traumatic brain injury. *American Journal of Physical Medicine Rehabilitation, 73,* 280–282.

Wehman, P. H., Kreutzer, J. S., West, M. D., Sherron, P., Zazler, N. D., Groath, C. H., Stonnongton, H. H., Burns, C. T., & Sale, P. R. (1990). Return to work for persons with traumatic brain injury: A supported approach. *Archives of Physical Medicine and Rehabilitation, 71,* 1047–1052.

Wehman, P. H., West, M. D., Kregel, J., Sherron, P., & Kreutzer, J. S. (1995). Return to work for persons with severe traumatic brain injury: A data-based approach to programme development. *Journal of Head Trauma Rehabilitation, February,* 27–39.

Weinberg, K. (1997). Communication outcome and quality of life one year post stroke. Unpublished undergraduate research project, University of Cape Town.

Weisbroth, S., Esibilln, R., & Zuger, R. (1971). Factors in the vocational success of hemiplegic patients. *Archives of Physical Medicine and Rehabilitation, Oct,* 441–446.

Wertz, R. T. (1983). A philosophy of aphasia therapy: Some things that patients do not say but that you can see if you listen. *Communication Disorders, 8,* 109–125.

West, M., Wheman, P. H., Kregel, J., Kreutzer, J., Sherron, P., & Zasler, N. D. (1991). Cost of operating a supported work programme for traumatically brain injured individuals. *Archives of Physical Medicine and Rehabilitation, 72,* 127–131.

World Health Organization (1997). International Classification of Impairment, Disability and Handicap—2. *http://www.who.ch/programmes/mnh/mnh//ems/icidh/icidh.htm.*

Wrightson, P., & Gronwall, D. (1990). Time off work and symptoms after head injury. *Injury, 12,* 445–454.

YOU (1998). (April) Surviving a stroke. Republican Press: South Africa.

*8*

# Forging Partnerships with Volunteers

## Linda E. Worrall
## Edwin Yiu

**Volunteers have a special role in functional communication therapy and are increasingly being used to supplement, rather than replace speech-language pathology services. The literature surrounding the effectiveness of volunteer-administered therapy on functional communication outcomes is reviewed. The advantages and disadvantages of using volunteers are described with the conclusion being reached that partnerships with volunteers must occur if the wider community is to play a part in the rehabilitation of people with a communication disorder.**

## Introduction

The topic of the use of volunteers to provide therapy to people with a communication disorder has been controversial (Lalor & Yiu, 1997). This chapter aims to explore the issues surrounding the controversy, describe some different ways in which volunteers are being used to facilitate functional communication, examine the literature that has evaluated these approaches, and finally weigh the advantages and disadvantages of promoting the involvement of volunteers with clients. The chapter concludes that partnerships between speech-language pathologists and volunteers are essential if clients are to achieve communication goals that enable them to participate in society.

The service provided by volunteers has particular relevance to functional communication. Everyday communication is more transparent to volunteers who have no training in the detail and intricacy of speech and language impairment. Functional communication is more readily understood by nonprofessionals and more likely to be targeted or valued in a service provided by volunteers. In addition, the value of many of the volunteer services that provide socialization opportunities to communication disordered individuals are now being understood and appreciated.

Aphasiology has been the primary area in which volunteer-administered therapy has been explored. There has been a long history of volunteer schemes in aphasia rehabilitation, particularly in Britain where a reported 48% of aphasia therapists make use of volunteers for aphasic clients (MacKenzie et al., 1993). The controversy surrounding the use of volunteers for aphasia therapy has been based fundamentally on the fear that nonprofessional staff will replace professional staff. Speech-language pathologists have often observed managerial decisions based on economic rationalist approaches, therefore studies that suggest that volunteers can make as much gains as speech-language pathologists have fueled some fears. Yet, there is little evidence to date that volunteers have replaced speech-language pathologists, even in areas where volunteer schemes for aphasic people are particularly well developed. Hence, despite the presence of volunteer schemes for several decades, and some literature that promotes the effectiveness of volunteer-administered therapy programs, there is little evidence to suggest that payers are replacing professional staff by nonprofessional staff. It is hoped that this is because there is a realization that volunteer schemes need to be established in partnership with professional help. When volunteer schemes act as supplements to professional speech-language pathology services, volunteer schemes add more cost to an existing service because volunteers require training, supervision, and coordination (Wade, 1983).

The issue has been examined in narrow terms in the literature to date with little recognition that in reality, many people with a disability have people who volunteer their time to help them. Some are in organized schemes, others are friends of the family or a local person who just wants to help out. Taking an even broader view that fits with the notion that functional communication extends into the Participation dimension of the ICIDH-2, many support organizations (e.g., International Aphasia Association, Action for Dysphasic Adults, National Aphasia Association) rely on volunteer help. These organizations play a major role in encouraging society to be more inclusive of its members and hence enabling greater participation of communicatively disabled people. In broadening their own role, speech-language pathologists need to tap into these resources in an effort to strengthen the support for people with communication disorders.

## Models of Facilitating Functional Communication by Volunteers

Volunteers operate in various settings and with a variety of disabilities. The most prevalent description of volunteer use comes from the aphasiology literature, however, volunteers have also been part of communication programs for healthy older people (Worrall et al., 1998), traumatic brain injury (Freeman, 1997; Moreci, 1996) or for nursing facility residents (Jordan et al., 1993), to name a few. In aphasiology, volunteers may provide individual treatment in the person's home (Marshall et al., 1989; Meikle et al., 1979; Worrall & Yiu, in press) in community centres (Kagan & Gailey, 1993; Lesser & Watt, 1978), and in hospitals (David et al., 1982). Service delivery can either be within a group setting or on an individual basis.

The effectiveness of volunteer-provided therapy for people with aphasia has been reviewed in this chapter because aphasiology has been the most keenly studied.

Volunteer treatment, like treatment provided by speech-language pathologists, can target the Impairment, Activity, or Participation level of the ICIDH-2 [World Health Organization (WHO), 1997]. In the following section of this chapter, several studies of the effectiveness of volunteer-administered therapy have been reviewed to determine if volunteers have a role in facilitating functional communication. The studies are categorized as impairment-based, activity-based, or participation-based studies on the basis of each study's focus of intervention. Studies in which the therapy has targeted the impairment level, but the effect has been measured in terms of a functional communication assessment have been included in the review as these are seen as interventions that facilitate functional communication.

### Volunteers Working at the Impairment Level

Intervention programs that target the impairment level implicitly carry the expectation that the intervention will generalize and affect everyday communicative activities and participation. However, not all studies measure the effect of impairment-based therapy on functional communication. Only studies that have evaluated impairment-based volunteer programs in terms of functional communication assessments were considered for this review. Studies such as those by Lesser et al. (1986), Meikle et al. (1979), and Shewan and Kertesz (1984) have therefore not been included because they use only impairment-based measures as outcome measures. Geddes and Chamberlain (1994) failed to include the results of the functional outcome measure, the Edinburgh Functional Communication Profile (Skinner et al., 1984) because of a high amount of missing data. Marshall and Sacchett (1996) rightly refute the Frenchay Activities Index (Wade et al., 1985) as a measure of social recovery or quality of life for people with aphasia. Therefore, the study by Geddes and Chamberlain (1994) was also not included. The only known study that has measured the impact of impairment-based therapy on functional communication was the Veterans Administration Cooperative Study, which compared clinic, home, and deferred language treatment for aphasia (Wertz et al., 1986)

As part of the Veterans Administration Cooperative Study, Marshall et al. (1989) explored the issue of home treatment by trained nonprofessionals in more detail. The volunteers in this study were called home therapists to include the relatives, friends, and volunteers who conducted therapy and about half of the home therapists did in fact reside in the same environment as the participant with aphasia. The communication outcome measures were the Porch Index of Communicative Abilities (Porch, 1967), the Communicative Abilities in Daily Living (Holland, 1980), Reading Comprehension Battery for Aphasia (LaPointe & Horner, 1979) and the Token Test (Spreen & Benton, 1969). Home therapy consisted of 8–10 hours of treatment each week for 12 weeks by the home therapist in the client's own home. Each home program was designed, explained, and demonstrated by the speech-language pathologist who then supervised the home therapist for the duration of the program. While the responsibility of the content of the program was at the discretion of the supervising speech-language pathologist, it appears that all modalities were treated and that criterion levels were established for tasks. While this does not exclude the possibility of functional communication therapy being conducted, it is more likely that the treatment targeted the impairment of aphasia. The primary result was that although the home therapy group made greater improvement than the no treatment phase of the deferred group, this did not reach statistical significance. When compared to the treatment provided by speech-language pathologists, there was no significant difference between professional and nonprofessional delivery of treatment. The results of the functional communication assessment, the Communicative Abilities in Daily Living (CADL), showed that scores improved after home therapy (mean difference = 15.03/130) but there was no significant difference between groups. That is, there was no significant difference between the home treatment, deferred and speech-language pathology treatment in terms of improvement on the CADL. The authors conclude with a statement that there is no evidence to suggest that treatment by nonprofessionals is efficacious. They acknowledge, however, that for patients who cannot financially afford professional services or who are geographically unable to access those professional services, treatment by trained and closely monitored nonprofessionals may be considered.

Hence, in this study in which the target of therapy was impairment-level tasks, there was little evidence to support the use of volunteers for people with aphasia. The difference between the no-treatment phase and home-treatment phase was not significant. The authors, however, point to the greater proportion of clients who improved on tests such as the CADL following home therapy compared to the group who had deferred treatment (i.e., the no-treatment group). They indicate that the use of volunteers might be an option in light of diminishing resources. However, it must be remembered that there was a high degree of supervision and guidance provided by professional speech-language pathologists in this study.

The approach used by Marshall et al. (1989) could be thought of as a "volunteer-as-therapist" model. In this model, the volunteer acts under the direction of the speech-language pathologist and performs impairment-based tasks that might have been performed by the therapist. The study by Marshall et al. suggests that this is not effective and does not improve functional communication.

### Volunteers Working at the Activity (Disability) Level

Activity-level treatment lends itself to being provided by volunteers. Everyday communicative activities are more transparent and familiar to volunteers. Volunteers also bring considerable experience in everyday communicative activities to the therapeutic situation.

There have been three studies that have deliberately or inadvertently targeted the activity level in treatment. None of these studies have the rigor or statistical power of the Marshall study, but nevertheless show that volunteer-provided therapy at the activity level has potential. The first was an opportunistic attempt to evaluate the proliferation of volunteer schemes in the United Kingdom. Lesser and Watt (1978) compared pretreatment and post-treatment measures on 16 people with aphasia who attended the Newcastle Speech-After-Stroke Clubs. Hence, this was an evaluation of group treatment in which volunteers were instructed to provide natural settings for encouraging communication, give social confidence for tasks such as shopping and using buses, and provide enjoyment for members and respite for relatives. The results indicated that while there were no significant differences on the 25 subtests of the Boston Diagnostic Aphasia Examination (Goodglass & Kaplan, 1972), 14 of the 16 participants showed improvement on the Functional Communication Profile—FCP (Sarno, 1969). There was no statistical comparison of the FCP scores. While the authors discuss many of the difficulties they encountered in measuring the effects of treatment, particularly in measuring functional outcome, they encourage the development of volunteer schemes concurrent with existing speech-language pathology services.

Again in the United Kingdom, David et al. (1982) conducted a large-scale comparison of the results achieved by speech-language pathologists and the results achieved by volunteers for people with aphasia. Outcome was measured by the FCP (Sarno, 1969) and this was the only assessment information made available to the volunteers. Hence, it is likely that the treatment that occurred for 2 hours per week over a 15- to 20-week interval was predominantly functional. It is not known what the exact nature of treatment would have been, however, for either group, since the content of therapy was left to the individual speech-language pathologist or volunteer therapist. Treatment was conducted in the hospital as an outpatient. This may have mitigated against a functional focus to treatment. Nevertheless, although there was a significant improvement for both groups, there was no significant difference between the groups. There was no comparison to a no-treatment group. The authors conclude by asking "If treatment works, does it matter who gives it?" (David et al., 1982, p. 960). They also emphasize that the volunteers had access to full and frequent speech-language pathology assessment results and worked within the speech-language pathology department at the hospital. In support of the argument that this study does not lend support to the notion that volunteers can replace speech-language pathologists, Wade (1983) points out that there were additional costs rather then a reduction of costs in administering such a scheme. He notes that the support of volunteers is time-consuming for speech-language pathologists as each volunteer is enrolled, given training, and matched with a suitable client with aphasia. Language assessment information is provided to the volunteer by the speech-language pathologist and a therapy program is devised, often with considerable input by the speech-language pathologist. Should difficulties arise, the speech-language pathologist is often called upon as a troubleshooter. Hence, the time commitment by the speech-language pathologist to the volunteer scheme must be high and this is translated into additional cost. Many schemes use a volunteer coordinator (Meikle et al., 1979; Lesser & Watt, 1978) and incur volunteer transport costs (Eaton Griffith & Miller, 1980)

To further determine the effectiveness of aphasia therapy delivered by volunteers, a recent Australian study compared functional communication therapy to recreational therapy, both delivered by volunteers (Worrall & Yiu, in press). The predominant aim was to determine if volunteers could make some functional gains when they used a specially developed program, the *Speaking Out* program. It was envisaged that the *Speaking Out* program would mainly be used in the rural and remote areas of Australia where face-to-face access to speech-language pathology services is difficult, but telephone access is more feasible. The program might also be used by established stroke volunteer organizations that provided a service to people in their own homes in metropolitan areas. Many people with long-standing aphasia cannot attend group programs because of transport difficulties, lack of interest in groups, or nonsuitability for group therapy. Financial constraints often preclude their ability to access private speech-language pathology services, hence, there is a need to establish home-visitor volunteer schemes for these people, even in areas where speech-language pathology services are well established. The question of whether people with aphasia would make greater gains with a speech-language pathology service rather than a volunteer service was not asked in this study.

In this study, it was considered important to compare the gains made using the *Speaking Out* program to a type of placebo in which volunteers would visit the person with aphasia and play card games or other nonlanguage activities. It was also important to compare the gains made by the functional communication therapy program to the gains made during a period of nonintervention. The Wertz et al. (1986) concept of deferred treatment was therefore used to obtain a no-treatment phase. Recognizing the limitations of comparative group studies to evaluate the efficacy of aphasia treatment, a research design was chosen that would allow intragroup comparisons as well as intergroup comparisons. Outcomes were measured using a battery of tests that reflected the Impairment, Activity limitations, and Participation restrictions of aphasia. Hence, outcomes were measured by assessing the participants at 10 weekly intervals on the Western Aphasia Battery—WAB (Kertesz, 1982), the American Speech-Language-Hearing Association's Functional Assessment of Communication Skills for Adults—ASHA FACS (Frattali et al., 1995), the Communicative Effectiveness Index—CETI (Lomas et al., 1989), the Everyday Communicative Needs Assessment—ECNA (Worrall, 1995), and the Short Form-36—SF-36 (Medical Outcomes Trust, 1994) for the aphasic and spouse participants.

The *Speaking Out* program consisted of ten modules each focusing on a particular aspect of everyday communication (e.g., use of the telephone, financial matters, leisure activities—going out). This program was delivered during a 2-hour weekly visit to the aphasic participant's home by the volunteer. The volunteers received 2 hours of training on the nature of aphasia generally and the *Speaking Out* program more specifically. Volunteers completed a questionnaire at the completion of each week's session and were supported by a speech-language pathologist for the duration of the program, mostly by telephone.

The results were mostly positive. The group who had the *Speaking Out* program after the recreational therapy program had more significant changes. Gains for this group were made on the WAB and the ASHA FACS following the *Speaking Out* program and the gains made during the program were better than the gains made during the recreational program and the nonintervention period. In terms of clinical significance, the statistically significant gains made for this group were a mean change of 3.14 AQ points on the WAB and a mean change of 0.19 on the overall communicative independence mean score on the ASHA FACS. While these gains were relatively small, it must be remembered that these participants were over 12 month post onset and the intervention period was only two hours each week for 10 weeks. There were also some participants who benefitted substantially from the program.

In summary, results for the effectiveness of volunteer-administered treatment at the Activity level are encouraging. While methodological difficulties continue to be present in these studies, evidence is beginning to accumulate that confirm that volunteers can provide effective functional communication therapy for aphasia. While the model of "volunteer-as-therapist" has been used to some degree in these studies, a more equal partnership is being crafted in which the everyday communicative experiences of the volunteer are being utilized to assist the person with aphasia in everyday communicative activities.

### Volunteers Working at the Participation Level

A recent development in aphasiology has been a strong interest in the use of non-professional volunteers to facilitate participation by people with aphasia. One of the models of best practice of this approach is the Aphasia Center in North York, Ontario, Canada. Kagan and Gailey (1993) have described their approach as analogous to providing wheelchair ramps to physically disabled people. At the Aphasia Center, they attempt to provide "communication ramps" so that people with aphasia can access the communicative life of a community. To do this, they train volunteers to be skilled conversation partners. Rather than be "teachers" of people with aphasia, volunteers are encouraged to perceive themselves as communication facilitators. Volunteers work with small groups of people with aphasia at the Aphasia Center and have professional training and support on hand. As Kagan and Gailey note, the low ratio of professional staff to aphasic people, enabled by volunteer staff, makes for an economical service.

Kagan (1998) has provided preliminary evidence of the effectiveness of the program by showing that training volunteers as conversational partners improves the interactional and transactional participation in conversation. However, evaluating the effectiveness of the program using the Participation dimension of the ICIDH-2 as a whole, has yet to be studied.

Providing an opportunity for social interaction is not, however, a new goal for many traditional aphasia groups. The presentation of this goal within a well-established theoretical framework has, however, legitimized this as a role for speech-language pathologists. In addition, the staff, volunteers, and aphasic individuals at the Aphasia Center have developed a program that is well-structured and well-resourced and this has encouraged other facilities to develop similar facilities in other countries of the world.

As noted earlier, taking a broader view of volunteers means the inclusion of support organizations. Organizations such as the National Aphasia Association or Action for Dysphasic Adults and its many equivalents in other parts of the world (Klein, 1996) or support associations for other communication disorders such as head injury, Parkinsons Disease, and Multiple Sclerosis often depend upon volunteer support. In the case of the aphasia associations, it is often the aphasic people themselves or their families that establish the associations. Indeed it is often the experienced aphasic people who volunteer their time to establish these connections.

The role of support organizations could be considered to be within the Participation dimension. Support groups certainly work to educate society about the disabilities of the group members and are often active lobbyists at a policy level within governments and peak bodies. They promote a message that encourages society to be inclusive of their members and may fight for social justice on behalf of their members. While these organizations need to be driven by nonprofessionals, they deserve the support of speech-language pathologists. They provide an invaluable resource for new clients as well as for professional staff new to the area, and provide a service that complements that of speech-language pathologists. It would seem that there is a common value shared by support associations and speech-language pathologists—the right of an individual to communicate in society. To achieve such a partnership, speech-language pathologists may wish to consider being a catalyst for the formation of such groups within their local area.

In summary, while speech-language pathology services continue to expand into the Activity and Participation dimensions of the ICIDH-2, the role of others in the community, such as volunteers, is unclear. Much research is needed to explore the role of volunteers at the Activity and Participation dimensions. The profession should broaden its outlook by moving away from the "volunteers-as-therapists" model to one in which volunteers are valued partners in facilitating the functional communication goals of clients.

Rigorous evaluation of the effectiveness of volunteers with communication-disordered clients is still required. Studies that demonstrate the clinical or social significance of the service are particularly needed, in addition to those that demonstrate statistical significance. While functional communication measures continue to be developed that will assist in the evaluation of such services, it is likely that qualitative research methods will play a more prominent role in evaluating the effectiveness of volunteer services, particularly at the Participation level.

### Factors Affecting Partnerships with Volunteers

Speech-language pathologists have tended to view volunteers as a threat rather than a opportunity. If the profession considers moving toward a mutually satisfying arrangement in which all stakeholders gain, then it must weigh the advantages and disadvantages of moving toward a partnership arrangement with volunteers. The advantages and disadvantages of a partnership arrangement are as follows:

Advantages:

1. *Extension of speech-language pathology services*: At a facility level, volunteers can provide an outreach service. An example of this is the *Speaking Out* program mentioned previously. Speech-language pathologists recruit, train, and supervise volunteers to go into the client's own home. The volunteer may be a fam-

ily member or friend who has become the home therapist (Marshall et al., 1989). Also at a facility level or regional level, speech-language pathologists may wish to develop the model used by the Aphasia Center in Ontario in which volunteers are recruited, trained and supervised by speech-language pathologists to facilitate communication in a group setting. Alternatively, speech-language pathology facilities may encourage the formation of support groups which eventually act relatively independently of the facility.

2. *Integration with community for clients*: Volunteers are perhaps more natural communication partners than speech-language pathologists. While speech-language pathologists are generally sensitive to the cues of a communicatively disordered speaker and are experts at accommodating any potential break-downs within a communication exchange, volunteers are more diverse in their ability to accommodate speaker's communicative behaviors. People with communication disorders can therefore practice their communication skills with a more diverse set of communication partners. Volunteers can therefore play a role in any generalization program. Consistent with Kagan and Gailey's notion of "communication ramps," volunteers who are skilled conversational partners can facilitate an individual's links to society. The role of the volunteer in this instance may simply be to provide some pleasurable social interaction with a client therefore fulfilling a need for social affiliation. Alternatively, professionals such as lawyers or medical practitioners who undergo training to communicate well with communication-disordered clients may be able to open up doors and provide access to services that have not been previously available to them.

Disadvantages:

1. *Cost:* Developing a volunteer scheme involves a degree of cost. This is a view supported by others such as Marshall et al. (1989) and Wade (1983). The costs can be financial (e.g., many schemes employ a dedicated volunteer coordinator, some pay for the transport costs of the volunteers) or they can be considered in terms of staff time (recruitment, training, and supervision by existing staff). While the cost–benefit ratio may be good, particularly once the scheme has been established with a core of volunteers, an established training program and an efficient method of supervision, many institutions have considerable financial or staffing restraints. The reality of establishing a volunteer scheme is in contrast to the myth that it will reduce costs. It may be a cost-effective way to extend a service or provide a new service, but it is unlikely to reduce the costs of an existing professional service.

2. *Partnership difficulties:* Moving into uncharted territory can be fraught with obstacles and it may require several excursions to establish an established pattern of practice. Speech-language pathologists who undertake to develop partnerships with volunteers need to understand the difficulties inherent in establishing this relationship. Apart from a substantial degree of commitment by speech-language pathologists, it may require additional effort over and above normal duties. There may be skepticism by colleagues who fear that handing over a therapeutic role to volunteers will result in poor-quality ser-

vice or that the introduction of volunteers will lead to a deprofessionalization of services generally. These are some of the uphill struggles that face a speech-language pathologist who is interested in supplementing an existing service with volunteers.

## Toward Best Practice

Speech-language pathologists should consider enlisting the help of volunteers. For clients, volunteers can improve their access to relevant services, improve their communication skills, and facilitate their participation in society. For speech-language pathologists and managers, volunteers can improve throughput in their facilities, extend the type of services that they can offer and provide a different perspective to communication and a different paradigm of care. For a volunteer, the benefits include insights into new domains and relationships with new people. It is a win–win situation for all stakeholders.

Rather than being an inexpensive alternative to speech-language pathology services, volunteer schemes require additional resources to establish and maintain. Recruiting good volunteers, developing effective training programs and providing support to volunteers who are working with clients requires a substantial amount of commitment by speech-language pathologists. Some agencies employ volunteer coordinators to conduct this important role. Given the choice, most volunteers want to work in partnership with speech-language pathologists. It is in the profession's best interests to initiate a partnership arrangement, rather than to be fearful and defensive of such a partnership.

If a value of the profession is that all people should have access to services that help them achieve their communication goals, then the profession needs to recognize the important service that volunteers can provide. The profession also needs to continually remind itself that clients do not communicate just with speech-language pathologists. They also communicate with family, friends, colleagues, neighbors, ministers of religion, and total strangers. The role of the speech-language pathologist is to ensure that these social networks are maintained if possible and to create new ones if needed. It is only through enlisting the help of members of society, of which volunteers can play a vital component, will speech-language pathologists move towards being recognized as an essential and highly relevant professional. To this end, speech-language pathologists need to reach out and enthuse a wider population about the centrality of communication in society and seek support for those members of society who are communicatively disadvantaged.

## References

David, R., Enderby, P., & Bainton, D. (1982). Treatment of acquired aphasia: Speech therapists and volunteers compared. *Journal of Neurology, Neurosurgery and Psychiatry, 45,* 957–961.

Eaton Griffith, V., & Miller, C. L. (1980). Volunteer stroke scheme for dysphasic patients with stroke. *British Medical Journal, 281,* 1605–1607.

Frattali, C. M., Thompson, C. M., Holland, A. L., Wohl, C. B., & Ferketic, M. M. (1995). *ASHA Functional Assessment of Communication Skills for Adults (FACS).* Rockville, MD: American Speech-Language-Hearing Association.

Freeman, E. A. (1997). Community-based rehabilitation of the person with a severe brain injury. *Brain Injury, 11*, 143–153.

Geddes, J., & Chamberlain, M. (1994). Improving social outcome after stroke: An evaluation of the volunteer stroke scheme. *Clinical Rehabilitation, 8*, 116–126.

Goodglass, H., & Kaplan, E., (1972). *Assessment of aphasia and related disorders*. Philadelphia: Lea & Febiger.

Holland, A. L. (1980). *Communicative abilities in daily living*. Baltimore: University Park Press.

Jordan, F., Worrall, L., Hickson, L., & Dodd, B. (1993). The evaluation of an intervention programme for communicatively impaired elderly. *European Journal of Disorders of Communication, 28*, 63–85.

Kagan, A. (1998). Training volunteers as conversation partners using "Supported conversation for adults with aphasia": An efficacy study. Paper presented at the 8th International Aphasia Rehabilitation Conference. Kwa Maritane, South Africa, August, 1998.

Kagan, A., & Gailey, G. F. (1993). Functional is not enough: Training conversation partners for aphasic adults. In A. L. Holland and M. F. Forbes (eds): *Aphasia treatment: World perspectives* (pp. 199–226). San Diego, California: Singular Publishing Group.

Kertesz, A. (1982). *Western Aphasia Battery*. New York: Grune and Stratton.

Klein, K. (1996). Community-based resources for persons with aphasia and their families. *Topics in Stroke Rehabilitation, 2*, 18–26.

Lalor, E., & Yiu, E. (1997). Current issues in the use of volunteers in aphasia therapy: An Australian perspective. *Asia Pacific Journal of Speech, Language and Hearing, 2*, 195–201.

LaPointe, L. L., & Horner, J. (1979). *Reading Comprehension Battery for Aphasia*. Tigard, OR: CC Publications.

Lesser, R., Bryan, K., Anderson, J., & Hilton, R. (1986). Involving relatives in aphasia therapy: An application of language enrichment therapy. *International Journal of Rehabilitation Research, 9*, 259–267.

Lesser, R., & Watt, M. (1978). Untrained community help in the rehabilitation of stroke sufferers with language disorder. *British Medical Journal, 14*, 1045–1048.

Lomas, J., Pickard, L., Bester, S., Elbard, H., Finlayson, A., & Zoghaib, C. (1989). The Communicative Effectiveness Index: Development and psychometric evaluation of a functional communication measure for adult aphasia. *Journal of Speech and Hearing Disorders, 54*, 113–124.

MacKenzie, C., Le May, M., Lendrum, W., McGuirk, E., Marshall, J., & Rossiter, D. (1993). A survey of aphasia services in the United Kingdom. *European Journal of Disorders of Communication, 28*, 43–63.

Marshall, J., & Sacchett, C. (1996). Does the Volunteer Stroke Scheme improve social outcome after stroke? A response to Geddes and Chamberlain. *Clinical Rehabilitation, 10*, 104–111.

Marshall, R. C., Wertz, R. T., Weiss, D. G., Aten, J. L, Brookshire, R. H., Garcia-Bunuel, L., Holland, A., Kurtzke, J., La Pointe, L., Milinti, F., Brannegan, R., Greenbaum, H., Vogel, D., Carter, J., Barnes, N., & Goodman, R. (1989). Home treatment for aphasic patients by trained non-professionals. *Journal of Speech and Hearing Disorders, 54*, 462–470.

Medical Outcomes Trust (1994). *SF-36 Health Survey*. Boston, MA.

Meikle, M., Weschler, E., Tupper, A., Benenson, M., Butler, J., Hulhall, D., & Stern, G. (1979). Comparative trial of volunteer and professional treatments of dysphasia after stroke. *British Medical Journal, 2*, 87–89.

Moreci, G. (1996). A model system of traumatic brain injury peer support importance, development and process. *Neurorehabilitation, 7*, 211–218.

Porch, B. E. (1967). *Porch Index of Communicative Ability*. Palo Alto, CA: Consulting Psychologists Press.

Sarno, M. T. (1969). *The Functional Communication Profile: Manual of directions*. (Rehabilitation Monograph No. 42). New York: New York Institute of Rehabilitation Medicine.

Shewan, C. M., & Kertesz, A. (1984). Effect of speech-language treatment on recovery from aphasia. *Brain and Language, 23*, 272–299.

Skinner, C., Wirz, S., Thompson, I., & Davidson, J. (1984). *Edinburgh Functional Communication Profile*. Winslow Press: Winslow, Buckingham.

Spreen, O., & Benton, A. (1969). *Neurosensory Comprehensive Examination for Aphasia*. Victoria, BC: Neuropsychology Laboratory, Victoria University.

Wade, D. T. (1983). Can aphasia people with stroke do without a speech therapist? *British Medical Journal, 286*, 50.

Wade, D. T., Legh-Smith, J., & Langton-Hewer, R. (1985). Social activities after stroke: Measurement and natural history using the Frenchay Activities Index. *International Rehabilitation Medicine, 7*, 176–181.

Wertz, R. T., Weiss, D. G., Aten, J. L., Brookshire, R. H., Garcia-Bunuel, L., Holland, A. L., Kurtze, J. F., LaPointe, L. L., Milianti, F. J., Brannegan, R., Greenbaum, H., Marshall, R. C., Vogel, D., Carter, J.,

Barnes, N. S., & Goodman, R. (1986). Comparison of clinic, home, and deferred language treatment for aphasia: A Veterans Administration Cooperative Study. *Archives of Neurology, 43,* 653–658.

World Health Organization (1997). *ICIDH-2: International Classification of Impairments, Activities and Participation. A manual of dimensions of disablement and functioning, Beta-1 draft for field trials.* Geneva: World Health Organization.

Worrall, L. (1995). The functional communication perspective. In D. Muller and C. Code (eds): *Treatment of aphasia* (pp. 47–69). London: Whurr Publishers.

Worrall, L., Hickson, L., Barnett, H., & Yiu, E. (1998). An evaluation of the *Keep on Talking* program for maintaining communication skills into old age. *Educational Gerontology, 24,* 129–140.

Worrall, L. E., & Yiu, E. (in press). Effectiveness of functional communication therapy by volunteers for people with aphasia following stroke. *Aphasiology.*

# 9

# Finding, Defining, and Refining Functionality in Real Life for People Confronting Aphasia

## JON G. LYON

The urgency for speech-language pathologists to define and develop treatments that yield life-altering differences in the daily lives of people confronting aphasia has never been more apparent. This chapter provides a rationale and plan of intervention that speaks to an ongoing, collaborative rather than directive approach when working with those individuals we hope to assist. Treatment targets emanate from wanting to enhance participation in life for all affected parties through improved social connections, feelings about self and others, and activities of choice.

## Introduction

Speech–language pathologists who treat people with aphasia are finding their past therapeutic roles endangered (Hersh, 1998; Petheram & Parr, 1998). In today's managed-care environment, only a fraction of former rehabilitative services remain. We, *as providers*, are being forced to ponder what benefits we can assure under highly curtailed treatment durations and reimbursement schedules (Frattali, Chapter 5). We are being told by those who control the purse strings, the *payers*, that the only treatments that are apt to endure are those that result in rapid, substantial gains in functional activities of daily life, ones that impact quality of life and further longevity and good health (Frattali, 1996; Frattali et al., 1995; Warren, 1996). We are being urged to expand our search for methods and measures that yield and verify functional outcomes (Frattali, 1998). In the ensuing shuffle to achieve more with less, those confronting life's differences due to aphasia, the *consumers,* are being asked to assume more responsibility for their own care with less assistance from us and other rehabilitation specialists.

## The Elephant

These divergent concerns and realities about the management of aphasia are reminiscent of three blind men groping the outer surface of an elephant from separate points of origin. All three perceivers (provider, payer, and consumer) are fully consumed in their own perceptions, but with a limited sense, dialogue, or investiture in knowing the entirety of each other's views, or more importantly, in determining the animal's true identity.

As we know only too well, speech–language pathologists (SLPs), the *providers,* find themselves in a desperate, uphill struggle to retain even a semblance of past roles or practices. Under current managed-care guidelines, our professional ability to provide prompt and effective "life-altering" services to adults with aphasia is considered suspect by the system that funds us, and is increasingly devalued. Once a mainstay of hospital in- and out-patient caseloads, aphasia rehabilitation has been diminished from a twice-a-day, 5-days-a-week, 3-month proposition to a total of 20 to 50 sessions, consummated in a matter of weeks post injury. More alarming than the reduction in service, is the increasing evidence of people with aphasia entering and leaving acute care without ever being diagnosed or referred for communication rehabilitative services (Gonzales-Rothi, 1996).

Health-care insurers, the *payers,* on the other hand, are minimally oriented toward the retention of past services, whether efficacious or not. Their prime "objective" is to find and implement a management formula that stabilizes cost (Iskowitz, 1998). To these ends, they have attempted to restrict reimbursement to life-sustaining options that yield immediate and lasting returns. Not only must interventions produce quick and enduring change, they must dramatically impact the actual living of life. Most importantly, reimbursable care must serve to keep recipients from returning to an already overburdened delivery system again and again.

People confronting aphasia, the *consumers,* have begun to sense their own vulnerability in this provider/payer crossfire of medical haves and have nots. Previously, they knew the type and probable duration of rehabilitation services and outcomes. More importantly, there was enough time and a sense of continuity of care to begin to understand aphasia's chronic nature and how life might "be" after treatment ended. In contrast, they now enter today's managed-care system with a dialogue about discharge within hours or days, not weeks or months. As a consequence, consumers tend to leave formal care confused about the moment, uncertain about the future, and panicked as to where to turn next. In the absence of viable, funded alternatives, they have begun pursuing legal and political ways to challenge the limited offerings and actions of HMOs (Gorman, 1998).

## Identifying the Elephant

Earlier in this volume, Frattali (Chapter 5) offered recommendations to assist SLPs in remaining active providers in today's health-care environment. She urges therapists to familiarize themselves with the guidelines of managed-care and craft outputs to maximize reimbursement. She notes, as well, that "unworkable systems" can be changed. If an equitable, comprehensive, long-term plan for assisting people confronting aphasia is ever to emerge, it will require reform by all involved parties (provider, payer, and consumer). Coming to define such an operable middle ground requires a bolstering of shared values while accounting for, yet deemphasizing, unshared ones.

For *providers*, such reform means that we must make fundamental and rapid shifts in our roles, perspectives on treatment, and responsibilities. As part of this revision, we must know when to don and when to shed our clinical white coats, when to prescribe and when to collaborate in our treatments, and when to seek functional independence in the injured person and when to foster interdependence with others. One reality, though, is indisputable: we can no longer wait to someday address treatments that stand to make a difference in everyday lives. We must address real-life therapy at once, and we must do so with conviction, vigor, and insight. Even though the efficacy of these new methods may seem more mysterious than proven at first, now is not a time to simply retreat from or acquiesce to payer-driven dictates. To forego our view of the elephant at a time when payers seemingly control access to the animal's entire surface not only perpetuates their biases but further constrains the much needed input from consumers. Unfulfilled needs of consumers still abound in confronting daily life in aphasia's wake, and it is our professional duty to see that this void is not overlooked or forgotten.

For *payers*, such reform means recognizing aphasia's chronic nature and accepting responsibility for a fair service delivery to address it. This physiological disruption in life is not simply about reacquiring lost linguistic and communicative functions in an injured adult. It is, instead, about an enduring, many-faceted remaking of daily processes that extend across key life domains and to persons intimately connected to and dependent on that individual's pre-injured self. If documentable interventions can effectively and efficiently yield life-altering differences while remaining fiscally responsible and consumer-sensitive, then payers must honor and be held responsible for ensuring the part they play in standard health care. Payer perceptions must extend not only to cost containment, but to searching out quality services that do alter and substantially improve the lives of those they serve, the consumers.

For *consumers*, such reform means realizing that ongoing services depend on their ability to assume responsibility for and to sustain life-altering differences in everyday life. Beyond a certain point of intervention, it may necessitate that consumers be willing to bear some or all of the cost for such services. However, when they must bear the burden of payment for desired services, it must be within their fiscal ability to do so. In other words, payment must be adjusted to the consumer's ability to pay. By assuming responsibility for the quantity and cost of therapy, consumers should gain broader access to all treatment options and services that speak to their own idiosyncratic needs and not have them preempted by prior payer exemptions or exclusions. Consumers of aphasia services must possess the right and freedom to sign up for the full gamut of long-term care after injury, not before.

In summary, it is essential to realize that the animal in front of the provider, payer, and consumer is the same beast, although individual perceptions may suggest otherwise. Accomplishing this will require everyone to make modifications, changes that may seem dramatic and sometimes even unacceptable either individually or collectively. However, each perceiver's perceptions can only be validated if all parties are willing to discover the animal's true and complex identity. The inherent challenge for each party is not simply avoiding the myopia of perceiving the issue from one view or perspective. The challenge, as well, is avoiding the blindness of abdicating one's own view and giving in to the views of others. If providers give up providing simply because it is not reimbursable at this point in time, one vital link in uncovering the accurate and authentic identity of this animal has been lost. We, as providers, cannot ensure that either payers or consumers will do their part. We can only be responsible for doing our own part. However, if we do it quickly and well, we stand the best chance to influence the proper overall identification of the elephant, and to help define future treatment opportunities for those challenged by chronic aphasia.

### Redefining Our Therapeutic Roles and Responsibilities

The common tenet shared among provider, payer, and consumer rests in promoting optimal functionality in real life. This means supporting treatments designed to make life and the daily living of it better, irrespective of aphasia's severity or chronic nature. The first difficulty in finding such treatments is agreeing on what functionality is. Elman and Bernstein-Ellis (1995) noted that SLPs typically see the term "functionality" as meaning augmentative ways of communicating when speech is not viable, or retooling targets toward thematic or real-life applications. In contrast, payers view functionality along a normative scale of how much basic function is necessary to allow daily life to work. As such, reimbursement need only pay for acquiring rudimentary skills and satisfying basic needs. Consumers, though, likely see functionality more globally. To them, the concept means returning communication and the living of life to what it was prior to injury. Thus, this term, functionality, conjures up many different notions and therapeutic expectations depending on the party defining it.

Regardless of the discrepant definitions of functionality, there is a tacit assumption by all parties that purposeful, meaningful participation in life is a desirable management objective as long as treatments remain cost-effective and consumer-driven. What is further assumed about this common ground is that treatments must not only reclaim function in treated specialty areas (e.g., language and communication), they must reclaim function and quality in daily life. Thus, functionality in real life as it applies to treating aphasia is not simply about making language or communication better in natural settings. It is about restoring life processes that typically go awry because of aphasia's ongoing presence and the restrictions it imposes.

### Our Therapeutic Past in Relationship to Real-Life Functionality

From the modern-day origins of aphasia rehabilitation, clinical researchers have long sought to determine ways to establish effective use of communication in real-life settings (Eisenson, 1946; Schuell et al., 1964; Wepman, 1951). Although these researchers prescribed forms of language remediation that emerged from hospital settings, their purpose was not to make people with aphasia better communicators with clinicians behind closed doors. Rather it was to make treated recipients better communicators in everyday life and with those people who mattered the most. The unforeseen obstacle was that clinically acquired communication strategies did not readily transfer to everyday life (Kraat, 1990; Simmons-Mackie & Damico, 1997; Thompson, 1989). Until recently, though, this shortcoming did not impact our delivery of services. In a fee-for-service system, payment was never questioned as long as therapeutic gains surpassed those of untreated controls (Wertz et al., 1986).

Clinical researchers have known about the limited transfer of clinical gains to natural settings for some time (Simmons-Mackie & Damico, 1997; Thompson, 1989). Furthermore, clinical investigators have made concerted efforts to search out and remedy this therapeutic dilemma (Kearns, 1989). So far, their success in discovering how to do so has been limited. In spite of their inability to uncover an enduring solution, their view of the problem has remained consistently narrow in focus. Most investigative efforts have focused on furthering the repair or circumvention of the language/communication breakdown in the injured adult in clinical settings. Little time or effort has been devoted to identifying either the variables or the steps in establishing communication in real-life settings and with those individuals with whom that use matters the most: spouse, caregiver, family, close friends, and co-workers (Kagan & Gailey, 1993; Lyon, 1992).

Over a decade ago, Davis and Wilcox (1985) wrote that communication is not an entity in and of itself. These authors stressed that communication is instead a medium, one through which we naturally share life's experiences, happenings, and outcomes as well as our ideas and feelings about them. Communication stripped of its real-life contexts is entirely devoid of purpose or form. Thus, to think that we can find enduring formulas for real-life functionality outside of natural environments, contexts, and interactants defies common sense (Duchan, 1997; Fujiki et al., 1996; Lubinski, 1981). Although a majority of clinical researchers of aphasia, among them Davis and Wilcox (1985), Holland (1982), and Thompson (1989), have long known or suspected this, the complexity of this enigma and a way to scientifically evaluate the worth of contextual treatments has kept investigators at bay (Damico et al., 1995; Elman, 1995). Not until recently have researchers begun turning to methods of qualitative inquiry that rely on rigorous documentation and validation, yet allow for, and actually depend upon, the naturalness and complexity of everyday life to help define what we should and need to attend to in our treatments (Parr et al., 1997; Oelschlaeger & Damico, 1998; Simmons, 1993).

It is not that our study of aphasia treatment to date has been without merit. After a half century of inquiry, we know a great deal about the repair of language and communication in clinical settings, knowledge that will serve us well in many natural applications. We also know, however, that attention to clinical repair alone has not been enough to support real-life use. To ensure the latter, we must better understand how clinical repair relates to outside world applications or, more importantly, what other real-life variables we must include (Darley, 1991; Holland, 1996; Lyon, 1992). One conclusion from the data so far is unmistakable: enduring therapeutic benefits, if attainable, are inseparably bound to the people, places, and reasons for communicative use in everyday life. Thus, we cannot hope to find lasting solutions without planning for and including real-life contexts.

## Finding and Defining Real-Life Functionality Today

Facilitating meaningful participation in life depends on more than considering the impact of natural contexts on communication. Worrall, in Chapter 1, provided an overview of the World Health Organization's (WHO) model for describing chronically disordered states (1980, 1997). The terms impairment (bodily loss or abnormality), disability (the personal restriction or inability that results), and handicap (the disadvantage to the person in fulfilling his/her "normal" role) are soon to be altered. As Worrall detailed, the WHO will retain the term, "impairment," while using the terms "activity" instead of "disability," and "participation" instead of "handicap."

These forthcoming shifts in terminology clarify former distinctions by using more neutral language that is less about "disabling" than "abling." "Activity" accentuates the nature and extent of functioning at the level of the person, while "participation" addresses the nature and extent of a person's involvement in life situations. While these changes represent significant improvements, the main contribution of the WHO model remains its unwavering inclusion of long-term consequences of injury as an integral part of, not separate from, the original disordered state.

Applying the WHO framework to aphasia, then, means that aphasia is more than the acute disruption to language and communication. Once the permanence of aphasia becomes apparent, it reveals a unique set of barriers to living life, challenges to daily activity and participation that are not confined to the person with aphasia but affect all persons closely bound to this individual's uninjured self. These consequences are no less of the whole of aphasia than the original impairment in language (Sarno, 1993). Furthermore, they are no less of what we, as providers, must carefully plan for and resolve in our therapies if we hope to enact life-altering change (Worrall, 1992).

Besides legitimizing the whole of chronically disordered states, the WHO model provides another important benefit. It helps structure where and how we might find and restore real-life function. In this regard, a common clinical misperception is that functional aphasia therapies should primarily target minimizing the disability. While Worrall noted that the term "functional" is predominantly associated with the disability level, she also cited researchers who relate the term to impairment and handicap as well.

Whereas the WHO defines disability as the performance restrictions consequent to impairment, it does not follow that all functional deficits occur at this level. The impairment and handicap influence real-life function, and it is the latter's effects that are most often obscured and frequently overlooked. Not wishing to communicate at the dinner table, over the phone, or with close friends are commonly cited disabling features in adults with nonverbal aphasias. Yet it is well known that clinically established and proven strategies do not ensure real-life use (Holland, 1982; Kraat, 1990; Simmons-Mackie & Damico, 1997). When such strategies fail to work in life, it may not be due so much to an inability as to a personal choice not to make use of them. When people view themselves as socially inappropriate, reliant on substandard forms of expression, or uncertain that interactants understand their true intent, lack of communication implies more than the need to restore activity. It suggests a need to examine individuals' perceptions of self and whether or not workable augmentations and alternatives fit their perceived images, needs, and skills. Before communication can work, there must be a perceived sense that its form and content matter to those involved. In this respect, communicative use depends as much on the perceptions of use as use itself. Issues of self-concept likely overlay nonfunction as much as ability. Therefore, sorting out real-life functionality requires conscious attention not only to disabling features, but to internal perceptions and feelings about participation.

Forthcoming revisions to the WHO model that incorporate "activity" instead of "disability" and "participation" instead of "handicap" should help clarify past misinterpretations about real-life functionality. These shifts in terminology from negative to neutral terms begin to address what Ryff and Singer (1998) have described as positive contours of health. These authors contend that good health involves more than the removal of negative symptoms; it necessitates the inclusion of essential features of wellness, both physical and psychological. The former focus and dependency on disability and handicap only serve to allow the enumeration of the negative correlates of disordered states instead of identification of correlates that promote well-being. For instance, the aphasia literature abounds with descriptions of handicapping aspects (Gainotti, 1997; LaPointe, 1996; Sarno, 1991). With few exceptions, these references revolve around in-depth discussions of situational or physiological depression. Whereas depression can and does appear as a common dysfunctional sequelae of aphasia, its absence is not an indicator of a good or successful lifestyle, or more importantly, that further treatment is unnecessary.

Ryff and Singer (1998) maintain that psychological well-being in daily life, in brain injured and nonbrain-injured people, depends on much more than the absence of negative consequences. These researchers suggest that positive states of psychological wellness depend on: (a) definitive purpose and direction for living, and (b) strong social connections with others who matter. From these, other vitally important features of well-being emerge, features like self-love and acceptance, autonomy, and mastery over one's environment. If the living of a good lifestyle depends on the presence of these positive elements, then a lack of depression is, by no means, a sufficient indicator that wellness exists. Not until meaningful direction and connections with others evolve are our treatments apt to be maximally effective. Within this context, the WHO's concept of "participation" better defines what our treatments should include and where they need to proceed.

In summary, real-life functionality, as it pertains to treating aphasia, is not reducible to any single WHO realm. Instead, it is a gradual, dynamic blending of WHO components that depend on the perceptions and reactions of those people most affected by aphasia's ongoing influence. At onset, it is not unusual to find patient and caregiver only cognizant of the language impairment, although other disabling features abound. Compared with having suddenly lost one's ability to talk at all, not conversing over the phone or interacting freely with friends seems unworthy of mention. At onset, loss of activity and participation are apt not to impact the operations of daily life as much as the impairment itself. Against a backdrop of lifelong verbal competency, it may take months of attempted repair or continuous experience with minimal speech before the realities of life without talking emerge. Even so, the delayed and individualized patterns of these aspects of chronically disordered states do not negate the importance of paying attention to, planning for, and beginning to treat real-life functionality from the beginning. Fundamentally, unless our treatments are targeted toward, and ultimately yield, life-altering change, they likely will not endure.

## Merging Our Views of Real-Life Functionality with Payer and Consumer Perceptions

The payer perspective regarding real-life functionality seems to have an evolution of its own. The initial dictates of managed care came from wanting to achieve an accountable system for health care by curtailing reimbursement services to proven real-life outcomes. Over time, though, and in the ensuing pressure to cut costs, it has become apparent that capitated rates do not always conform to or depend on such data. This discrepancy seems to have led some providers to feel that pursuing therapeutic methods that yield stronger, real-life returns are not truly valued or rewarded by payers. It is important that we not allow these temporary injustices to influence our own course and action. Consumers of all health-care services are beginning to become more vocal in their protest of denied yet justified services. Although their complaints may take time to change the current system, the indication is that more and more payers will be asked to account for their actions, legally and politically (Gorman, 1998).

Turning to the consumer's perspective, Parr et al. (1998) have recently sampled the opinions of 50 adults with aphasia regarding their feelings about aphasia and its remediation. All participants in this qualitative investigation were at least 5 years post onset, had aphasia ranging in severity from mild to severe, and were between 26 to 92 years of age. Topics of inquiry included family and personal circumstances surrounding stroke, the immediate aftermath and consequences of their injury, first perceptions and later consequences of aphasia, health care, access to information, and understanding of aphasia and disability. Findings indicated a broad swath of real-life disruption from aphasia. Simultaneous breakdowns occurred across multiple domains of social experience and personal relationships. Aphasia was commonly viewed as a bewildering phenomenon that transformed one's sense of self, consequences that these authors termed "system-based, contextualized, long-term and dynamic."

When asked what aphasia therapy should address and provide, these respondents collectively indicated that it should: (a) respect individual interpretations and beliefs, (b) acknowledge the complexity of aphasia and the multiple contexts in life that it influences, (c) be sustained and sustainable, (d) address life systems, as well as individual impairments, (e) educate and train others, (f) affirm individual, social, and collective identities, (g) promote social change, (h) provide relevant and accessible information, and (i) promote autonomy and self-help. What was most striking about their joint desires, after 5 years of confronting life with aphasia, was the minimal emphasis on individual language repair. Rather, the therapeutic focus these participants wanted was on establishing social and life systems that extend beyond the impairment of aphasia, and ensure activity and participation in daily life.

Parr et al.'s findings are not singular in the literature. LeDorze and Brassard (1995) examined the consequences of aphasia by analyzing the personal accounts of nine dyads (a person with aphasia and a significant other). Besides validating the long-term impact of aphasia, these researchers specified the varied effects of disabling and handicapping consequences on the living of daily life. For both parties, life was forever altered and coping effectively with its changed form required much more than simply coming to understand the problem. For these adults, it required ongoing personalized exploration and assistance. Just recently, Garcia et al. (1998) queried people with aphasia, employers, and SLPs about their perceptions of obstacles preventing a person with aphasia from returning to work. Noteworthy was the divergence of thought and perceptions. Most people with aphasia felt they could still do portions of their former jobs although they recognized task and productivity limitations. Employers lacked fundamental knowledge of aphasia and it consequences, and cited organizational and societal barriers for not permitting more return-to-work options. SLPs perceived barriers to rest within the injured person's disordered language and communication, and with societal attitudes, and seldom saw or sought solutions within the organization. Thus, people with aphasia desired a chance "to try" to doing something of worth, employers wanted to know more about how they might facilitate such a process, and SLPs appeared minimally oriented or trained in how to address such issues as a facilitator within existing organizational structures.

These consumer accounts point to distinct treatment objectives for restoring real-life functionality. People confronting aphasia are seeking more from rehabilitation than simply repairing language. With awareness and acknowledgment of permanent loss and dysfunction, they want services that address and restore some purpose and direction in daily life, and supply some sense of meaningful connections with others, services unavailable in today's health-care system. Until we focus our energies on methods that provide these outcomes, the constraints of managed care are not even of issue. It is our responsibility to attempt to define and to refine the definition of the part of the elephant before us. It is time to do so, and then to advocate for a conceptualization of the entire animal that keeps our vision intact.

## Treatment of Real-Life Functionality

The immediate dilemma is how to go about implementing real-life modifications in our treatment. How do we do more in a health-care system and era that provide less? An obvious concession from the outset is that we cannot preserve a semblance of what we once did and still attend to all that remains undone. To ensure a viable role as a provider, we must recast a traditional model of care while recognizing what we have done in the past. Table 9–1 distinguishes the prime constructs that underlie these changes.

Table 9–1. Redefining Our Roles, Services, and Outcomes

| *Historical Role: Therapist* | *Proposed Role: Facilitator* |
| --- | --- |
| **Duties**: Devise, direct, and oversee a restorative process | **Duties**: Assist, advise, empower others to act in their own behalf with existing capabilities; secondarily augmenting those skills with individualized strategies |
| **Target**: Repair and circumvent language and communication deficit(s) | **Target**: Enhance the living of daily life |
| **Recipient of services**: Injured adult | **Recipient of services**: Individuals most affected by aphasia's daily presence and constancy (person with aphasia, caregiver, significant others) |
| **Environment**: Clinic (hospital or rehabilitation settings) | **Environment**: Natural settings (where daily life occurs) |
| **Prognostic indicator**: Stimulability and variability in performance in treated language and communication contexts | **Prognostic indicator**: Willingness and dedication to strive for change in participation in daily life |
| **On-line indicator**: Increased accuracy, completeness, efficiency, and promptness of targeted language/ communication responses | **On-line indicator**: Increased comfort, function, involvement, and pleasure in daily life |
| **Agent of change**: Frequent and therapist-controlled amounts of stimulation, exercise, and practice | **Agent of change**: Guidance in matching existing skill with life challenges; informed and supported participant-determined decisions about continuing, modifying, or discontinuing services |
| **Method of change**: Encouraging multi-modality language stimulation or diagnostic isolation of primary deficits within language or communication; retarget alternative, supportive ways of resuming lost or disrupted functions | **Method of change**: Isolating preferred areas of living life that remain dysfunc-tional; probing options for making change (modality, methods, etc.); assessing real-life worth; continually modifying the variables until workable solutions prove valuable |
| **Therapeutic discord**: An Oops!!! Problem in design, delivery, implementation, or patient-potential | **Therapeutic discord**: Expected!!! A natural consequence of interacting in real-life contexts with people to effect change |
| **Outcome**: Quantifiable changes in language and communication skills; more functional independence of the injured adult | **Outcome**: Enhancing participation in life; increased personal pleasure, comfort, and well-being; "flow"; more functional interdependence with others and life's environments/contexts |

Summarized, Table 9–1 details a facilitative rather than prescriptive focus of change in those we treat. Along with being more assistive, advising, empower-ing, and collaborative, we need to search for methods that enhance participation in real-life by all parties affected by the daily presence of aphasia. This focus would supplant our former goal of merely fostering functionally independent communication within the injured adult in hopes of promoting communicative success in daily life. To achieve these newer participatory ends, we must pursue a service delivery model of functional interdependence; one that, while assuring cost-effectiveness, still allows provider and consumer to co-design and determine a long-term course of aphasia management based on change in life systems and overall enhancement of comfort, function, involvement, and pleasure in daily life. As long as consumers are willing to assume more responsibility for enacting change over time and providers' roles become more consultative in nature, then termination of service should rest more with the consumer and less with a third-party payer.

Thus, our most pressing professional obligation at the moment is to design and perfect real-life treatment protocols that, over time, will move us closer toward such outcomes. Even though it is unclear now how such services may qualify for reimbursement, we need to look for ways within, and when possible, outside existing delivery systems to move us in these treatment directions. The more effective our methods are at restoring function to disrupted real-life processes, the more likely payer perspectives may change. Realistically, we not only need to make a difference within the tight reimbursement constraints we now face, but we need to be creative in our use of other resources including university clinics, and in our continuing proactive thought. Change will not come because of us alone, but also because of consumer demands that health-care organizations be more responsive to *their* health-care needs and priorities. When the tide of service delivery shifts to a consumer-driven format, SLPs need to ensure we are still visible as providers by having honed an arsenal of life-altering therapies.

### Real-Life Treatment Protocols

Because reimbursable aphasia treatment has dwindled rapidly to end within 30 to 60 days post onset, we must begin retooling our treatment endeavors at once. The recommended shift in focus may seem subtle because much of early formal care still needs to address the repair of the language impairment. In those first moments following injury, no consequence exists beyond the injury itself. However, with such a narrow window to plan and prepare for the magnitude, complexity and duration of the what lies ahead, it is important that we assume a long-term perspective early on.

In this 1 to 2 month interim, caregivers must be afforded equal concern and attention, if not equal time. It is essential to prepare them informationally as well as psychologically for what they will soon need to know and likely encounter. Setting the proper stage does not so much mean telling them of aphasia's irrevocable presence in life, but providing broad real-life guidelines and temporal yardsticks by which they might judge their progress and status (Lyon, 1998b). Foremost, we need to start explaining the long path of aphasia's recovery, not just rehabilitation's formal efforts to repair dysfunction, but how life with aphasia is not without hope or merit. We are the only ones who can advise that it requires time post injury to internalize and understand their own altered daily profiles and how these differences will influence daily life for them. It is at the time of injury, perhaps not the beginning days, but in the subsequent weeks of acute and subacute care that caregivers must learn and begin to understand the long-term picture of what recovery from aphasia means.

Besides informing individuals about the lengthy process of recovery and assisting them in looking ahead, we must facilitate another important modification to past practices. It involves supporting those we treat by advocating for reimbursement from the health-care system, not simply to repair language, but instead to provide a skeletal framework against which we might conduct the remodeling of disrupted life systems because of injury. To do so, however, we first need to establish a viable means of linkage over time that permits long-term access to individuals confronting aphasia in order to intervene. Such intervention, again, would not be to continue to repair the impairment but would be to identify and modify life-oriented breakdowns associated with "activity" and "participation" as they begin to surface. To achieve these ends, we must pursue treatment methods and protocols that, in a cost-efficient manner, allow us to transfer more of the burden of "doing" to the consumer yet, over time, craft real-life differences and augment real-life processes in ways that truly matter.

### A Long-Term Treatment Plan for Aphasia

Once people confronting aphasia leave formal care, they begin to forge their own realities of life after injury. It often takes actual physical and emotional acts of living daily life with altered states of being to permit absorption of what does or does not need further attention. In such a climate, individuals begin to explore what, if anything, within their own knowledge base, past life experiences, and current coping mechanisms allows for the lessening of current dysfunction. It is within this transitional framework of building meaningful, functional adjuncts to daily life that our careful attention and input are most likely to yield outcomes that can and likely will yield life-altering differences.

The treatment protocols designed for these ends are only beginning to evolve (Elman, 1999; Hickey et al., 1998; Kagan, 1998). The remainder of this chapter details those that are currently under consideration, use, and refinement at Living with Aphasia, Inc. By no means do they represent the gamut of possibilities to be explored. In fact, it would be accurate to say that much more lies unexamined than has been discovered or refined so far. We are in but the beginning of this essential therapeutic transformational process.

### What We Do in Treatment

Living with Aphasia, Inc. is a nonprofit agency dedicated to restoring purpose, direction, meaning, comfort, and pleasure to the daily lives of people confronting aphasia. The clientele have been referred after having been discharged from formal care. We contract with a social service agency in the Madison, WI area, called Supportive Elder Services, Inc., to help provide an initial in-depth evaluation of real-life functionality. This means not simply looking at the viability of communication in the home, but also at daily life systems and their potential to improve. Probing the latter begins with several open-ended meetings where a SLP pairs with a person with aphasia, and a social worker talks separately with the prime caregiver. Each professional attempts to determine current strengths, weaknesses, needs, and unfulfilled aspirations. As an integral part of that evaluation, today's functionality is compared with what existed prior to injury. To assess this, the caregiver, and if possible, the person with aphasia are asked to supply four

Table 9–2.  Distribution and Percentage of Allotted Time to Free and Obligated Activities of Daily Life for Person with Aphasia Prior to Onset and at Present

| *Prior to Onset* | |
|---|---|
| *Free/10–20%* | *Obligated/80–90%* |
| • Playing and walking the dog<br>• Reading books and magazine<br>• Travel within the United States with spouse<br>• Bridge; poker; gin rummy; nightly game of spite and malice<br>• Theater and movies | • Dialysis—M, W, F; 3 pm<br>• Office/work: 9:30–12 weekly<br>• Golf—9 holes M,W,F; 18 holes T, Th, Sat, Sun<br>• Weekly mtg with salesmen—M<br>• Paid all household bills/expenses. Did all banking and monthly checkbook accounting<br>• Took care of doctor and dentist appointments (did blood sugar testing) |
| *At Present* | |
| *Free—85%* | *Obligated—15%* |
| • Lunch with friends when they are available (summer months)<br>• TV-sporting events and the news<br>• Napping<br>• Vegetating | • Listening occasionally to "talking books"<br>• Home exercise program . . . walking daily<br>• Dialysis—T, Th, Sat<br>• Personal hygiene and dressing<br>• Cleaning off table after eating; unloading dishwasher; taking out trash and papers<br>• Bowling group—every other Friday |

lists of daily activities: two with reference to the lifestyle of the person with aphasia (Table 9–2) and two pertaining to the lifestyle of the caregiver (Table 9–3).

The first list of activities for each participant describes typical daily occurrences prior to injury while the second list contains comparable information about life at the moment. Besides noting type and frequency of activities, clients are asked to categorize entries under "obligated" and "free-time" headings. Obligated activities refer to required or mandatory occurrences while free-time activities pertain to open-ended or spontaneous happenings, relaxation, or personal pleasure. Next, each participant estimates the average percentage of daily time devoted to each: obligated and free time.

What is most significant about the profiles in Tables 9–2 and 9–3 are the dramatic differences in lifestyles pre and post injury. Prior to injury, the adult with aphasia spent a majority of his daily time with work or committed tasks (80 to 90%). Only a small portion of time was unobligated or free (10 to 20%). Now most of his daily life is open or unstructured (80 to 90%) and there is little meaningful committed time (10 to 20%). For the caregiver, an opposite pattern appears. Prior to injury, she or he enjoyed a more equal balance between obligated and free activities. Following injury, she or he now possesses no free time and daily routines have become overloaded with obligatory tasks. Such shifts in life "activity" profiles are not uncommon, especially in the early stages of coping with the chronicity of aphasia.

The target of therapy is not to restore the daily patterns of either person to former, pre-injury specifications, although such an option may remain possible for

Table 9–3.   Distribution and Percentage of Allotted Time to Free and Obligated
Activities of Daily Life for Caregiver Prior to Onset and at Present

| Prior to Onset | |
| --- | --- |
| *Free—50%* | *Obligated—50%* |
| • Volunteer at local hospital; 4½ hours weekly—coffee shop<br>• Luncheon dates; club meetings—play cards weekly<br>• Theater: Season tickets, symphony, opera, traveleagues, theater; road show plays and movies<br>• Bridge with another couple after having dinner together<br>• Small dinner parties at home; 6–8 people | • Managing household: Marketing; meal planning; cooking and baking; laundry |
| At Present | |
| *Free—0%* | *Obligated—100%* |
| | • Transport spouse to dialysis; attend to medications for week; Order medications when needed; Take blood sugar levels daily; insulin injections daily; administer medications daily; pay bills and handle finances; select spouse's clothes for the day; tie shoes<br>• Managing household: Marketing; meal planning; cooking and baking; laundry |

the caregiver. For the person with aphasia, though, such a transformation is not likely, nor even desirable with existing skill levels. What may be attainable, instead, is the gradually returning of the pair to relative percentages of obligated and free time that existed prior to injury. The object is not to reinstitute the particulars of life as they were before; it is to establish a familiar, comfortable flow to daily routines. What is essential to accomplishing this outcome is not simply changing the daily routine of the person with aphasia, but that of the caregiver as well. For the uninjured caregiver, it typically means relinquishing or reassigning some responsibilities, those either inherited or transferred at time of injury. For the person with aphasia, it typically requires concentrated attention and assistance in two realms: meaningful communication with others and participation of choice outside the home.

### Meaningful Communication with Others

It has long been the domain and prime therapeutic aim of SLPs to make the person with aphasia more functionally independent as a communicator in everyday life. It may seem dubious to suggest that promoting real-life functionality means identifying a different therapeutic target for communication. Rather than singling out treatment criteria that speak solely to the accuracy, completeness, efficiency, and promptness of information exchanged, communication in real-life relies as much, if not more, on methods that keep those people who must confront its challenges together socially, emotionally, and interpersonally. For communication to work in the real world, it must do more than allow for an exchange of information. The act of communicating must bond, secure, and ensure that the requisites of personal dignity, respect, and parity underlie its intent. If communication occurs, but is devoid of personal honor, power and import, little of meaning has truly transpired.

Simmons (1993) and Simmons-Mackie and Damico (1997) used ethnographic methods to examine the form and uses of communication strategies of two adults with moderate to severe aphasia in their natural settings. This method entailed the videorecording, review, and analysis of conversations on a broad range of topics, with a variety of interactants, and in a number of natural settings. Of their revealing findings, many spoke dramatically to the qualities that define real-life communication. First, a wide range of natural communication strategies were used by both adults with aphasia depending on the interactant, situation, and topic of discussion. Second, the communicative strategy used was often idiosyncratic to the user or specialized for a particular topic or situation. Third, much of what occurred communicatively seemingly originated from personal preferences or behaviors that existed prior to injury. Fourth, frequently used strategies were automatic or easily prompted. Fifth, there was little evidence of communication strategies previously trained by the SLP. Sixth, a majority of attempts by these adults to initiate conversation originated from a need to remain socially bonded, rather than to simply convey information.

Although based on only two in-depth cases of adults with aphasia communicating in their natural settings, Simmons-Mackie and Damico's (1997) findings are profound in terms of their inferences for understanding and defining treatment targets in real-life. Even more significant than telling us, as providers, that clinically trained communicative strategies are not likely to find their way into real-life use, these results suggest that we must focus on and include other variables in our treatment if we hope to enact enduring change. In this expanded view, it would seem that we must devise methods that allow for and promote the idiosyncratic strategies that people bring on *their own* to communiqués. As well, we must support strategies that come to be used automatically and ones that speak as strongly to keeping interactants connected as people who care for one another as they do to exchanging information.

Such a therapeutic challenge may seem overwhelming, especially when the person with aphasia is verbally restricted, and repairing speech seems to be the most paramount need. When the return of speech appears minimal, however, and when augmentative means of communicating are appropriately addressed, treatment goals broaden. In an extensive review of the use of alternative and augmentative communication (AAC) systems for people with minimal verbal output, Light (1988) lists four purposes of AAC: (a) to communicate wants and needs, (b) to transfer information, (c) to develop and maintain social closeness, and (d) to maintain social etiquette. It is not happenstance that the first two items are targeted at enhancing informational exchange, while the latter two are more socially focused. In fact, Kagan (1995) notes that when verbal output is minimal, we are told repeatedly by those we treat that they value the return of talking *more* than anything else. Kagan maintains that without it, one's social competency in life is constantly under review or question. Not surprisingly, then, a prime focus of restorative communicative treatment has been to either fix verbal output or circumvent the lost output with other nonverbal communication options.

This constant weighing of the relative communicative values of information with social bonding, of meaning with feeling, and of thought with personal respect have been defined by linguists as distinctions between "transactional" and "interactional" components of communication (Brown & Yule, 1983; Schriffin, 1988). Transaction speaks to exchanging information while interaction refers to staying personally and socially bonded. What severe aphasia adds to this equation is the loss of a commonly and easily shared way to exchange information, one we often use to establish a topic or referent around which to interact. Without that, the ability of interactants to make use of transactional or interactional possibilities is taxed.

In the rush to remediate, it seems that providers have inferred that the fullness, richness, and quickness of exchanging information must precede any hope of socially or emotionally connecting. Certainly, it is true that some transactional structure must exist for communication to occur, and the need for a variety of well-designed and researched AAC methods is unquestionable (Fox & Fried-Oken, 1996; Garrett & Beukelman, 1992; Kraat, 1990). What is not as clear is that real-life communication requires only a minimal level of transactional ability and skill for interactants to begin constructing a strong and viable interactional framework. In my therapeutic experience, functionality in everyday life demands that as much attention be paid to keeping people meaningfully linked as to crafting more effective ways of exchanging information. If taken to an extreme, transactional proficiency can promote an atmosphere of interactional exclusion, rather than inclusion. Augmentative techniques such as picture/word boards and booklets that rely almost entirely on transactional formats, unless they serve to support an interactional system of choice, tend not to work on any enduring basis in real life. Their failure is not due solely to normal, naive interactants not knowing how to use such tools, but rather to their sterile rigidity in not allowing any true human, social, or personal equality or connectedness. By their very form, nature, and reliance on the same sequential skills lost in aphasia, they typically inhibit free, interactive, and mutually participatory interactions.

In the wake of aphasia's communicative obstacles, meaningful exchanges must permit the broadest, most natural gamut of interactiveness to occur without the processes themselves becoming the object of the interaction. It is not that augmentation of communication serves no purpose; it is essential. On the other hand, if an augmentative system becomes the entirety upon which the exchange is based, then little of its form is apt to endure or to work in the real world. The success of reciprocal, communicative turn-taking must guide our treatment efforts as much as, if not more than, the extent, accuracy, or completeness of information exchanged. This does not mean that the content of messages accounts for nothing in the exchange; it simply means that the process of interacting cooperatively and well, or interdependently must take precedence, and must precede any subsequent enhancement in transactional methods (Holland, 1998). Once again, it takes only a small amount of transactional skill, as long as both parties are willing to devote the necessary time and effort, to build a mutually gratifying interactional outcome: to communicate meaningfully in everyday life.

Understandably, though, the ease and effectiveness with which communication is exchanged becomes more challenging as severity of the aphasia increases. However, it is not simply how independently the person with aphasia can participate in communicative exchanges, but rather how interdependently the dyad can cooperate to make communication work, both transactionally and interactionally (Goodwin, 1995). When aphasia is moderate to severe, the mode and manner of communicating become even more important to achieving real-life functionality.

COMMUNICATIVE DRAWING

A multitude of augmentative means exist to facilitate everyday communication in adults with severe aphasia (Collins, 1986; Hux et al., 1994; Kraat, 1990). Many of these alternative forms of expression have been refined to provide individualized plans and partner training (Fox & Fried-Oken, 1996; Garrett, 1996). Unfortunately, however, most such AAC methods require ongoing manipulations in either the selection or ordering of graphic or iconic symbols, processes of prime dysfunction in people with aphasia. Even though such symbols may aid simple or redundant interactions in daily life, their usefulness in facilitating the complexities and demands of real-life contexts and topics falls short and for much the same reason that speaking does not work—aphasic limitations to symbol-selection and ordering.

Communicative drawing offers a different kind of supplement to interaction because, when properly used, it relies more on a conceptual, visual whole than on isolated parts, or individual symbols. Because core ideas of people with aphasia are characteristically preserved, this form of expression provides a more direct linkage to unaltered states of thought. It is important to realize, however, that people with aphasia do not draw normally, and typically do not draw on command. Rather, they require the presence of established communicative and interactant-drawn contexts into which to insert their often unclear pictorial details of key notions and ideas. Such insertions are not part of a drawing task. They are, instead, part of a communication process that includes close proximity, warm affect, gesture, vocalization, and any other communicative means available to either party. Even though the line-drawn additions of aphasic interactants may be indistinguishable at the moment they appear, they often are interpretable through questions, enlargement of key components, or further interactive drawing between participants. Thus, drawing by itself is not an augmentative tool of much communicative merit. Its use is only within an established communicative context and an interactant-initiated depiction that allows for a completeness and comfort of interaction not often possible otherwise.

Communicative drawing as a treatment protocol has been detailed elsewhere (Lyon, 1995a, 1995b; Lyon & Sims, 1989). However, there are six key principles that underlie its therapeutic use. They are: (1) have paper and pencil always at hand, (2) do not begin interactions with requests that the aphasic partner draw, (3) embed drawing in your own communication, (4) take the first turn by drawing a context, and then encourage mutual turn-taking, (5) do not expect drawings of the person with aphasia to be distinguishable or complete, and (6) use what is indistinguishable as a way of interacting further. If these principles are followed, drawing often adds to communicative clarity, completeness, and connectedness.

## CYCLIC REFINEMENT OF REAL-LIFE USE OF COMMUNICATION

Besides finding an effective route around limited verbal expression, sustainable real-life use demands much more. Simmons-Mackie and Damico (1997) have suggested that strategies must come with ease and contain naturalness to remain a functional part of everyday life. If they are inherently difficult, depleting, or incongruous with the personalities and personal preferences of those using them, they are not apt to endure. Due to the need to make strategies conform to the communicative and life systems of those we treat, it would seem that we should begin by carefully examining what is and is not working in natural settings, what might augment that, and what of the latter would be the most simple and complementary, yet most sustainable and reinforcing among the options available.

It is important to note that simple and complementary options do not exclude the consideration and use of nonstandard strategies such as drawing. In everyday communication situations devoid of ready access to spoken words, nothing need be deemed unnatural until it is tried and found to be so. Determining what is natural in a highly unnatural set of circumstances and environments is neither automatic nor certain. It depends on carefully examining the ease with which alternative ways for communicating might become sustainable. When they do not work quickly or automatically, then one must assess their potential for subsequent adoption, and the loss to the person if they are not continued. Although the latter process of elimination should rightly influence treatment decisions and revisions, it is more the former observation of inclusion that should govern them. In other words, chosen strategies must show strong signs of becoming a natural part of communication in real life shortly after their introduction. If they do not, it is not the people we treat who must change, but rather the options we provide.

Thus, promoting real-life communicative use and effectiveness among people who rely on augmentative, nonverbal options requires a collaborative search. It requires an active and cyclic exploration of possibilities and their complementary fit with those individuals who must adopt and use them. Given the complexities of abilities and tolerances of the people involved, it is unlikely that initially targeted strategies will become adopted in full. Instead, a series of refinements must occur. Such shifts in focus to find the right fit should not be viewed as failures, but rather as necessary steps in incorporating what is now known into an individualized, usable and sustainable communication system.

Lyon (1998a) has detailed a treatment case of real-life communicative use in a couple confronting severe aphasia. He presented an intervention involving six cycles of revision over a period of 3 months, each helping to move toward this couple communicating better at home. At first, the cycles involved sorting through personal and communicative abilities to find a reliable way of inputing information to the wife with severe aphasia, while the last two cycles of modification addressed output options in the home. With weekly sessions of an hour to an hour and a half, communication strategies were progressively modified, first toward a target of documentable use at home, and second, toward sustained applications in that environment.

Starting from a written choice format to aid auditory input, revisions followed to accommodate personal and communicative preferences. Without question, the wife's comprehension of exchanged content was aided at times by the addition of printed cues. However, that communicative boost depended on familiarity with the topic and an involved set of individual and interactional variables. For instance, she was highly sensitive and attuned to any failure on her part in the exchange, while her husband struggled to learn to curtail his verbal and printed cues to key concepts and words. If too much verbiage or printed cueing occurred, his wife was likely to abandon the topic, or even the interaction. Thus, we cooperatively modified treatment options until an operable, comfortable, and somewhat automatic means of interacting emerged, not because this configuration captured the best way of exchanging information, but because it produced signs of constancy and genuine communicative use.

A similar treatment scenario followed for finding ways that might permit this woman with aphasia to express her basic desires at home. Once again, what was the most communicative means for exchanging content in the clinic was not the most successful in real life. Instead of pointing to printed preferences on cards or in a booklet, which was both possible and often more complete in its specificity, she preferred pointing to the locations of desired objects and activities on hand-drawn maps of rooms in her home. Once an area in the house was designated, the method allowed her husband to then supply a more specific list of things or actions to be found or accomplished there.

The therapeutic assertion here, therefore, is that real-life functionality, as it relates to communicative use, and especially when it involves an interactant with severe aphasia, depends on more than simply teaching an assortment of augmentative methods for exchanging information. Sustained use in real life requires finding which of these augmentative methods naturally brings interactants together in a turn-taking process that personally binds and strives to provide parity in personal value and power. Success is not solely about which augmentative methods best promote an exchange of information. Rather, a successful method of facilitating transactional aspects of communication is one that permits and promotes an enduring interactional exchange, and is sustainable over time.

## Participation of Choice Outside the Home

Within the scope of making life more harmonious, it is crucial that we help to facilitate activities that promote purpose, direction, and meaningful ties with others. This important part of treatment ensures that there is a self-selected and valued context within which and about which interaction even matters (Marshall, 1993; Sarno & Chambers, 1997). For this reason, we begin our treatment of real-life functionality by examining personal profiles of activities in daily life for the person with aphasia and the caregiver. We do this in an attempt to restore the relative amounts of obligated and free time in daily life to levels that existed prior to injury. By making such modifications in life systems, we purposefully merge communicative and participatory treatment targets. It is crucial to understand that one is not more important than, nor need precede, the other. Whereas some mutually shared means of coding information is essential in the beginning, taking actions of choice and gradually assuming control over life's options are essential catalysts in restoring self-worth. Such life experiences permit a gradual recalibrating of what is and may be possible in daily life. With increased cause and confidence to participate again in life, the reason to interact with others heightens. Thus, while one may initially want to find a bridge by which to contact those who matter most in life, until engaged in activities of choice and pleasure, there may be little of importance about which to communicate (Chapey, 1992).

The therapeutic processes of reinvolving people with aphasia in activities of choice in daily life have been described in depth elsewhere (Lyon, 1996, 1997; Lyon et al., 1997). While these treatment steps will not be detailed here, it is important to clarify their role as they relate to restoring real-life functionality. In this regard, personal emptiness and dissociation from others frequently dominates the lives of people with aphasia. It is the presence of these features that Ryff and Singer (1998) see as obstructional to positive contours of good health. Whereas the daily constraints imposed on life by aphasia are many and varied, it is the misperception of life's options afterward that most interferes and ultimately undermines meaningful reinvolvement outside the home.

People with aphasia whose impairment is confined to just that, are able to do almost every activity, "in kind," that they did prior to injury. This potential reclamation in life's offerings exists even for more severely impaired adults. What is usually different, of course, is the level of one's ability to perform such activities. No longer is it possible to perform with the same ease, proficiency, efficiency, or completeness. When daily life skills are curtailed, either because of real or perceived deficits, the natural tendency for all responsible parties is to cautiously assess, and grossly underestimate the possibilities. This theorem holds true not only for family, friends and society, but the patient, and the medical and social support staff. As a result, even being allowed to act in one's own behalf is commonly questioned. Instead of carefully exploring what might be possible within existing skill levels, daily responsibility for life's form and action shifts to others. When a person with aphasia is not granted legitimacy in daily life, either by self or others, to consider, decide, and act on one's own preferences, it is not surprising that self-worth, esteem, and confidence suffer.

Overcoming misperceptions about what is possible underlies treatment targets here. Moving from inactivity to engagement in life comes next. Csikszentmihalyi (1990, 1993, 1997) has extensively studied and written about a phenomenon of optimal experience, which he refers to as "flow." It is a process of becoming so absorbed in the act of "doing" a pursuit of choice that one totally "forgets" self, time, outcomes, or even potential benefit. According to Csikszentmihalyi's numerous accounts, people in flow become so lost in participating in the experience of the moment that all else vanishes from one's conscious mind. It is the act or action itself that dominates over the actor and his/her abilities.

The concept of flow is most pertinent to the topic of reinvolving people with aphasia in daily life. Flow does not depend on skill or ability to act. Anyone able to act at any level of proficiency is able to experience flow. According to Csikszentmihalyi, it comes from matching skill with challenge. If, for example, someone is ordered to parachute from a plane in an hour, the real or perceived challenge before the person is apt to far exceed his/her abilities, and anxiety and fear will ensue. If, on the other hand, someone is asked to sort thousands of pennies into equal stacks of ten, skill far outdistances the challenge, and boredom is likely to occur. But when the challenge matches skill, regardless of where that skill level may be, flow is a possible outcome. It depends not so much on one's ability to act, but on his/her capacity to become totally absorbed in the act of acting, to the extent that such involvement precludes any thought of self.

It may seem that when skill levels are severely curtailed, as they may be for people with severe aphasia, flow is not an option. Yet, according to Csikszentmihalyi (1993), Special Olympic athletes sacrifice nothing in terms of access to or quantity of flow when compared with their official Olympic counterparts. How well one runs, jumps, swims, dives, sails, or skis has nothing to do with whether or not such individuals can become totally consumed in the act of doing. What sets people with aphasia apart from Special Olympic athletes is that they have accrued two or more generations of experience and knowledge about living life as daily performers with much better and more refined skills. Many must confront a paralyzing fear that no worthwhile skill remains or, at least, none that is personally or socially acceptable. It is not strange in this real-life context that refusal to act is a common occurrence. Every act, especially in the early stages of redefining one's changed self, serves as a vivid reminder of what does not work, rather than what does.

What is often misunderstood about this struggle to move forward with meaningful reinvolvement in life is that the battle is not so much against one's past as it is for one's present and future. People with aphasia often doubt whether properly restructured challenge (clear goals with unambiguous feedback within existing skill levels) can yield outcomes of preference and pleasure in real life. They must often be shown convincingly and repeatedly that such doors exist and that entry is neither as formidable nor as adverse as they may envision, before they are apt to make a concerted effort.

Often the key to bringing people with aphasia to the threshold of participating in real life is to focus their complete attention on the contrast between doing and not doing any modified skill, challenge, or activity of interest. It is crucial to deemphasize the importance of current skill levels, other than to say that whatever exists is adequate. For many people, and for reasons just alluded to, it is impossible to conceive that such diminished participation could hold any personal worth. Only when they have had the opportunity to experience the actual act of doing, with their altered states of function, are they able to internalize a sense that acting in life, even at reduced levels of skill, is preferable to not participating at all. The bitter scenario faced by each person is either remaining before a TV screen through much of the day (where skill exceeds challenge . . . and thus, boredom is guaranteed) or risk re-involvement in life (where skill is thought to rest below an acceptible challenge . . . and thus, anxiety or fear is guaranteed).

Flow, no matter how diminished one's skills, is not out of reach. What may be blocked is one's perception of life's worth when one must face it with current skill levels. Besides focusing the person with aphasia on the act of doing something of personal choice, our treatment must pay careful attention to well-specified goals that equate current skills with reasonable and attainable challenge. As well, there needs to be constant and unequivocal feedback about performance within this operative framework and certainly, not about performance with reference to what once was. It is unlikely that the past can, or should be, totally expunged from the current equation. However, it deserves and requires only an occasional acknowledgment. Years after working hard to perfect a golf swing with only one hand (due to hemiparesis, dyscoordination, and bodily instability), a formerly "par" golfer with aphasia proudly asserted that hitting a consistently straight shot of 100 yards took far more skill than hitting a two-handed shot of 250 yards before. More importantly, when the current challenge was his focus, he frequently still "lost himself" in the act of playing golf.

Flow, too, is not simply a treatment target for the person with aphasia. It must be a frequent part of the daily life and routines of the caregiver. Attempting to restructure both partners' personal profiles to the earlier balance between obligated and free time, does more than evoke some sense of normalcy in daily routines. It often inadvertently serves to give caregivers permission to release themselves from undue duties, burdens, and responsibilities involving the person with aphasia that they may have unknowingly assumed in the beginning stages of dysfunction. Often their states of flow are bound indirectly to their loved one's perceived status and ability to function independently in daily life. When the latter is restricted, it is important in treatment to find effective ways for the caregiver to escape. Whether through work, planned respite, or time with others, flow must not be the hope of just the person with aphasia. It must be a frequent part of the life of the caregiver and ultimately part of their lives together.

Real-life functionality cannot be reduced, then, to the presence or absence of independence of communicative use in the person with aphasia. It is more broadly based and dependent on life systems that effectively address a communal sense of wellness in spite of the chronic nature of aphasia. It depends on isolating and implementing effective ways of restoring purpose, meaning, and ties with others in life more than on just remediating the functional breakdowns in communication.

### It "IS" an Elephant

It may seem of late as if this animal's identity has already been clearly and indisputably reduced and defined from a single perspective. In practical terms, it seems as if it is whatever payers are willing to let providers or consumers think it is. At this auspicious moment in health-care history, the payers control reimbursement and seemingly all avenues to it. As a result, we are left with the meager form of today's service delivery and treatment outcomes. It would be a grave mistake, though, to confuse the perceiver who currently has dominion over input into this animal's identity with what that identity truly is.

We, as providers, have long known that we must pursue and produce life-altering differences, functional differences that impact quality of life in those we treat. This chapter has provided theoretical and practical statements as to how we might wish to proceed. Currently, people confronting aphasia are leaving formal care with less attention to and care addressing the remediation of the underlying linguistic and communicative deficits. As well, they are leaving with less information about what aphasia is. Most alarming, they are leaving without a sense of what they did not receive, that is, what specifically is needed, what might be done to make their altered lives more productive and comfortable, and what is worthy of their further effort and attention.

We know from consumers who have endured this process and have been asked to reflect on their plights and outcomes that treatments need to be highly idiosyncratic, life-oriented and altering, sustainable, and accessible over time (Parr et al., 1998). It is our systematic attention to these therapeutic outcomes in a cost-effective manner that will most influence whether we continue to be an invited guest at this table of inquiry. For in the near future, it will not be just the payer who rules over what is or is not provided; it will likely be the consumer. To the degree we are able and ready to provide what consumers want, we will procure a stable position and role at this table. Rest assured, though, the animal before us is an elephant and as long as we do our part, its proper identity will emerge.

## References

Brown, G., & Yule, G. (1983). *Discourse analysis.* New York: Cambridge University Press.

Chapey, R. (1992). Functional communication assessment and intervention: Some thoughts on the state of the art. *Aphasiology, 6,* 85–94.

Collins, M. (1986). *Diagnosis and treatment of global aphasia.* San Diego: College-Hill Press.

Csikszentmihalyi, M. (1990). *Flow: The psychology of optimal experience.* New York: HarperCollins Publishers.

Csikszentmihalyi, M. (1993). *The evolving self.* New York: HarperCollins Publishers.

Csikszentmihalyi, M. (1997). *Finding flow: The psychology of engagement with everyday life.* New York: HarperCollins Publishers.

Damico, J. S., Simmons-Mackie, N., & Schweitzer, L. A. (1995). Addressing the third law of gardening: Methodological alternatives in aphasiology. In M. L. Lemme (ed): *Clinical aphasiology,* Vol. 23 (pp. 83–93). Austin, TX: Pro-Ed.

Darley, F. L. (1991). I think it begins with an A. In T. Prescott (ed): *Clinical aphasiology,* Vol. 20 (pp. 9–20). Austin, TX: Pro-Ed.

Davis, G. A., & Wilcox, M. J. (1985). *Adult aphasia rehabilitation: Applied pragmatics.* San Diego, CA: College-Hill Press.

Duchan, J. F. (1997). A situated pragmatics approach for supporting children with severe communication disorders. *Topics in Language Disorders, 17,* 1–18.

Eisenson, J. (1946). *Examining for aphasia.* New York: The Psychological Corporation.

Elman, R. J. (1995). Multimethod research: A search for understanding. In M. L. Lemme (ed): *Clinical aphasiology,* Vol. 23 (pp. 77–81). Austin, TX: Pro-Ed.

Elman, R. J. (ed). (1999). *Group treatment of neurogenic communication disorders: An expert clinician's approach.* Boston: Butterworth-Heinemann.

Elman, R. J., & Bernstein-Ellis, E. (1995). What is functional? *American Journal of Speech Language Pathology, 4,* 115–117.

Fox, L., & Fried-Oken, M. (1996). AAC Aphasiology: Partnership for future research. *Augmentative and Alternative Communication, 12,* 257–271.

Frattali, C. (1996). Clinical care in a changing health system. In N. Helm-Estabrooks, A. L. Holland (eds): *Approaches to the treatment of aphasia* (pp. 241–265). San Diego, CA: Singular Publishing Group.

Frattali, C. (1996). Measuring disability. *Asha Special Interest Division 2—Neurophysiology and Neurogenic Speech and Language Disorders, 6,* 6–10.

Frattali, C., Thompson, C. K., Holland, A. L., et al. (1995). *Functional assessment of communication skills for adults.* Rockville, MD: Speech–Language–Hearing Association.

Fujiki, M., Brinton, B., & Todd, C. M. (1996). Social skills of children with specific language impairment. *Language, Speech and Hearing Services in Schools, 27,* 195–201.

Gainotti, G. (1997). Emotional, psychological and psychosocial problems of aphasic patients: An introduction. *Aphasiology, 11,* 635–650.

Garcia, L., Barrette, J., & LaRoche, C. (1998). *Perceptions of the obstacles to work reintegration for persons with aphasia.* Presentation at the Clinical Aphasiology Conference, Asheville, NC.

Garrett, K. (1996). Augmentative and alternative communication: Applications to the treatment of aphasia. In G. Wallace (ed): *Adult Aphasia Rehabilitation* (pp. 259–278). Boston: Butterworth-Heinemann.

Garrett, K., & Beukelman, D. (1992). Augmentative communication approaches for persons with severe aphasia. In K. Yorkston (ed): *Augmentative Communication in the Medical Setting* (pp. 245–338). Tucson, AZ: Communication Skill Builders.

Gonzales-Rothi, L. (1996). The compromise of aphasia treatment: Functional and practical but realistic. *Aphasiology, 10,* 483–485.

Goodwin, C. (1995). Co-constructing meaning in conversations with an aphasic man. *Research on Language and Social Interaction, 28,* 233–260.

Gorman, C. (1998). Managed care 1998: Playing the HMO game. *Time, 152,* 22–27.

Hersh, D. (1998). Beyond the 'plateau': Discharge dilemmas in chronic aphasia. *Aphasiology, 12,* 207–217.

Hickey, E., Alarcon, N., Rogers, M., et al. (1998). *Social validity measures for family-based intervention for chronic aphasia (FICA).* Presentation at the Clinical Aphasiology Conference, Asheville, NC.

Holland, A. L. (1982). Observing functional communication of aphasic adults. *Journal of Speech and Hearing Disorders, 47,* 50–56.

Holland, A. L. (1996). Pragmatic assessment and treatment for aphasia. In G. Wallace (ed): *Adult aphasia rehabilitation* (pp. 161–173). Boston: Butterworth-Heinemann.

Holland, A. L. (1998). Why can't clinicians talk to aphasic adults? Comments on supported conversation for adults with aphasia: Methods and resources for training conversational partners. *Aphasiology, 12,* 844–846.

Hux, K., Beukelman, D., & Garrett, K. (1994). Augmentative and alternative communication for persons with aphasia. In R. Chapey (ed): *Language Intervention Strategies in Adult Aphasia,* 3rd ed. Baltimore: Williams & Wilkins.

Iskowitz, M. (1998). Preparing for managed care in long-term care. *Advance for Speech–Language Pathologists and Audiologists, 8,* 7–9.

Kagan, A. (1995). Revealing the competence of aphasic adults through conversation: A challenge to health professionals. *Topics in Stroke Rehabilitation, 2,* 15–28.

Kagen, A. (1998). Supported conversation for adults with aphasia: Methods and resources for training conversation partners. *Aphasiology, 12,* 816–830.

Kagan, A., & Gailey, G. (1993). Functional is not enough: Training conversational partners for aphasic adults. In A. L. Holland, M. M. Forbes (eds): *Aphasia treatment: World perspectives.* San Diego: Singular Publishing Group.

Kearns, K. (1989). Methodologies for studying generalization. In L. V. McReynolds, J. Spradlin (eds): *Generalization strategies in the treatment of communication disorders* (pp. 13–30). Toronto: BC Decker.

Kraat, A. (1990). Augmentative and alternative communication: Does it have a future in aphasia rehabilitation? *Aphasiology, 4,* 321–338.

LaPointe, L. L. (1996). Adaptation, accommodation, aristos. In L. L. LaPointe (ed): *Aphasia and related neurogenic language disorders,* 2nd ed. New York: Thieme.

Le Dorze, G., & Brassard, C. (1995). A description of the consequences of aphasia on aphasic persons and their relative and friends, based on the WHO model of chronic diseases. *Aphasiology, 9,* 239–255.

Light, J. (1988). Interaction involving individuals using augmentative and alternative communication systems: State of the art and future directions. *Augmentative and Alternative Communication, 4,* 66–82.

Lubinski, R. (1981). Environmental language intervention. In R. Chapey (ed): *Language intervention strategies in adult aphasia* (pp. 223–248). Baltimore: Williams & Wilkins.

Lyon, J. G. (1992). Communication use and participation in life for adults with aphasia in natural settings: The scope of the problem. *American Journal of Speech–Language Pathology, 1,* 7–14.

Lyon, J. G. (1995a). Drawing: Its value as a communication aid for adults with aphasia. *Aphasiology, 9,* 33–50.

Lyon, J. G. (1995b). Communicative drawing: An augmentative mode of interaction. *Aphasiology, 9,* 84–94.

Lyon, J. G. (1996). Optimizing communication and participation in life for aphasic adults and their prime caregivers in natural settings: A use model for treatment. In G. Wallace (ed): *Adult aphasia rehabilitation* (pp. 137–160). Boston: Butterworth-Heinemann.

Lyon, J. G. (1997). Volunteers and partners: Moving intervention outside the treatment room. In B. Shadden, M. T. Toner (eds): *Communication and aging* (pp. 299–324). Austin, TX: Pro-Ed.

Lyon, J. G. (1998a). Treating real-life functionality in a couple coping with severe aphasia. In N. Helm-Estabrooks, A. L. Holland (eds): *Approaches to the treatment of aphasia* (pp. 203–239). San Diego, CA: Singular Publishing Group.

Lyon, J. G. (1998b). *Coping with aphasia.* San Diego, CA: Singular Publishing Group.

Lyon, J. G., Cariski, D., Keisler, L., et al. (1997). Communication partners: Enhancing participation in life and communication for adults with aphasia in natural setting. *Aphasiology, 11,* 693–708.

Lyon, J. G., & Sims, E. (1989). Drawing: Its use as a communicative aid with aphasic and normal adults. In T. Prescott (ed): *Clinical aphasiology,* Vol. 18. (pp. 339–356). Boston: College-Hill Press.

Marshall, R. C. (1993). Problem-focused group treatment for clients with mild aphasia. *American Journal of Speech–Language Pathology, 2,* 31–37.

Oelschlaeger, M., & Damico, J. (1998). Joint productions as a conversational strategy in aphasia. *Clinical Linguistics and Phonetics, 12,* 459–480.

Parr, S., Byng, S., Gilpin, S., et al. (1997). *Talking about aphasia: Living with loss of language after stroke.* London: Open University Press.

Parr, S., & Byng, S., & Pound, C. (1998). *Perspectives, partnerships, practicalities and policies: Developing a sustainable service for people with aphasia.* Presentation at the Clinical Aphasiology Conference, Asheville, NC.

Petheram, B., & Parr, S. (1998). Diversity in aphasiology: A crisis in practice or a problem of definition? *Aphasiology, 12,* 435–446.

Ryff, C. D., & Singer, B. (1998). The contours of positive human health. *Psychological Inquiry, 9,* 1–28.

Sarno, J. (1991). The psychological and social sequelae of aphasia. In M. Sarno (ed). *Acquired aphasia* (pp. 499–519). San Diego: Academic Press.

Sarno, M. T. (1993). Aphasia rehabilitation: Psychosocial and ethical considerations. *Aphasiology, 7,* 321–334.

Sarno, M. T., & Chambers, N. (1997). A horticultural therapy program for individuals with acquired aphasia. *Activities, Adaptation and Aging, 22,* 81–91.

Schiffrin, D. (1988). Conversation analysis. In F. L. Neumayer (ed): *Linguistics: The Cambridge survey IV, Language: The sociocultural context.* Cambridge: Cambridge University Press.

Schuell, H., Jenkins, J. J., & Jiménez-Pabón, E. (1964). *Aphasia in adults: Diagnosis, prognosis and treatment.* New York: Harper and Row Publishers.

Simmons, N. (1993). An ethnographic investigation of compensatory strategies in aphasia. Ann Arbor, MI: University Microfilms International.

Simmons-Mackie, N., & Damico, J. (1997). Reformulating the definition of compensatory strategies in aphasia. *Aphasiology, 8,* 761–781.

Thompson, C. K. (1989). Generalization research in aphasia. A review of the literature. In T. Prescott (ed): *Clinical aphasiology,* Vol. 18 (pp. 195–222). Boston: College-Hill Press.

Warren, R. (1996). Outcome measurement: Moving toward the patient. *Asha Special Interest Division 2—Neurophysiology and Neurogenic Speech and Language Disorders, 6,* 5–6.

Wepman, J. M. (1951). *Recovery from aphasia.* New York: Ronald Press.

Wertz, R. T., Weiss, D. G., Aten, J. L., et al. (1986). Comparison of clinic, home, and deferred language treatment for aphasia: A Veterans Affairs cooperative study. *Archives of Neurology, 43,* 653–658.

World Health Organization (1980). *International Classification of Impairments, Disabilities, and Handicaps.* Geneva, Switzerland: Author.

World Health Organization (1997). *International Classification of Impairments, Activities, and Participation (ICIDH-2).* Geneva, Switzerland: Author.

Worrall, L. (1992). Functional communication assessment: An Australian perspective. *Aphasiology, 6,* 105–110.

# 10

## *Social Approaches to the Management of Aphasia*

## NINA N. SIMMONS-MACKIE

**A social approach is one that promotes an individual's participation in a social world and contrasts to the more traditional medical model of aphasia rehabilitation. Nine principles that guide a social approach to intervention in aphasia are described, and interventions such as conversation therapy, partner training, and developing "prosthetic communities" are detailed. Broader aspects to intervention such as institutional and societal changes are also explored.**

The past decade has witnessed significant progress toward socially motivated intervention models for aphasia (e.g., Armstrong, 1993; Parr, 1996; Simmons, 1993; Simmons-Mackie, 1993, 1994). A social model of aphasia management is designed to reduce the social consequences of aphasia and promote social communication within natural contexts. Furthermore, a social model is designed to promote the individual's participation in a social world and reduce barriers to participation. Based on this definition of a social model, it is clear that the concept conforms to the broad definition of a functional approach to management—targeting "real life" communication. Thus, the social model addresses outcomes at the "participation" level of the World Health Organization (WHO, 1997) classification of Impairments, Activities, and Participation (formerly impairment, disability and handicap; WHO, 1980).

Social approaches have arisen in part to address the need for improved functional outcomes in aphasia therapy. Although traditional aphasia research has defined treatment efficacy as intervention resulting in desired modification of a target behavior, "effective treatments" can be irrelevant when the changes fail to make a difference in the life of the individual. Improved ability to communicate does not necessarily guarantee improved participation in communication events (e.g., Parr et al., 1997; Simmons, 1993). As Penn (1998) notes ". . . improvement on standard measures often have little clinical relevance in the broader context of the patient and his or her life." Therefore, pressures for evidence that aphasia therapy makes a difference in the lives of people with aphasia have arisen from funding sources and from our own ranks. The expected outcome of a social approach is to make a difference in the individual's quality of life, to make living with aphasia more satisfying, and to decrease social isolation.

Another motivation for social intervention relates to the significant pressures from shrinking health-care funding. With cutbacks in the amount of time and money available for treatment of aphasia (Gonzales-Rothi, 1996), alternative service delivery systems must be explored. The social model of treatment provides a philosophical context and clinical rationale for nontraditional intervention approaches and alternative service delivery.

Perhaps the most compelling pressure for attention to a social model of intervention has arisen from the voices of people with aphasia and their families (LeDorze & Brassard, 1995; Parr et al., 1997). The reality of unmet needs among our consumers is difficult to ignore. Interviews with people with aphasia describe discrimination, social isolation, exclusion from work, education and leisure pursuits, and limited community support and benefits (Parr, 1996; Parr et al., 1997). While these pressures to examine traditional intervention methods have been uncomfortable, they have provided an opportunity to explore new models and practices, and strengthen the movement toward more functional, socially motivated management in aphasia.

### Shifting from the Medical to the Social Model

A social model of intervention requires a philosophical shift away from the traditional medical model. Traditional aphasia management follows a structured sequence similar to medical care including assessment, diagnosis, treatment, and discharge. Terminology is borrowed from medicine. For example, people receiving aphasia therapy are often called "patients." Aphasia is viewed from the perspective of an illness, and intervention is geared toward recovery from illness. This focus on "recovery" suggests that people with aphasia will recover. Unfortunately, full recovery is rarely the outcome. Usually discharge from treatment occurs in spite of residual impairments and limitation in activities and participation (Hesch, 1998).

The social model moves away from a focus on illness and toward a focus on health. The social model views aphasia from the "long-term" perspective. There is sensitivity to the chronicity of aphasia—that is, living with aphasia. Within a social model there is no specific "termination" point in the road toward autonomy. Thus, services are likely to be a continuum along which various forms of intervention are available with the ultimate outcome of social membership dictating the services. The service delivery system and individuals with aphasia evolve. While it might be appropriate for assessment and treatment to be directed at specific impairments and performance of daily activities, a social model requires that goals must enhance the individual's participation in their social community to the extent that the individual desires.

### Principles of a Social Model

A social approach to aphasia management is based on a set of principles that extend beyond traditional impairment-based models. The following principles might be considered relevant to a social approach (Simmons-Mackie, 1993, 1994, 1998a,b). Social approaches should:

1. assume that communication is designed to meet dual goals of social interaction and transaction of messages;
2. view communication as a flexible, dynamic, multidimensional activity;
3. emphasize authentic, relevant, natural contexts;
4. consider conversation as a primary site of human communication;
5. focus on communication as a collaborative achievement;
6. focus on the social and personal consequences of aphasia;
7. focus on adaptations rather than impairments;
8. emphasize the perspectives of the person with aphasia; and
9. embrace qualitative as well as quantitative measures of outcome.

The following sections will address each of these driving principles of a social approach to intervention.

COMMUNICATION SERVES DUAL GOALS

Traditionally aphasiology has advanced an "information exchange" definition of communication. That is, communication has been defined as the ability to receive or convey messages in any way possible (Davis, 1993; Hough & Pierce, 1994). While information exchange is a highly significant goal of communication, most communication is designed not only to transact an exchange of messages, but also to fulfill social needs (Brown & Yule 1983; Goffman, 1967; Gumperz, 1982; Tannen, 1984, 1986). Human communication is an intensely social activity. Through communication we affiliate with other people, assert our individuality, demonstrate our competence, form and maintain relationships and gain membership in social circles. Thus, communication serves dual goals—transaction (the exchange of information) and interaction (the fulfillment of social needs) (Simmons, 1993; Simmons-Mackie & Damico, 1995). When communication fails, ones ability to exchange messages is reduced, but perhaps more importantly, ones participation as a member of a social group is often compromised. A social model is designed to address these dual goals of transaction and interaction.

COMMUNICATION IS FLEXIBLE AND DYNAMIC

Traditional, impairment-based approaches to aphasia tend to view the aphasic speaker in relation to an "idealized normal" speaker. In other words, clinicians compare the language of each client to the expected performance of nonaphasic speakers. This assumes a sort of invariance or static quality to communication that fails to account for the remarkable variation typical of natural communication. For example, informal social conversation is replete with hesitations, dysfluencies, word production errors, sentence fragments, and incomplete propositions (Button & Lee, 1987; Shiffrin, 1987). The following excerpt is a standard speaker conversing with a colleague.

> *Oh yea . . mhm . . but like I say for some people . . . . for me even . . for some . . might not be willing to you know to do to do that cause it requires to be willing, to take time and you know sort of like a a a a game out of it or someba . . something.*

This excerpt would be considered "deviant" when measured according to traditional standards. Yet these "deviations" are typical of "normal" speakers during informal interactions. Do we hold our clients up to higher standards than we ourselves meet in conversation?

Because impairment-based approaches focus on "normal" language, accuracy and efficiency of communication is measured relative to an expected level. Unfortunately this does not account for the flexible and creative use of language to perform various *social* functions. For example, Goodwin (1987) examines the use of "forgetfulness" (such as forgetting a name) as a strategy used by nonaphasic couples to engage their partners in interaction. Thus, a husband telling a story about a family vacation to a group of friends might "forget" the name of a city and look to his wife to enter the conversation to provide the name; the husband's strategy elevates his wife from a listener to a participant in telling the story. The involvement of his wife promotes affiliation, demonstrates respect and solidarity, and paves the way for social participation. "Forgetfulness" is viewed as a resource to promote social participation rather than a response deviation.

A social model takes into account the flexibility of communication and requires that communication be viewed from the perspective of achievement of social and communicative goals. It accepts that norms are relative to the situation and the goals of the moment. This requires a philosophical shift away from a traditional normative view of communication to a *flexible and context-driven* view of communication. This certainly does not mean that the aphasiologist should abandon measures of impairment or forsake consideration of appropriate versus inappropriate behavior. Rather, a social model begs for expansion of assessment to include consideration of individual social actions, communicative goals, vagaries of informal talk, and flexible functions of behavior.

## EMPHASIS ON AUTHENTIC, RELEVANT, NATURAL CONTEXTS

Much traditional aphasia therapy is conducted in relatively controlled contexts in which the clinician presents stimuli (such as pictures) and elicits responses from the person with aphasia. While this controlled context allows the clinician to manipulate variables believed to influence language, it replaces the rich social context typical of natural, interactive communication. In fact, research has suggested that there are specific therapy discourse structures that differ markedly from natural, social conversation (Simmons-Mackie & Damico, 1997b, 1999). Clearly, traditional therapy, including activities such as picture description or "set up" conversation, does not simulate the demands of natural communication outside of therapy. In fact, some clients demonstrate different communicative strategies outside of therapy when confronted with social demands (Simmons, 1993). The communication differences between therapy contexts and other social contexts must be studied lest we assume that improvements in the traditional context represent the entire constellation of behaviors that constitute social interaction. Furthermore, improvement should be judged relative to the positive changes made in natural, relevant contexts.

A FOCUS ON CONVERSATION

While there has been a growing emphasis on functional communication treatment, natural conversation seems to have been largely ignored in aphasia therapy. In fact, research has suggested that therapists often view conversation as taking a break from the real work of treatment (Armstrong, 1989). Assessment tools rarely sample authentic, natural conversation and few traditional approaches directly target natural conversation. The apparent neglect of conversation in both assessment and treatment is surprising considering the functional relevance of this pervasive communicative event. Each of us would probably freely admit that most of our daily communication is "conversation"—authentic, spontaneous communication associated with social interaction. Our "activities of daily living" are enriched by social conversation. For example, ordering in a restaurant is an important "functional" task, but the enjoyment of dining out is probably more closely related to chit chatting with our dinner partners. In fact, the literature sites conversation as the fundamental site of language use in Western cultures (Clark & Wilkes-Gibbs, 1986). All other forms of communication such as lectures, writing, or interviews are secondary. As Holland (1998) so picturesquely asks "What relegates conversation to some sort of sleazy, shady, unreimbursable Neverland that must perforce either precede or follow the real goods—the therapy?"

Perhaps one answer traces back to traditional impairment-based therapy that focuses on restoring language by working on components such as naming or formulating simple sentences. Impairment-based therapies have typically assumed that improving the individual elements of language results in overall improvement in communication. Improvement is typically measured on standard tests that measure the "components." When spontaneous communication is measured, traditional approaches generally pick out linguistic components such as the number of content words or grammatical completeness. These approaches measure the traditional linguistic aspects of communication, but fail to look at the social devices and strategies that help us craft social interaction. Thus, tradition has focused aphasiologists away from considering communication in its most natural and whole form—social conversation.

FOCUS ON COMMUNICATION AS A COLLABORATIVE ACHIEVEMENT

Research has repeatedly demonstrated that natural conversation is a co-constructed activity in which participants endeavor to make each other understand with as little effort as possible (e.g., Clark & Wilkes-Gibb, 1986; Goodwin, 1996;

Milroy & Perkins, 1992). In addition to sensitive negotiation of meanings, this collaboration involves intricate social negotiations to affiliate or maintain distance, preserve identity, and maintain face (Goffman, 1967; Gumperz, 1982; Tannen, 1984, 1986). Speakers continually modify their speaking style, content, opinions, and discourse structure to accommodate to speaking partners, to context and to communicative goals (Bell, 1984; Giles et al., 1973). Viewing communication as a collaborative achievement forces us to look beyond the individual with aphasia. The locus of the problem is shifted from the individual to the interaction. Responsibility for a successful exchange is placed on speaking partners as well as on the individual with aphasia. This contrasts with impairment-based therapies that focus on the individual with aphasia. The social model shifts the focus to the collaborative nature of communication and away from the concept of achieving independence. Rather there is an emphasis on mutual dependence or interdependence within the social structure of communication (French, 1993; Holland, 1998; Oelshlager & Damico, 1998; Parr & Byng, 1998; Pound 1998).

## FOCUS ON THE SOCIAL CONSEQUENCES OF APHASIA

A social model of intervention is concerned with the consequences of aphasia. Individuals will vary greatly in how they experience aphasic impairments and disabilities. Thus, one individual with Broca's aphasia might find the impairment creates significant vocational, emotional and social problems, while another individual with an identical impairment might experience minimal impact in life. To insure that intervention is efficient and socially valid, the consequences for each individual and their loved ones must be evaluated. This requires sensitivity not only to individual social consequences of aphasia, but also to the social consequences of our therapy.

Much aphasia therapy has focused on improving the individual's ability to get ideas across in any way possible. Thus, people with aphasia have been trained to use gestures, written cues, picture boards, and drawing to compensate for linguistic deficits. The assumption has been that improved ability to get ideas across will be rewarding to the person with aphasia. Unfortunately, such practices have to some degree failed to take into account social expectations and cultural norms. For example, Simmons (1993) discovered that clients failed to use learned compensatory strategies during situations when the behaviors would be considered "stigmatizing." Most people with aphasia want to look and act like everybody else—to fit into their social community. While some trained behaviors might be stigmatizing, other successful communication behaviors are too time-consuming to be socially effective. For example, in studies of literacy practices of people with aphasia, Parr (1996) noted that some preferred to delegate literacy activity rather than struggle to do it themselves. The social and personal consequences outweighed the benefits of independence. In addition, the consequences of aphasia on the family and friends of the person with aphasia must be accounted for; consequences such as excess energy consumption or social stigma can impact speaking partners. Again, successful outcomes must be measured relative to reducing personal consequences of aphasia. Thus, intervention is designed to promote communication and quality of life.

In addition to viewing consequences relative to the person with aphasia, it is important to view consequences of aphasia from the perspective of social barriers. Barriers to participation for individuals with disabilities are often created by society (Finkelstein, 1991; LeDorze, 1997; Parr, 1996; Pound, 1998). These barriers represent ignorance of the disorder, lack of appropriate community resources, and lack of skill in facilitating communication. Thus, the "handicap" is a societal problem more than an individual problem. Again, a social approach requires that the focus be shifted away from the individual to the community.

### A FOCUS ON ADAPTIVE BEHAVIORS

When communication is disrupted, the communicative skills of the individual often are adapted to compensate. Newhoff and Apel (1990) suggest that some identified "deficits" (such as pragmatic deficits) in aphasia might be compensatory mechanisms or adaptations for dealing with reduced linguistic abilities. For example, a client with severe aphasia was judged by her clinician to be "pragmatically impaired" because she failed to "look at" or exchange greetings with acquaintances in public (a marked change from premorbid behavior). Interviews and observations revealed that the client used these "pragmatic compensations" to avoid being placed in a position where she might have to talk—and fail—resulting in embarrassment to the acquaintance and herself (Simmons, 1993). Thus, the "deficit" was actually a social adaptation to the impairment. Certainly if the person with aphasia is expected to communicate in spite of an impaired language system, then communicative behaviors that are atypical must be expected. A social perspective that focuses on an individual's adaptation to impairments, must shift to a more open minded perspective in which each behavior is viewed in relation to the pragmatic purpose served and the available alternatives.

The tendency to judge behaviors as either appropriate/normal or inappropriate/abnormal is evident in the cataloging of linguistic impairments. For example, "processing delays" such as hesitations on word retrieval have been discussed as sensitive indicators of aphasic deficits (e.g., Porch, 1981). Thus, a client who says "*uh uh uh pen*" to identify an object can be viewed as having a word retrieval delay—a problem. This identification of a processing deficit helps to focus restorative therapy. However, a social approach emphasizes attention to adaptations. In the example of word retrieval delay a social approach might focus on the "*uh uh uh*" as a floor-holding strategy. The floor-holding adaptation is a resource that helps the client stay in the speaker role by alerting the listener that a word search is underway. Because aphasia tend to be a chronic disorder in which most clients retain some degree of impairment, it is important to maintain sensitivity to what is "right" as well as what is "wrong" (Armstrong, 1993; Weniger & Sarno, 1990).

In addition, because many compensations or adaptations tend to be idiosyncratic, each individual is likely to demonstrate unique or individualized patterns of compensation (Simmons-Mackie & Damico, 1997a). Therefore, behavior might be viewed for its purposeful potential rather than relative to a norm or expectation. For example, the aphasic speaker with severely limited ability to elaborate on topics might use "inappropriate topic shifting" as a method of participating in the conversation, exerting conversational control and preserving face. Should this behavior be judged as inappropriate or as a successful social adaptation? A social model requires that behaviors be viewed from an "adaptive" perspective.

Addressing adaptations is nothing new in aphasia management. Compensatory strategies have been touted for years. However, many approaches tend to emphasize what's wrong so that compensations can be devised to overcome the problem. Trained compensatory strategies tend to focus on "clinician" chosen behaviors that assist in getting ideas across (Simmons, 1993). While these methods certainly have value, research and experience suggest that many trained compensations are not used (e.g., Thompson, 1989). Perhaps we need to revise our conceptions of compensatory training to focus on enhancing what is already going on naturally (Armstrong, 1993; Ferguson, 1994; Weniger & Sarno, 1990; Simmons, 1993; Simmons-Mackie & Damico, 1997a). A social approach builds on existing adaptations and social skills. Furthermore, focusing on ability instead of disability can enhance self-concept as well as function.

Finally and perhaps most importantly, adaptation is not unique to the individual with aphasia. In the process of communicating with people with aphasia, speaking partners adapt to the communicative differences. The adaptive skills of all parties involved in an interaction will determine the success and satisfaction of the exchange. Therefore, clinicians must consider creating a "compensatory" environment that supports communication rather than simply focusing on changing the individual with aphasia.

THE PERSPECTIVE OF THE PERSON WITH APHASIA

As many have pointed out, aphasia management must reflect the customer's perspective of the disability and focus on consumer satisfaction (Frattali, 1992; Parr, 1996; Worrall, 1992). This concept of autonomy and personal choice is a basic tenet of a social model (French, 1993; Parr & Byng, 1998). For example, an individual who is trained to use an augmentative communication device might opt *not* to use the device when there is potential for social stigma even though it might enhance independence. Clinicians tend to identify "lack of generalization" as therapy failure. When clients choose to avoid communication rather than face embarrassment, this is a personal choice consistent with social needs and social sensitivity. Considering these choices to be "failures" to communicate demonstrates a bias toward the clinician perspective; it allows the clinician to define "success." This does not mean that the social approach takes a hands-off attitude and lets "people be." Rather, it starts with a respectful consideration of the individual and family's social and communicative perspective, then works to build communication and quality of life within that perspective. Instead of dispensing with the idea of training an augmentative system, the therapist would identify the social barriers that inhibit its use outside of therapy and address these barriers.

A FOCUS ON QUALITATIVE AS WELL AS QUANTITATIVE MEASURES

A social model focuses on the *experience* of a communication disorder rather than the measurement of linguistic performance. The perspective of a social model is decidedly subjective. It requires shifting from a clinician-driven emphasis on objective measurement to a client-centered focus on subjective experience. Behaviors are viewed relative to the individual's own abilities and purposes rather than in relation to an objective norm. Because the emphasis is upon quality of life and social membership, measurement does not fit well into traditional quantitative paradigms. Quality of life measures, qualitative approaches, and satisfaction assessment are potential tools for monitoring social intervention.

## Implementation of a Social Approach

Hopefully the preceding discussion provided a philosophical context within which the clinician can construct interventions to minimize participation limitations of people with aphasia. Because a social approach is a philosophical construct and a clinical undertaking, the following section will provide suggestions for implementation. Specific objectives of a social approach might include:

1. increasing conversational skill;
2. increasing communicative supports;
3. increasing opportunities for participation in relevant activities;
4. maximizing a healthy identity and promoting empowerment; and
5. promoting advocacy and social action.

Intervention need not be restricted to the "handicap" or participation level to fulfill social goals. Rather, goals are cast in relationship to what is required to enhance participation and membership in the community. Direct intervention might involve focusing at any of the WHO levels including the impairment level, functional activity level (disability) or participation level (see Chapter 1). However, the goal is for the individual to participate as a functioning member of society. The implementation of a social approach will vary considerably depending on the personal goals of the client and family, time post onset, the characteristics of the aphasia and the service provider. It is important that attention to the social outcome *not* be relegated to the "end" of rehabilitation or when traditional therapy is completed.

CONVERSATION AS THE FOCUS OF INTERVENTION

One objective of a social approach is for those affected by aphasia to experience improved social communication. In some cases, this will entail work at the level of conversation. Although aphasia clinicians seem comfortable with defining goals, choosing appropriate stimuli and manipulating language behavior within the context of impairment-based therapy, many seem confused by conversational management. Perhaps the confusion arises because "conversation" can be the goal, the stimulus, and/or the approach. It has not been clear if conversation therapy refers to therapy that improves conversation or therapy that involves conversation. In this chapter, the term *conversation therapy* will be reserved for "working on conversation"; in other words, conversation therapy is direct, planned therapy that is overtly designed to enhance conversational skill and confidence. Conversation therapy does not necessarily require "having a conversation" with the client, although conversational stimuli are probably most appropriate.

Direct conversation therapy can be contrasted with simply "having a conversation" with a client. The goal of *working on conversation* (conversation therapy) is to improve ones skill and confidence as a conversational participant. The goals of *having a conversation* are to exchange messages and fulfill social needs. Clients might need both of these. In other words, they profit from working to enhance their conversational skills through conversation therapy, and they also need opportunities to participate in satisfying social conversations. While these goals are distinctly different, socially responsible intervention requires that aphasiologists address both of these needs by improving the individual's conversation skill and by reducing barriers to participation in actual conversations. Therefore, the clinician might work on providing *conversation opportunities* for people with aphasia. Successful conversation participation is facilitated when opportunities include appropriate communicative supports. *Supported conversation* involves promoting successful participation by providing supports such as trained partners. On occasion these conversation approaches will overlap such as using *supported conversation* to carry-over *conversation therapy* goals, to practice specific communicative devices or to build interactive confidence.

To work at the level of conversation, conversation must be defined. Based on research findings and intuitions as language users, it is clear that the structure of most traditional, impairment-based therapy is not typical of satisfying adult, social conversation. The phrase "adult, social conversation" is used somewhat loosely to refer to authentic, spontaneous communication associated with social interaction—the everyday, ordinary talk that serves dual goals of exchanging messages and fulfilling social needs. Typically this implies that all parties engaged in social conversation have the potential to offer topics, introduce content, take turns and structure the participation framework. This conversational parity does ***not*** mean that each person has to share the same amount of information, take the same turn lengths or get an equal number of turns. Rather it means that participants have the power and ***opportunity*** to craft a conversational format that they desire. There is collaboration in how the conversation is negotiated. Defining conversation in this way is not meant to imply invariance in the structure of social conversation. Rather, the phrase "social conversation" is being used to contrast with other forms of discourse such as interviews, teaching, and lectures. Although one might argue the huge range of styles, power balances, and structures of social conversation, the primary goal in this chapter is to provide a frame of reference for evaluating interventions.

Comparison of therapy discourse with natural conversation suggests that the structure of most traditional therapy tasks and much therapy "conversation" does not provide clients with experience in generating and structuring natural social discourse. For example, research indicates that a pervasive discourse structure in therapy is the Request–Response–Evaluation (RRE) triad (Simmons-Mackie & Damico, 1997b; Simmons-Mackie & Damico, 1999). This adjacency structure begins with a therapist request to perform (e.g., "What is the name of this?"), followed by a client response (e.g., "cup"), followed by a therapist evaluation (e.g., "good"). This structure is typical of therapy and teaching discourse, but is not typical of adult social conversation. Also, "conversation" that precedes and follows didactic therapy tasks is often structured like "interviews" with therapists asking questions and clients responding to questions (Silvast, 1991; Simmons-Mackie & Damico, 1997b; Wilcox & Davis, 1977). Thus, the structure of traditional impairment-based therapy tend to place clients in a passive role and limit their power as conversation partners. There is little opportunity to practice strategies for controlling discourse, initiating varied structures, using creative devices and varying social stances. In contrast, a social approach to aphasia intervention should provide the client with the skills and confidence to negotiate social conversations.

Study of discourse structure and characteristics of social conversation will assist clinicians in tailoring therapy to more closely approximate natural conversation. For example, for those interested in moving away from the rigid structure of traditional therapy, identifying RRE sequences can signal therapist-centered discourse structure versus more natural interaction. The following examples contrast a traditional RRE-structured naming task to a task more characteristic of conversational interaction.

Ten pictures of common food objects are arranged in front of the client.

#1      Request–Response–Elaboration:

Clinician:   *What is this?* (points to a picture of sandwich)

Client:      *Sandwich*

Clinician:   *Good*

#2      Question–Answer–Comment:

Clinician:   *Which of these do you like to eat for lunch?*

Client:      *Sandwich* (pointing to picture)

Clinician:   *Oh, I like sandwiches too.*

The first example is a structured RRE sequence that is closed by clinician reinforcement of the correct response. The RRE structure places the client in a passive discourse role—simply filling the "response" slot within the dependency structure. The second example includes a clinician request for information and the final clinician turn constitutes a comment rather than a direct evaluation. While the clinician is clearly still in control of the discourse format, the interactive features are slightly more natural. When appropriate to the goals, such simple variations in discourse structure allow clients to engage in more varied discourse experiences within intervention. Thus, similar to the fading of prompts and cues in traditional stimulation therapy (e.g., Davis, 1993), the informed clinician can gradually fade control of discourse and participation structures. Awareness of the structure of discourse within and outside of our sessions can help us move clients toward more discourse variety and control.

CONVERSATION THERAPY

Certainly, the overall goal of conversation therapy is to enhance conversational skill; however, each individual should have goals based on specific skills and strategies needed to manage social conversation. Intervention to increase the client's skill and confidence as a conversationalist emphasizes transactional and interactional skills and strategies. These goals are specific to the individual's residual abilities and to the desired outcome. The literature has widely addressed the first of these goals: message transmission (e.g., Davis, 1993; Davis & Wilcox, 1985). Treatment approaches such as Promoting Aphasic's Communicative Effectiveness (Davis & Wilcox, 1985) provide a semistructured approach to encouraging clients to get ideas across and utilize compensatory strategies. Far less emphasis has been placed on enhancing "interactive" skills. Although clients with aphasia are usually considered to be fairly intact interactively, they acquire aphasia with little prior practice in dealing with significant communicative breakdowns. A social approach assists the client in achieving the most effective social strategies. This might include evaluating the effects of message exchange strategies (such as gesture, writing) within real social interaction. It also involves enhancing interactive strategies. For example, one person with aphasia might work on strategies for initiating topics and holding on to turns, while another individual might work on strategies for shifting turns to the speaking partner. Continuers (such as head nods) or interest markers (such as *oh really, mhm, nice*) can encourage the speaking partner to do the talking and prevent exhaustive rounds of repairs (Simmons-Mackie & Damico, 1996b). The social communication resources of speaking partners will also markedly affect the quality of the interaction. Communication specialists must understand, reinforce, and expand on discourse devices and promote communication that is socially and contextually appropriate. Also, goals should reflect the outcome choices of the individual with aphasia. While the therapist might deem "conversational assertiveness" to be important relative to a particular client's ability to enter conversations, the client might prefer a more passive, listener role. The perspective of the client is critical in insuring success of a social approach. A social model must assist clients in maximizing communication and participation *as defined by the client.*

When improved conversation is the target, actual conversational stimuli are appropriate, such as using group discussion as the medium for therapy. In addition, direct training of specific component skills or strategies might be appropriate for enhancing ones skill as a conversationalist. The caveat of course, is that skills learned in didactic tasks might not integrate easily into the context of natural social interaction. Thus, the more conversational the medium of therapy, the more likely that the skills will be applicable. In addition, impairment-based approaches run the risk of placing the client in a disempowering interactive arrangement that could undermine social goals. The following sections will present several contexts for introducing conversational goals.

### Group Therapy

Group therapy is an excellent context for conversational intervention. However, groups must be structured to promote conversation, to address communication goals, and to enhance conversation strategies. Considerable skill is required to ensure that group interactions are "conversational" and not simply traditional therapy overlaid into a multiparty context. The components of interactive group therapy and the potential benefits are reported elsewhere (e.g., Elman, 1999; Elman & Bernstein-Ellis, 1999).

**Scaffolded Communication**

The child language literature discusses the use of "scaffolded" communication as a method of increasing communication skills (e.g., Damico, 1992). This approach is simply an extension of therapist cueing and facilitation (common in aphasia therapy) into an interactive, conversational framework. The client is placed in an activity requiring conversation, and the therapist provides cues or mediates within context. Criteria for promoting a scaffolded conversation include the following (Damico, 1992):

1. The interaction is client focused rather than clinician focused. In other words, the clinician does not control the topics or rate of the session. Rather the clinician expands on the client's contributions.
2. Conversation evolves out of a meaningful activity.
3. Feedback is situationally appropriate. Rather than rewarding successful productions with *"good"* or *"Wait, say it like this,"* the therapist responds with natural, conversational contingencies including sustaining the talk, elaborating or asking for clarification when something is not understood.
4. The client and clinician work toward specific goals such as improving the ability to elaborate on topics or increasing conversational participation.

Scaffolding is particularly useful when integrated into group therapy or used in role play activities. If properly done, it provides a bridge between clinician controlled therapy discourse and the give and take of natural interaction.

**Conversational Coaching**

Another method of working on conversational skills is to use conversational coaching as suggested by Holland (1991). The therapist acts as a "coach" providing the client an opportunity to practice a communication "scenario" with support and guidance. This approach can help individuals deal with specific problem situations. For example, a client who attended frequent cocktail parties with her husband felt dependant upon her husband to help her out of communication breakdowns and was embarrassed by her failure at "party talk." Conversational coaching focused on strategies for dealing with small talk. Thus, scenarios were developed and scripted to practice specific interactive routines. Rather than concentrating on "improving language," therapy focused on developing strategies for fitting in and preventing failure such as using practiced topic starters, using turn-shifting strategies, and using context to support talk (e.g., using the buffet table to generate talk). These sessions also revealed situational barriers that inhibited this client's participation in the talk. For example, holding a wine glass inhibited her use of gesture. Thus, barriers could be identified and reduced wherever possible.

Armstrong (1993) uses an approach similar to conversational coaching in which scripts or texts are used to focus on both the social functions and forms of discourse. Her approach is anchored in Halliday's (1985) systemic-functional grammar framework that takes into account linguistic and social aspects of communication. Clients work on various forms such as questioning and requesting at the discourse level, as well as narrative skills such as telling stories. Such a focus is important because people with aphasia have reported problems with aspects of interactive discourse such as telling stories, relating a piece of gossip, lodging complaints, or participating in arguments (e.g., Parr et al., 1997).

### Strategies for Engagement

Promoting conversation as a therapy medium can be challenging. As noted above many speech–language pathologists use "interview" style discourse to interact with people with aphasia. The following suggestions might promote social interaction, distribute the "power" to negotiate discourse more equitably, and serve as the stimuli for conversation therapy. Using a story prompt, suggested in the child language literature (McCabe, 1994), is one excellent means of starting conversation. The therapist or group leader tells a story such as an embarrassing or scary incident. This often "prompts" others to share similar stories resulting in a round of stories, comments, and sharing. For maximum effectiveness the story prompt should be introduced in a natural, spontaneous fashion—"*Wow, guess what happened to me*" versus "*let me get everyone started talking.*" Topics that promote listings (e.g., "*What I did on the weekend,*" trip descriptions) are less successful in promoting the give and take of conversation (McCabe, 1994). Other potential conversation stimuli include discussion of television shows, jigsaw barrier tasks, and discussion webs (Damico, 1992), and diaries, photo albums, or remnant books (Bernstein-Ellis & Elman, 1995). These activities serve as "stimuli," which evoke interaction. It is then the therapist's job to scaffold, coach, or facilitate achievement of individual conversational goals within this interactive context.

### Adjusted Compensatory Training

Training in compensatory strategies dates to the origins of intervention in aphasia (e.g., Goldstein, 1939; Zangwill, 1947). The approach is well founded in theory and practice. A social approach extend the focus on compensation to emphasize socially relevant and flexible use of strategies that enhance information exchange and social interaction. Thus, compensatory strategy training is expanded from training specific behaviors to developing creativity, generativity, and interactivity. For example, the individual does not simply learn a set of gestures, but works on *generating and creating* gestural communication within the context of conversational interaction. Approaches such as Lyon's (1995) interactive drawing and Demchuk's (1996) drama therapy are good examples of techniques that build compensation within an interactive and dynamically social framework. For example, Demchuk describes use of a group setting in which the clinician begins acting out a scenario (such as a teenager asking to use the family car) and engages clients in participating in a dramatic role-play. Creative body language, facial expression, pantomime, intonation, vocalizations, and speech are encouraged. The goal is to build skill and confidence in creatively generating ideas and interacting with others.

Compensatory training should focus on strategies that are flexible, identity enhancing, face saving, and socioculturally appropriate for the individual. Finally, compensatory training should be integrated into authentic contexts and take into account the need for speaking partners to collaborate in constructing compensations.

## Increasing Participation: Supported Conversation

Ultimately, skills and strategies must be used in the flexible and dynamic context of real conversation. This provides opportunity for practice and confidence building as well as fulfillment of social needs. A subsequent section will address various outlets for increasing the success of and opportunity for communication including training partners to provide support, to provide resources, and to enhance opportunities to participate in relevant activities.

### INCREASING COMMUNICATIVE SUPPORTS: PARTNER TRAINING

Beyond ensuring that conversational behaviors of the person with aphasia are maximized, a social model of aphasia intervention must promote successful communicative collaboration between people with aphasia and their communication partners. Communication is inherently "interdependent" (e.g., Holland, 1998; Oelschlaeger & Damico, 1998; Parr & Byng, 1998; Simmons, 1993). Thus, lack of partner skill and support is a barrier to participation for people with aphasia. Conversely, a partner who is skilled in facilitating interaction can enhance the communicative success of the dyad and increase the opportunity for successful social interaction. In fact, research repeatedly demonstrates that training communication partners of people with aphasia improves communication within the dyad (Alarcon et al., 1997; Boles, 1997; Lyon, 1997; Lyon et al., 1997; Simmons et al., 1987). For example, Simmons et al. (1987) demonstrated that the communication between a person with aphasia and his spouse improved after the spouse was taught strategies to facilitate communication, even though the individual with aphasia did not participate in the training. Lyon (1997) demonstrated increased scores on a functional communication measure after intervention targeting the interaction between a person with aphasia and spouse. Garret and Beukelman (1995) demonstrated that varying the type of partner "support" changed the interactive patterns of an individual with severe aphasia. Kagan (1998) is accumulating data demonstrating that training of volunteers to interact with people with aphasia results in increased communication ratings for both the volunteer and the individual with aphasia. The accumulated evidence indicates that training of communicative partners and focusing on communicative collaboration can be effective in improving communication in aphasia.

Partner training serves several goals. First, it provides a potential source of conversational interaction for the person with aphasia. Second, a trained partner is likely to promote a more satisfying and successful communicative exchange, thereby increasing the likelihood that the parties will continue the relationship. Third, the training often decreases negative perceptions about aphasia. "Lay people" sometimes believe that people with aphasia are incompetent, deaf, or mentally ill (Kagan, in press; Parr et al., 1997). The aphasic speaker's communicative breakdowns and use of stigmatizing strategies probably reinforce these attitudes (Goffman, 1963). Training has the potential for revealing to the partner that the person with aphasia is a competent human being who enjoys social contact. Fourth, a skilled partner can encourage the use of unusual, but successful compensations by capitalizing on the tendency for speakers to accommodate to each other's speaking style. When people with aphasia interact with nonaphasic people, the nonaphasic partner typically uses the auditory-verbal mode of communication and is unlikely to write or use a picture board to get their ideas across. It is natural for the speaker with aphasia to accommodate to the prevailing "expected" auditory-verbal mode rather than introduce a novel form of communicating (Giles et al., 1973). When speaking partners introduce multi-modal communication, this minimizes the responsibility on the person with aphasia and reduces a potential barrier to participation (LeDorze, 1997; LeDorze et al., 1993; Simmons-Mackie, 1998b).

### Training Regular Partners

Because communication is a co-constructed event, enhancing the interaction of people with aphasia and their customary communication partners is an appropriate goal of intervention. Thus, family members and friends of people with aphasia can be identified and brought into training.

### Expanding Social Networks

For many people with aphasia former jobs or hobbies are no longer viable activities and the associated social relationships are forfeited. Thus, they experience a significant reduction in the number of people that they communicate with on a daily, weekly, or monthly basis. In some cases the nuclear family can become the "focal point" of the person's social life. Training immediate family members does little to address this social isolation or expand the individual's social participation. Furthermore, expecting the family to fulfill social needs could actually increase the burden on an already stressed nuclear family. Thus, efforts might be directed at expanding the social network of the individual with aphasia (Simmons-Mackie & Damico, 1996a).

Expanding social networks involves identifying people with whom the client can establish an ongoing relationship, then working with the identified partner and person with aphasia to maximize their interpersonal communication. Of course the problem is often availability of partner "candidates." Candidates might include existing friends or acquaintances, individuals connected with existing social networks, volunteers, or peer mentors.

Existing family, friends, or acquaintances with the potential for a *more active relationship* might be recruited for partner training. For example, a client reported that an old friend had stopped calling. An interview with the "former" friend revealed that he felt uncomfortable with the client since the onset of aphasia. The friend agreed to be part of a "pilot" program aimed at improving the client's communication. In fact, this program focused on teaching the friend strategies for communicating with the client. The friend was amazed with the client's "improvement" and their relationship was renewed.

Individuals who are connected to existing social networks of the person with aphasia are also potential partners. For example, a friend at church who is willing to participate in training might recruit additional church members to expand the individual's trained social network.

Volunteers can serve as partners and social contacts (Jordan & Kaiser, 1996; Kagan & Gailey, 1993; Lyon et al., 1997). Lyon pairs people with aphasia with a volunteer and trains them to be an effective communicative dyad. Each volunteer's training is tailored to the style and skills of the individual with whom he/she is paired. Kagan and Gailey (1993) describe training of volunteers to interact with people with aphasia; however, this training is generic. That is, volunteers are taught general skills required of a good partner. A day-center context is provided in which the trained volunteers run conversation groups. Both approaches have significant benefit in that they expand the social participation of the individual with aphasia by providing supportive, skilled communication partners.

Finally, people with aphasia might serve as and profit from peer mentors trained as communication partners. Peer mentors are colleagues with aphasia who offer communication opportunities, serve as social partners, assist as advocates, or perform identified services. For example, two men with aphasia, G.R. and J.B., were paired as social partners. G.R. could drive a car, while J.B. could not. J.B.'s linguistic skills were superior to G.R.'s. Therefore, the two helped each other participate in community activities. G.R. provided the transportation, while J.B. ran "interference" when activities required higher level language. Peer support, peer counseling, and peer visitation as potential services for people with aphasia hold promise for expanding social networks (Cohen-Schneider, 1996; Jordan & Kaiser, 1996).

### A Trained Community

Although a daunting goal, the ultimate communication support system would include a knowledgeable, "prosthetic" community. While it is unlikely that we could train the world to facilitate interaction with people with aphasia, accepting responsibility for public education is a viable and worthy goal for speech–language pathologists and people with aphasia. Thus, community service programs could target generic partner training such as public service programs on television or free workshops at businesses, churches, or schools. Such programs are costly; however, they have the potential for enhancing client referral for funded services and expanding public support for services.

LOGISTICS OF PARTNER TRAINING

The key to successful partner training is to teach the partner *how to converse* rather than *how to work on conversation*. Thus, the partner and the person with aphasia learn to create a "seamless" interaction using all available modes. The partner's use of augmentative systems such as writing, pictures, drawing, and gesture establishes the appropriateness of alternate modes and reduces the potential of social stigma, failure, and embarrassment for the person with aphasia. Developing a skilled partner requires direct "hands-on" training that includes strategies that facilitate transaction and interaction. Counseling, observing therapy, or providing lists of dos and don'ts are not effective methods of training partners (Simmons et al., 1987). In fact, the common practice of having partners observe traditional didactic therapy can create "teacher" partners who engage in inappropriate communicative interactions such as asking for known information, requesting performance, and evaluating responses. The goal of partner training is to provide someone skilled at "having a conversation" with the person with aphasia, not to enlist another therapist. The approach to direct training will vary from "workshop" settings that train a number of partners in general strategies to dyad training in which a specific partner and individual with aphasia participate in intervention.

## Increasing Communicative Supports: Resources

Providing communicative support systems within a speaker's community can include not only skilled partners, but also access to communication resources. Resources include anything that will potentially enhance an individual's communication such as picture resource materials, paper and markers, remnant books, or alteration of physical surroundings (Lubinski, 1981). Materials that facilitate the exchange of information such as picture props, maps, communication boards, and books (Kagan et al., 1996a,b) can enhance interaction, particularly when the nonaphasic partner is skilled in the use of such resources. Similarly, a partner's use of written support such as "thematic written support" can increase the participation of the person in a conversational exchange (Garrett & Beukelman, 1995). Resources that provide a context for communication also are important. For example, LeDorze (1997) has noted that individuals confined to institutions such as nursing homes often have little shared information with caregivers. In such situations "life story" notebooks with a brief life history, family pictures, and relevant life events can provide a living, interesting identity to "the patient in bed 202" (LeDorze, 1997). Similarly, remnant books or photo albums can help initiate and sustain conversational interactions among individuals with aphasia (Bernstein-Ellis & Elman, 1995). These resources provide a shared context for conversation, and remove the burden for verbally introducing new information from the person with aphasia.

## Increasing Participation in Relevant Activities

"Communication is facilitated when peoples' contexts are rich in opportunities to communicate and be understood" (Ferguson, 1994, p. 9). Unfortunately many individuals with aphasia have few opportunities for communication due to decreased participation in relevant activities. Most conversations surround some activity of interest (e.g., eating, shopping, working, and playing cards), yet the number and variety of experiences and activities are often diminished for the individual with aphasia. A social approach facilitates participation in relevant activities.

If a social approach to aphasia management is designed to enhance "participation" in personally relevant activities, what relevant activities should be targeted? As in partner training, the contexts for participation must be defined with each individual by assessing current and past interests and activities and possibly identifying new activities. The target of intervention (or whether to intervene at all) is the choice of the client, not the clinician.

### Activity Focused Intervention

One approach is to support the client in identifying activities of interest, developing self-generated goals for participation in the identified activities, then facilitating participation in the identified activity (Fox, 1997; Lyon et al., 1997; Simmons, 1993). Pachalska (1993) introduces therapeutic outings as part of Social Communication Oriented Treatment (SCOT). These outings provide "real-life" opportunities for people with aphasia and their families to participate in community events and activities. Community volunteers can serve as liasons to enhance participation of individuals with aphasia in chosen community activities (Lyon, 1997; Lyon et al., 1997). Thus, the volunteer becomes a "partner" in promoting participation in a relevant activity. It is also possible for the clinician to work directly with the client to identify potential opportunities for expanding social participation. Activities might be an expansion of existing activities or an entirely new endeavor. Often clinicians find that clients simply shrug when asked in which activities they would like to participate. One possibility is to utilize resource pictures representing a large inventory of potential activities such as going to church, playing cards, sports, politics, painting, gardening, grooming pets, etc. The client then sorts the pictures into those that are appealing and those that are not. The stack of "preferences" can be used as a starting point for identifying potential intervention activities.

Once a potential activity is identified, then the clinician must "pave the way" for participation. Too often, activities are simply suggested—"Why don't you join the health club?" or "Why don't you volunteer at the garden center?" Experience suggests that this rarely results in increased participation. Rather, the clinician must identify the specific site(s), visit the site to identify and reduce barriers to participation, work with the client to develop participation goals, then facilitate participation. Similar to the concept of supported employment, "supported" participation in relevant activities must be provided. While activity-based intervention will extend the role of the speech–language pathologist beyond traditional clinical settings, this is a viable expansion of role. The speech–language pathologist is uniquely qualified to analyze the communication requirements of activities, identify potential communication adaptations, and collaborate with involved parties to enhance participation. For example, R.S., a man with moderate aphasia, wanted to participate in watching televised sports events at a local sports bar. Although frequently expressing interest in this activity, R.S. failed to pursue his interest. A visit to the event by his therapist revealed a number of inobtrusive compensatory adaptations to facilitate participation such as placing a blackboard with key words next to the television (e.g., team names, stadium name) and providing "team cards" listing players. Also the bartender, a former friend of R.S., was recruited to support participation. Finally, conversational coaching involved practicing possible communication scenarios to build R.S.'s confidence and skill. Thus, activity-based intervention overlapped with skill training, partner training, and providing resources.

DEVELOPING "PROSTHETIC COMMUNITIES"

In addition to facilitating participation in identified activities, programs can foster and support participation in social activities by providing supportive, "prosthetic" communities. For example, programs that provide aphasia therapy can also offer social activities to bridge intervention and social participation. The

Aphasia Center of California provides group therapy focusing on improving communication and also provides recreational activities and a social outlet for people with aphasia (Elman, 1998). Living with Aphasia, Inc. in Wisconsin (Lyon, Chapter 9) provides direct intervention at the level of social communication and also sponsors a theatre group and a bowling league for people with aphasia. The Pat Arato Aphasia Centre in Toronto provides conversation groups and recreational activities for adults with aphasia in a community center atmosphere, as well as opportunities to work on specific skills such as writing. The "clubhouse model" associated with traumatic brain injury provides a facility with a community center atmosphere as well as intervention. Such programs can potentially fulfill direct intervention needs and serve as a social "community" for people with aphasia.

In addition, existing community centers, recreational facilities, work training centers, and adult education should be made more accessible to individuals with communication impairments. Speech–language pathologists might serve as consultants to identify barriers to participation and adaptations. People with aphasia can form advocacy groups that work on paving the way for participation in community activities. Employees or volunteers of community facilities or programs can be trained to interact positively with people with aphasia and serve as advocates to assist in filling out forms, completing registration procedures, and meeting other participants.

### Identity and Membership

A basic tenet of the social model is that the individual with aphasia is a valuable member of society. Unfortunately, aphasia is often associated with a subtle (or not so subtle) constellation of disempowering events and attitudes that undermine this membership. The onset of aphasia often precipitates role changes; thus, a wage earner becomes "unemployed" or a club president becomes a "former" member. Our roles in society help us construct our identities, support healthy egos, and ensure social memberships. Loss of such roles can diminish perceptions of ones worth. Because membership in a social community is intricately tied to ones roles and personal identity, aphasia impacts roles, identity, and ultimately membership.

Although people with aphasia can acquire new roles, some of those associated with the onset of aphasia are not necessarily "identity enhancing." For example, Newhoff and Apel (1990) note that people with aphasia are often assigned a role as "the patient." This "incompetent patient" and inadequate communicator role is reinforced by communication failures (Newhoff & Apel, 1990; Simmons-Mackie & Damico, 1999). Also the "patient" role can be reinforced by traditional aphasia therapy, which often adopts procedures, jargon, and props from medicine (e.g., charts, diagnosis, prognosis, treatment recommendations). Traditional therapy is largely designed and controlled by the therapist (Simmons-Mackie et al., 1995). The clinician is the expert who is in control of tasks, stimuli, and discourse structures (Simmons-Mackie & Damico, 1999). The client learns quickly to acquiesce to the therapist's authority—"to take the cure." Although therapists attempt to support and encourage their clients, the traditional patient role is inherently associated with dependency and disempowerment. The emphasis is placed on impairments (what is wrong) and the client is reminded through intervention and assessment of the presence of aphasia. The semantics of incompetence (e.g., the aphasic, the patient, recovery, handicap) reinforce the client's diminished status. Once the client becomes skilled at the "patient role," then he or she is often ready for discharge. Hesch (1998) sites feelings of abandonment sometimes associated with discharge from aphasia therapy. As one man described "you work hard to get better, then you get dumped." Perhaps one aspect of this feeling of loss is that the client is losing yet another social role—that of "the good patient."

In addition to role changes, people with aphasia are exposed to patronizing and disempowering attitudes (Parr et al., 1997; Simmons, 1993). People often react with surprise or negative emotion to communication differences. Such reactions potentially create the stigma of aphasia and serve to further diminish feelings of self worth (Goffman, 1963). Kagan (1995) identifies communication as the means through which others judge our social, intellectual, and emotional competence. Thus, when communication is impaired, others might perceive the individual as generally incompetent. The effects on identity can be devastating. Analysis of therapy discourse has revealed that subtle attitudes communicated during aphasia therapy might also serve to disempower people with aphasia (Simmons-Mackie & Damico, 1999).

Therefore, a critical aspect of a social approach is to foster a positive identity (Parr, 1996; Pound, 1998; Simmons, 1993). This will necessarily involve a range of adjustments to traditional approaches. One adjustment requires that aphasiologists consciously accept responsibility for that gray area often called "psychosocial adjustment." Confidence as a communication participant and positive self-perceptions are intricately woven into the tapestry of communication success. We cannot continue to treat the impairment and "expect" the client and family to adjust to the disorder as though ones adjustment is separate and distinct from ones communication participation. Improved language without the confidence to participate in communication events is worthless. Therefore, a social approach must foster communicative confidence and empower speakers with aphasia.

Empowerment can be enhanced as therapists critically evaluate their attitudes and interactive behaviors. Perhaps we might redefine our role as "experts" and consider that the real expert on the consequences of aphasia is the client. As Finkelstein (1991) suggests, the professional should accept a role as a resource to the person with a disability rather than assuming the role of the specialist who assesses the client to determine the appropriate interventions. Existing therapies should be studied and practices that promote "incompetent" identities should be eliminated (Simmons-Mackie et al., 1995). Client strengths rather than "problems" can be emphasized; thus, clients can be provided a list of "great adaptations" instead of a catalogue of what's wrong. This is particularly important for the person with chronic aphasia who does not need a catalog of impairments— this individual has lived the disorder. A focus at this stage is on reinforcing and expanding positive adaptations. Another method of promoting empowerment is to eliminate jargon that implies helplessness, dependence, or inadequacy (e.g., patient, illness, treatment). For example, rather than admit people with aphasia to university clinics to serve as patients for students, we might consider designating these individuals "client-teachers" who are assuming a leadership role in helping train students. Certainly, they obtain a needed therapy service, but they also provide a service to training institutions. In other words, empowerment is advanced when we facilitate the client's focus on his or her uniqueness, importance, and individuality as a person.

In addition to examining our own practices and attitudes, services directed specifically at development of a robust identity with aphasia should be provided. Counseling and education are valuable services for people with aphasia beyond the acute phase (Brumfitt & Clark, 1983; Ireland & Wotton, 1993; Wahrborg, 1989). Counseling might be directed at positively emphasizing the individual's uniqueness as a person (e.g., lover of animals, religious believer, opinionated in politics) (LeDorze, 1997 ), as well as defining the personal meaning of aphasia (Parr et al., 1997). As Parr (1996, p. 425) explains "The changing interpretations brought to the impairment by the aphasic person and close family members and friends must be understood. Without this knowledge the clinician will not be able to support the chronically impaired person in moving towards a reconciliation of views and towards a strong new identity."

Self-help groups are another potential identity-enhancing service; individuals with aphasia become their own advocates. Finally, aphasiologists will be expected to practice our own preachings, and truly value the experience and perspective of individuals with aphasia. For example, people with aphasia can assume leadership positions to train volunteers and students, provide insights into the experience of aphasia at conferences, or through client-driven research (such as Parr et al., 1997), and participate in program evaluations or focus groups.

Identity work also involves changing "barriers" such as attitudes of others and enhancing membership. In a discussion of augmentative communication intervention, Ferguson (1994, p. 10) notes that practicioners tend to focus too much on "intervention" and focus too little on membership, "specifically participatory, socially valued, image-enhancing membership." Membership is enhanced by collaboratively creating cultural identities that attribute competence, individuality, value, and roles. It involves shifting the "problem" away from the person with aphasia and onto the barriers to participation created by society (Parr, 1996; Pound, 1998; LeDorze et al., 1993). Making "differences" commonplace can reduce stigma and attitudinal barriers (Goffman, 1963). This can be done by paving the way for clients to enter an activity, by training partners or by changes at the institutional and societal level (such as public education). Organizations such as the National Aphasia Association (United States) or Action for Dysphasic Adults (Britain) increase the level of public awareness of aphasia and thereby diminish the stigma and barriers.

## Institutional and Societal Changes

A social approach dictates that service providers serve as advocates for institutional and social change. If aphasia intervention is to fully address functional communication, then the long-term consequences and the availability of community resources, services, and financial support must be considered and addressed.

This will require considerable adjustment to the institutional structures and service delivery models in most countries.

In the United States the acute stage of aphasia is the locus of most intervention and unfortunately the shrinking health-care dollar continues to limit available services at this stage. Yet, it is during the chronic stage that individuals with aphasia often learn the personal meaning of being aphasic in a communicating world. If a social model is appropriate, then support for managing the long-term consequences of aphasia must be expanded. Systems promoting socially responsible outcomes must not terminate with discharge from acute stage intervention. Rather, Pound's (1998) suggestion of "therapy for life" must be considered as a model of service delivery; intervention and support are offered at relevant periods as the individual lives with aphasia and encounters barriers to participation.

This ongoing system of intervention and support might entail expanding the responsibility for aphasia management beyond health care and into the realm of social and community services. Thus, supporting life with aphasia becomes the domain of community centers, recreation facilities and adult education, as well as health-care facilities. Such an approach will entail a constellation of services, some recognizable within the realm of therapy, and others falling more appropriately in opportunities for supported participation. Elman (1998) describes the need for an array of services for aphasia from which the individual might pick and choose from choices such as individual therapy, group therapy, supported conversation, recreational classes, counseling, prevocational training, self-help groups, and advocacy groups. Thus, services could be selected to suit the individual's needs and desires at any given time, rather than following the traditional linear approach.

Clearly the role of the speech–language pathologist must expand beyond traditional confines. Roles as consultants and collaborators will be expanded. To advance social approaches, aphasiologists will necessarily work at the level of community reintegration and define communication in terms of participation.

### Effectiveness of Social Approaches

While the tenets of a social approach are intuitively appealing, it is imperative that any approach be subjected to rigorous testing. While evidence of the success of social approaches is accumulating, there is work to be done. Two potential aspects for judging functional intervention include: (1) the approach improves the persons ability to perform activities that reflect physical, psychological, and social well-being and (2) the approach is judged relative to client satisfaction with the outcome and the level of functioning (Frattali, 1997). In addition, functional intervention might be judged by measures of increased participation in relevant activities. Thus, the outcome of a social approach is to improve quality of life and enhance participation in a communicating society. It is important to advocate for services that effectively address the social needs of people with aphasia, and devise methods for judging the outcome of these services. Creative approaches for turning the health-care crisis into an opportunity for change are emerging around the globe (e.g., Elman, 1998; Kagan, 1998; Lyon, 1997; Parr, 1996). Aphasiologists must not be complacent and resigned to do more with less. The movement toward a technology and philosophy dedicated toward functional, social outcomes in aphasia promises an exciting future.

## References

Alarcon, N., Hickey, E., Rogers, M., & Olswang, L. (1997). Family based intervention for chronic aphasia. Presentation at the Nontraditional Approaches to Aphasia Conference, Yountville, CA.

Armstrong, E. (1989). Conversational interaction between clinician and aphasic client during treatment sessions. Presentation at the American Speech–Language–Hearing Association Convention, St Louis, MI.

Armstrong, E. (1993). Aphasia rehabilitation: A sociolinguistic perspective. In A. Holland, M. Forbes (eds): *Aphasia treatment: World perspectives* (pp. 263–290). San Diego: Singular.

Bell, A. (1984). Language style as audience design. *Language and Society, 13,* 145–204.

Bernstein-Ellis, E., & Elman, R. (1995). A picture's worth a thousand questions: The use of a photo event journal with a severely aphasic patient and his spouse. Presentation at the Clinical Aphasiology Conference, Sunriver, OR.

Boles, L. (1997). Conversation analysis as a dependent measure in communication therapy with four individuals with aphasia. *Asia Pacific Journal of Speech, Language and Hearing, 2,* 43–61.

Brown, G., & Yule, G. (1983). *Discourse analysis.* New York: Cambridge University Press.

Brumfitt, S., & Clark, P. (1983). An application of psychotherapeutic techniques to the management of aphasia. In C. Code, D. Muller (eds): *Aphasia therapy* (pp. 89–100). London: Whurr.

Button, J., & Lee, J. (eds). (1987). *Talk and social organization.* Clevedon, England: Multilingual Matters.

Clark, H., & Wilkes-Gibbs, D. (1986). Referring as a collaborative process. *Cognition, 22,* 1–39.

Cohen-Schneider, R. (1996). Peer support and leadership training program for aphasic adults. Presentation at the American Speech–Language–Hearing Association Annual Convention, Seattle, WA.

Damico, J. (1992). *Whole language for special needs children.* Buffalo, NY: Educom Associates.

Davis, A. (1993). *A survey of adult aphasia and related disorders.* Englewood Cliffs, NJ: Prentice Hall.

Davis, A., & Wilcox, J. (1985). *Adults aphasia rehabilitation: Applied progamatics.* San Diego, CA: College Hill Press.

Demchuk, M. (1996). Creative communication in aphasia. Presentation at the American Speech–Language–Hearing Association. Seattle, WA.

Elman, R. (1998). Memories of the plateau: Health-care changes provide an opportunity to redefine aphasia treatment and discharge. *Aphasiology, 12,* 227–231.

Elman, R. (ed). (1999). *Group treatment of neurogenic communication disorders: The expert clinician's approach.* Boston: Butterworth-Heinemann.

Elman, R., & Bernstein-Ellis, E. (1999). The efficacy of group communication treatment in adults with chronic aphasia. *Journal of Speech–Language–Hearing Research, 42,* 411–419.

Ferguson, D. (1994). Is communication really the point? Some thoughts on interventions and membership. *Mental Retardation, 32,* 7–18.

Finkelstein, V. (1991). Disability: An administrative challenge. In M. Oliver (ed): *Social work, disabled people and disabling environments* (pp. 19–39). London: Jessica Kingsley.

Fox, L. (1997). The power to choose: Returning control to people with severe aphasia. Presentation at the Non-traditional Approaches to Aphasia Conference, Yountville, CA.

Frattali, C. (1992). Functional assessment of communication: Merging public policy with clinical views. *Aphasiology, 6,* 63–85.

Frattali, C. (1997). Measuring functional outcomes. Presentation at the American Speech–Language–Hearing Association and Annual Convention. Boston, MA.

French. S. (1993). What's so great about independence? In J. Swain, F. Finklestein, S. French, M. Oliver (eds): *Disabling barriers—Enabling environments* (pp. 44–48). London: Sage Publications.

Garrett, K., & Beukelman, D. (1995). Changes in the interactive patterns of an individual with severe aphasia given three types of partner support. In M. Lemme (ed): *Clinical Aphasiology, Vol. 23* (pp. 237–251). Austin, TX: Pro-Ed.

Giles, H., Taylor, D., & Bourhis, R. (1973). Towards a theory of interpersonal accommodation through language: Some Canadian data. *Language in Society, 2,* 177–192.

Goffman, I. (1967). *Interaction ritual.* New York: Pantheon Books.

Goffman, I. (1963). *Stigma: Notes on the management of spoiled identity.* New York: Touchstone.

Goldstein, K. (1939). *The organism: A holistic approach to biology derived from pathological data in man.* New York: American Book Co.

Gonzales-Rothi, L. (1996). The compromise of aphasia treatment: Functional and practical but realistic. *Aphasiology, 10,* 483–485.

Goodwin C. (1987). Forgetfulness as an interactive resource. *Social Psychology Quarterly, 50,* 115–131.

Goodwin, C. (1996). Transparent vision. In E. Ochs, E. Schegloff, S. Thompson (eds): *Interaction and grammar* (pp. 370–404). Cambridge: Cambridge University Press.

Gumperz, J. (1982). *Language and social identity.* Cambridge: Cambridge University Press.

Halliday, M. (1985). *An introduction to functional grammar.* London: Edward Arnold.

Hesch, D. (1998). Beyond the plateau: Discharge dilemmas in chronic aphasia. *Aphasiology, 12,* 207–243.

Holland, A. (1998). Why can't clinicians talk to aphasic adults? Clinical Forum. *Aphasiology, 12,* 844–847.

Holland, A. (1991). Pragmatic aspects of intervention in aphasia. *Journal of Neurolinguistics, 6,* 197–211.

Hough, M., & Pierce, R. (1994). Pragmatics and treatment. In R. Chapey (ed): *Language intervention strategies in adult aphasia,* 3rd ed. (pp. 246–268). Baltimore: Williams & Wilkins.

Ireland, C., & Wotton, G. (1993). Time to talk. ADA counseling project. Department of health report. London: Action for Dysphasic Adults.

Jordan, L., & Kaiser. W. (1996). *Aphasia—A social approach.* London: Chapman & Hall.

Kagan, A. (1995). Revealing the competence of aphasic adults through conversation: A challenge to health care professionals. *Topics in Stroke Rehabilitation, 2,* 15–28.

Kagan, A. (1998). Supported conversation for adults with aphasia. Clinical Forum. *Aphasiology, 12,* 816–830.

Kagan, A., & Gailey, G. (1993). Functional is not enough: Training conversation partners for aphasic adults. In A. Holland, M. Forbes (eds): *Aphasia treatment: World perspectives* (pp. 199–226). San Diego: Singular.

Kagan, A., Winckel, J., & Shumway, E. (1996a). *Pictographic communication resources.* Toronto, Canada: Aphasia Centre North York.

Kagan, A., Winckel, J., & Shumway, E. (1996b). Supported conversation for aphasic adults: Increasing communicative access (Video). Toronto, Canada: Aphasia Centre North York.

LeDorze, G. (1997). Towards understanding communication in communication disorders such as aphasia. Presentation at the Nontraditional Approaches to Aphasia Conference, Yountville, CA.

LeDorze, G., & Brassard, C. (1995). A description of the consequences of aphasia on aphasic persons and their relatives and friends, based on the WHO model of chronic diseases. *Aphasiology, 9,* 239–255.

LeDorze, G., Croteau, C., & Joanette, Y. (1993). Perspectives on aphasia intervention in French-speaking Canada. In A. Holland, M. Forbes (eds): *Aphasia treatment world perspectives* (pp. 87–114). San Diego: Singular.

Lubinski, R. (1981). Environmental language intervention. In R. Chapey (ed): *Language intervention strategies in adult aphasia,* 1st ed. (pp. 223–245). Baltimore: Williams & Wilkins.

Lyon, J. (1995). Drawing: Its value as a communication aid for adults with aphasia. *Aphasiology, 9,* 33–94.

Lyon, J. (1997). Treating real life functionality in a couple coping with severe aphasia. In N. Helm-Estabrooks, A. Holland (eds): *Approaches to treatment in aphasia* (pp. 203–239). San Diego: Singular.

Lyon, J., Cariski, D., Keisler, L., et al. (1997). Communication partners: Enhancing participation in life and communication for adults with aphasia in natural settings. *Aphasiology, 11,* 693–708.

McCabe, A. (1994). Assessment of preschool narrative skills. *American Journal of Speech–Language Pathology, 3,* 45–56.

Milroy, L., & Perkins, L. (1992). Repair strategies in aphasic discourse: Towards a collaborative model. *Clinical Linguistics and Phonetics, 6,* 27–40.

Newhoff, M., & Apel, K. (1990). Impairments in pragmatics. In L. LaPointe (ed): *Aphasia and related neurogenic language disorders* (pp. 221–234). New York: Thieme.

Oelschlaeger, M., & Damico, J. (1998). Joint productions as a conversational strategy in aphasia. *Clinical Linguistics and Phonetics, 12,* 459–480.

Paschalska, M. (1993). The concept of holistic rehabilitation of persons with aphasia. In A. Holland, M. Forbes (eds): *Aphasia treatment: World perspectives* (pp. 145–176). San Diego: Singular.

Parr, S. (1996). Everyday literacy and aphasia: Radical approaches to functional assessment and therapy. Clinical Forum. *Aphasiology, 10,* 469–503.

Parr, S., & Byng, S. (1998). Breaking new ground in familiar territory. Clinical Forum. *Aphasiology, 12,* 847–850.

Parr, S., Byng, S., Gilpin, S., & Ireland, C. (1997). *Talking about aphasia.* Buckingham, UK: Open University Press.

Penn, C. (1998). Clinician–researcher dilemmas: Comment on supported conversation for adults with aphasia. Clinical Forum. *Aphasiology, 12,* 839–843.

Porch, B. (1981). *Porch Index of Communicative Ability, Administration Scoring and Interpretation. Vol. 2.* Palo Alto, CA: Consulting Psychologists Press.

Pound, C. (1997). Social model approaches to aphasia and disability. Presentation at the Nontraditional Approaches to Aphasia Conference, Yountville, CA.

Pound, C. (1998). Therapy for life: Finding new paths across the plateau. *Aphasiology, 12,* 222–227.

Shiffrin, D. (1987). *Discourse markers.* New York: Cambridge University Press.

Silvast, M. (1991). Aphasia therapy dialogues. *Aphasiology, 5,* 383–390.

Simmons, N. (1993). *An ethnographic investigation of compensatory strategies in aphasia.* Ann Arbor, MI: University Microfilms International.

Simmons, N., Kearns, K., & Potechin, G. (1987). Treatment of aphasia through family member training. In R. Brookshire (ed): *Clinical Aphasiology Conference Proceedings* (pp. 106–116). Minneapolis, MI: BRK.

Simmons-Mackie, N. (1993). Management of aphasia: Towards a social model. Workshop presented at the Julie McGee Lambeth Conference, Denton, TX.

Simmons-Mackie, N. (1994). Treatment of aphasia: Incorporating a social model of communication. Workshop presented at the Aphasia Centre North York, Toronto, Canada.

Simmons-Mackie, N. (1998a). A solution to the discharge dilemma in aphasia: social approaches to aphasia management. Clinical Forum. *Aphasiology, 12,* 231–239.

Simmons-Mackie, N. (1998b). In support of supported communication for adults with aphasia. Clinical Forum. *Aphasiology, 12,* 831–838.

Simmons-Mackie, N., & Damico, J. (1995). Communicative competence in aphasia: Evidence from compensatory strategies. *Clinical Aphasiology, 23,* 95–105.

Simmons-Mackie, N., & Damico, J. (1996a). Accounting for handicaps in aphasia: Communicative assessment from an authentic social perspective. *Disability and Rehabilitation, 18,* 540–549.

Simmons-Mackie, N., & Damico, J. (1996b). The contribution of discourse markers to communicative competence in aphasia. *American Journal of Speech Language Pathology, 5,* 37–43.

Simmons-Mackie, N., & Damico, J. (1997a). Reformulating the definition of compensatory strategies in aphasia. *Aphasiology, 8,* 761–781.

Simmons-Mackie, N., & Damico, J. (1997b). Support for nontraditional management of aphasia: Evidence from conversation analysis. Presentation at the Nontraditional Approaches to Aphasia Conference, Yountville, CA.

Simmons-Mackie, N., & Damico, J. (1999). Social role negotiation in aphasia therapy: Competence, incompetence and conflict. In D. Kovarsky, J. Duchan, M. Maxwell (eds): *Constructing (in)competence: Disabling evaluations in clinical and social interaction* (pp. 313–342). Mahwah, NJ: Erlbaum.

Simmons-Mackie, N., Damico, &., & Nelson, H. (1995). Interactional dynamics in aphasia therapy. Presentation at the Clinical Aphasiology Conference, Sunriver, OR.

Tannen, D. (1984). *Conversational style: Analyzing talk among friends.* Norwood, NJ: Ablex.

Tannen, D. (1986). *That's not what I meant.* New York: Ballantine.

Thompson, C. (1989). Generalization in the treatment of aphasia: A review of the literature. In T. Prescott (ed): *Clinical Aphasiology,* vol. 18 (pp. 195–222). Boston: College Hill.

Wahrborg, P. (1989). Aphasia and family therapy. *Aphasiology, 3,* 479–482.

Weniger, D., & Sarno, M. T. (1990). The future of aphasia therapy: More than just new wine in old bottles? *Aphasiology, 4,* 301–306.

Wilcox, J., & Davis, A. (1977). Speech act analysis of aphasic communication in individual and group settings. In R. Brookshire (ed): *Clinical aphasiology conference proceedings* (pp. 166–174). Minneapolis: BRK.

World Health Organization. (1980). *International classification of impairments, disabilities and handicaps.* Geneva: Author.

World Health Organization. (1997). ICIDH-2 international classification of impairments, activities and participation. [http://www.who.ch/programmes/mnh/mnh/ems/icidh/icidh.htm]. (Beta-1 draft for field trials.)

Worrall, L. (1992). Functional communication assessment: An Australian perspective. *Aphasiology, 6,* 105–111.

Zangwill, O. (1947). Psychological aspects of rehabilitation in cases of brain injury. *British Journal of Psychology, 37,* 60–67.

# SECTION 3

# *Assessment and Treatment of Functional Communication in Specific Populations*

# 11

# The Influence of Professional Values on the Functional Communication Approach in Aphasia

## LINDA E. WORRALL

**Aphasiology has a rich history of functional communication assessment and treatment. This chapter examines the professional values that guide a consumer-driven, goal-orientated functional intervention for aphasia. Shared decision-making, individualization, social justice, the strengths perspective and goal attainment scaling are all explored within the context of the phases of therapy. The profession of speech-language pathology needs to debate its professional values and these are offered as some of the principles of the functional approach.**

## Introduction

Functional communication assessment and therapy were described in Chapter 1 using the World Health Organization's (WHO's) International Classification of Impairments, Activities, and Participation—the ICIDH-2. The functional communication approach was seen to encompass two dimensions of the ICIDH-2, with the Activity and Participation dimensions being targeted. While many speech–language pathologists are familiar with assessment and therapy at the Activity level, working within the Participation dimension is less familiar. This chapter seeks to draw together elements of the Activity and Participation dimensions by incorporating several social model values into existing Activity-based functional communication assessment and therapy processes. The chapter therefore seeks to provide some guidelines on how an integrated mode of practice within functional communication can be achieved via a set of principles, values, or beliefs that guide the therapist along each step of the therapeutic process.

The process of functional communication therapy described in this chapter is a personal reflection on the underlying values that have guided the author's assessment and treatment of clients over the years.

The functional communication therapy described here is designed for individual clients. There are, however, many advantages to providing functional communication therapy in groups. Holland states that previously she considered group therapy as a useful adjunct to individual therapy, but now considers the reverse to be true (Holland & Ross, 1999). Ross, who co-authored the chapter and has aphasia himself, supports the need for group treatment by stating that he sensed that he did not get better until he met others with the same problem. He and his colleagues state that joining a group is the most important thing a stroke survivor can do. However, the clinician may deliberately choose to provide therapy on an individual basis because of the unique needs of the client or there may be practical constraints in a facility such as not enough suitable clients for group therapy. It is argued that a combination of group and individual therapy is ideal so that individual needs and group membership needs are met. The principles outlined in this chapter, however, are mostly appropriate for individual therapy.

This chapter draws heavily from the philosophy and value system of social work. It therefore seeks to apply many aspects of the social model to the discipline of speech–language pathology. The values of social work that will be explored within a functional communication context are: shared decision-making, individualization, social justice, and the strengths perspective (an approach in which the client's strengths are used to optimize therapy). Accountability will also be explored in the context of the consumer-driven goal-oriented therapy described in this chapter. These professional values will be discussed within the context of each phase of client management—goal setting, preservice evaluation, service provision and postservice evaluation. While the case examples in this chapter are of clients with aphasia, the principles of professional values should apply to other types of communication and swallowing disorders.

## Why Professional Values or Beliefs are Important to Functional Communication Therapy

Several authors of chapters in this book including Parr and Byng (Chapter 4), Lyon (Chapter 9), and Simmons-Mackie (Chapter 10) have argued for an increased understanding and adoption of the principles of the social model in speech–language pathology. One of the most convincing reasons for the inclusion of the social approach into speech–language pathology is that the social model of disability stems from the views of disabled people themselves.

It could be argued that professional values should guide speech–language pathology practice in a general sense, that is, they should not apply specifically to the functional communication approach. It is argued, however, that professional values are grounded in the Participation dimension of the functional communication approach. The Participation dimension of the ICIDH-2 encompasses societal values. Professional values stem from the social model of disability and therefore fit firmly within the Participation dimension. Therefore, the influence of professional values is more pronounced in, but not restricted to, the functional communication approach.

To illustrate the concepts within the social model, Jordan and Kaiser (1996) contrast the features of the social model with the more familiar medical model. The contrasting features begin with disability being seen as a "problem" in the medical model, whereas the social model views disability in a positive framework. The medical model infers that the main source of problems for people with a disability is their impairment, whereas the social model refers to a disabling society. That is, the problem rests with society in that it is not sufficiently inclusive of people with a disability. The focus of policy within a social model is equal opportunity for people with a disability and the focus of intervention is on removing barriers to participation. The medical model, however, emphasizes treating at the level of the impairment and improving functioning. A further contrast of the two approaches is how services are determined. Self-determination is valued highly within the social model, while in the medical model, the services are generally determined by the health professional.

Many speech–language pathologists have strong roots in the medical model and find that the social model challenges their attitudes and values. While it is important not to discard the benefits that a medical model brings to the profession, it is also vital that the profession adopts the social model to a far greater degree than it has to date. As Oliver (1996) notes, there has been limited impact of the social model of disability on the consciousness, let alone practice, of many professionals, apart from social work. Because the social model of disability stems from the views of disabled people themselves, it is imperative that this be a focus of any health system. To adopt the approach advocated by the disability movement, health professionals themselves must re-examine their own value system. It is for this reason that this chapter attempts to integrate social values with the conventional Activity-based functional communication approach.

Health professionals such as speech–language pathologists are not philosophers by nature, however because they enter into people's lives in a real way, they become involved in philosophical issues about the nature of human living (Biestek, 1961). Debate about the value system or philosophies of speech–language pathologists has not readily occurred, yet for many years, social workers have attached much importance to a set of principles that guide their practice and inform their decision-making. Hepworth and Larsen (1982) state that "Values of a profession refer to strongly held beliefs about people, preferred goals for people, preferred means of achieving those goals, and preferred conditions of life. Stated simply, values represent selected ideals as to how the world should be and how people should normally act" (p. 20). While it is not suggested that speech–language pathologists adopt another profession's values or even that all speech–language pathologists adhere to the same set of values, becoming explicit about an underlying value system can help elucidate the perspective and approach of the clinician.

The remainder of this chapter describes a set of values, beliefs, or principles that have guided my practice of the functional communication approach. These five beliefs have guided a type of functional communication therapy that is highly consumer-driven and goal-oriented. Each principle or belief is discussed

Table 11–1.   Guiding Principles for the Phases of Functional Communication Therapy

| Guiding Principles | Phases of Therapy | Description |
| --- | --- | --- |
| Shared decision-making | Goal setting | Therapist *facilitates* the client's own goal setting |
| Individualization | Preservice evaluation | Assessment of the performance of the client *on their stated goals* |
| Social justice and the strengths perspective | Service provision | Provision of treatment or a service aimed at *meeting the goals of the client* |
| Accountability | Postservice evaluation | Outcome measurement in terms of *whether the client's goals were met* |

within the phases of functional communication therapy outlined in Worrall (1995, 1999).

## Phases of Therapy

Worrall (1995) described a series of steps for planning functional communication therapy for individual clients. The steps involved were determining the everyday communicative needs of the client, collaborative goal setting, prioritizing their goals, observing and rating their performance in everyday communicative activities, profiling the results, implementing therapy and reassessing goals, and finally measuring the outcome or change to ratings. Taking into account the more recent emphasis on social models of disability, these steps have been revised and simplified into a four-step process. Table 11–1 describes each step and offers some guiding principles behind each step.

## Step 1: Goal Setting

As a general rule, speech–language pathologists have not viewed goal setting as the initial step and have proceeded directly to an initial communication or swallowing assessment procedure. Many speech–language pathologists, however, have recognized the value of involving the client directly in setting goals. This in turn directs the selection of assessment procedures. For example, if a client wishes to improve his or her speech or language skills, then impairment-based assessments should be included in the test battery. If the client wants to answer the telephone, then an Activity-based and Impairment-based measure might be used. If, on the other hand, a client wants to resume an active social life, then a measure of social participation as well as other measures would be essential. An issue that speech–language pathologists need to address in goal setting is whether we, as a profession, believe that our clients have a right to self-determination.

Self-determination dictates that the power of decision making rests with the person with a disability who may use the health professional as a resource. At the basis of this principle is the belief that clients not only has the right and need to make decisions that affect them, but also that self-determination can be extremely beneficial to the outcome of the service provided. As Biestek (1961) observed "casework treatment is (was) truly effective only when the client made his own choices and decisions" (p. 101).

Mindful of Meinhert et al.'s (1994) assertion that values are malleable and variable and that words and labels will vary in meaning from situation to situation and from person to person, it is important to differentiate some possible constructions of the term "self-determination" within the context of speech–language pathology. The speech–language pathology literature contains many examples of the assertion that a clinician must first assess the client's needs and involve the client in the discussion of these needs; however, it is suggested that this process is not an example of self-determination.

"Needs" in speech–language pathology have been determined through a variety of approaches. First, "needs" can be assessed at the impairment level via a standardized test. Impairment-level needs, such as the ability to name objects, comprehend sentences or produce intelligible polysyllabic words, could be determined to be the client's needs. This is discussed with the client to gain cooperation in the tasks that follow. This is definitely not self-determination. In this case, the power rests with the "expert" and the client undertakes a course of treatment prescribed by the clinician. Many speech–language pathologists will identify with this model of practice that is grounded in the medical model.

In an earlier publication (Worrall, 1995), a collaborative approach to functional communication was described. The assessment process was called the Everyday Communicative Needs Assessment (ECNA). The assessment process arose out of an earlier study (Smith, 1985) in which it was found that people with aphasia had many and varied everyday communicative needs or activities and skills that they wanted to resume. Hence, in the ECNA, the collaborative discussion of functional goals with the client was a move toward shared decision-making. Self-determination, however, had not been fully operationalized. In offering a menu of potential activities that the client may need to do, the ECNA had restricted the client's choice to a list of activities that were perceived to be relevant to the client. Hence, clinician bias was implicit in the assessment process.

Charles et al. (1997) use the term "shared decision-making" to describe the approach advocated in this chapter. It is a collaborative decision-making arrangement where power is shared between the clinician and the patient. They distinguish this approach from three other types of decision-making. The first is the paternalistic model in which the patient merely gives consent to a treatment with no recognition of the patient's wishes. The second, the professional-as-agent model, recognizes the input of the patient in the process but ultimately the outcome or decision is the responsibility of the clinician. The third, the informed-decision making model, is the closest concept to complete self-determination, where the patient is entirely responsible for making a decision once all the necessary information is provided. Shared decision-making, in which the clinician and client reach a consensus about the preferred treatment approach after information is shared between the two participants, is the closest model to the approach advocated here.

While shared decision-making could be described as power sharing in the relationship between clinician and client, in contrast, complete self-determination requires that the power in the relationship is shifted to the client. Coulter (1997) reviews the evidence for and against shared decision-making. In particular, Coulter examines claims that clients do not want to make decisions, that information about risks and uncertainties can be harmful, that providing relevant information to clients is too time-consuming and costly, and that some clients will demand too much in this process. While in general these concerns are not supported, Coulter also points to a lack of available evidence in many areas. For speech–language pathologists, it is noteworthy that age and educational qualifications are two criteria that affect client's preference for information and involvement in decision-making. Older clients are more willing to trust the decision-making ability of the clinician, while more highly educated clients will want greater involvement in decision-making.

In speech–language pathology, it is often difficult to facilitate decision making and to confirm decisions with people who have a speech and/or language impairment. With severely communication disordered individuals, there is sometimes the question of the client's competency to make decisions as result of accompanying cognitive deficits. As a general rule, however, competency should always be assumed unless evidence suggests otherwise. This is consistent with the approach advocated by Kagan and Gailey (1993), which is based on the belief that all people with aphasia are competent to make their own decisions in a "supported conversation" environment. Hence, the clinician who adopts the principle of shared decision-making must believe that his or her client is competent to determine goals of intervention and will provide the support necessary to enable this process.

It should be noted that shared decision-making does not restrict the person's goals to within a functional framework. It can include goals from the Impairment dimension as well. The principle of shared decision-making stems from a social model of disability but the outcome in terms of the type of intervention chosen by the client is not limited to any particular model or dimension.

In summary, a person with a disability must have the right to be involved in shared decision-making. Biestek (1961) goes so far as to suggest that "conscious, wilful violation of the client's freedom by a caseworker is an unprofessional act which transgresses the client's natural right and impairs casework treatment or make it impossible" (p. 101). Hence, one of the first questions that clients should be asked is "What do you want to achieve by coming here?" What follows in the interview is a probing of the client's values and preferences, information sharing about services, treatments and assessments, and negotiation about what will be provided or achieved. While some clients respond well to this form of interview, other clients prefer to be more passive recipients of treatment. This is their choice, and this too should be respected.

### Step 2: Preservice Evaluation

Another cardinal value of the social work profession is individualization. As Butrym (1976) points out, the principle is derived from the uniqueness of the individual. In practical terms, Butrym states that "failure to recognize that every human situation is also unique, that no two problems are alike, and to see that situation or problem through the eyes of the person who is experiencing it, constitutes a denial of that uniqueness and detracts from the respect due to the individual" (p. 50). In the following section, it will be proposed that conventional functional communication therapy does not accommodate individual differences particularly well.

In a conventional functional approach, a standardized measure of functional communication is generally administered first. However, in an audit of speech–language pathology files of people with aphasia in Brisbane et al. (1990) found that no standardized functional assessments had been administered to the 68 aphasic people in the study. Smith and Parr (1986) found that many therapists preferred to use informal observations of functional communication skills. This may reflect some of the limitations of standardized functional communication assessments for planning functional communication therapy for individual clients. Standardized functional communication assessments may not assess the ability of the client in his or her specific area of need. Communicative activities such as reading knitting patterns or chairing meetings are typically not included in standardized functional communication assessments because they are highly individualistic.

An approach that emphasizes individualism is to assess the performance of the patient only on tasks related to the stated goals of the patient. Hence, the items will vary from patient to patient. This consumer-driven approach is advocated by Beukelman et al. (1984) and Worrall (1995). The evaluation process of the Everyday Communicative Needs Assessment (Worrall, 1995), which later became the Functional Communication Therapy Planner (Worrall, 1999) is an example of this type of approach that responds to individual differences.

An example of the process behind the Functional Communication Therapy Planner—FCTP (Worrall, 1999) is provided by the following case example. One of our clients with long-standing aphasia who attends our university clinic, wanted to use public transport so that he was not housebound when his partner was at work. This was to become a major focus of therapy for a few months. To measure the outcome of therapy, it was inappropriate to simply rate his abilities on all 43 items of the ASHA FACS. It was also inappropriate to use the Communicative Abilities in Daily Living (CADL) or the Communicative Effectiveness Index (CETI) that does not include this scenario or item.

The logical pretreatment and post-treatment evaluation in this case was to assess this client's ability to take a return journey on a bus. Because the client still had some difficulties with balance and walked with a stick, we decided to simulate the tasks with real-life materials rather than assess in the real world although real-life observation is generally far more preferable. The goal was subdivided into a number of tasks: reading the bus schedule, waiting for the bus at the correct time at the correct place, identifying the correct bus destination, paying the fare, asking the driver to wait until he sat down before moving off, recognizing his destination, and indicating to the driver that he wished to get off. These tasks also had to be repeated for the return journey. We used materials familiar to the client and relevant to the task. The client brought in the local bus schedule and he selected the destination that he most wanted to reach. The client used his own money to pay the correct fare for the journey and maps were used as prompts for locations of bus stops. Each task was rated on a 7-point multidimensional scale of communicative effectiveness with the ratings from 4 to 7 representing adequate abilities (i.e., he was successful in the task) and ratings of <4 reserved for inadequate performance of the task. The difference between ratings was dependent upon the degree of independence shown, the efficiency of the performance, and the appropriateness of communication in the task.

This approach is similar to the situation-specific therapy described by Hopper and Holland (1998). They differentiated situation-specific therapy to the process-based approaches such as facilitating naming strategies. The measure chosen for the two single-subject experimental designs of Hopper and Holland (1998) included trained and untrained sets of pictures of emergency situations. The task was for the aphasic person to state the nature of the emergency to a stranger on the phone, replicating the local emergency or 911 procedure. Both subjects' ability to verbally express simulated emergencies on the phone improved over the 10 sessions of therapy. Hence, the evaluation procedure in this study was situation-specific and focused only on the target of treatment.

In summary, a preservice evaluation that focuses on the individual goals of clients recognizes and respects the principle of individualism. The FCTP (Worrall, 1999) describes one method whereby specific communicative activities of clients can be determined, evaluated, treated, and re-evaluated.

## Step 3: Service Provision

Within the treatment phase, there are two principles that guide intervention: the "strengths perspective" and the principle of social justice. While the strengths perspective can be applied to the Activity and Participation dimensions of the ICIDH-2, the principle of social justice drives the Participation dimension in particular.

### The Strengths Perspective

The strengths perspective (Saleeby, 1997) is another guiding philosophy of social work that may be useful to speech–language pathologists. Saleeby states that the strengths perspective is when everything you do in practice is focused on "helping to discover and embellish, explore and exploit clients' strengths and resources in the service of assisting them to achieve their goals, realize their dreams, and shed their irons of their own inhibitions and misgivings" (p. 3). This positive approach to service provision epitomizes the flexible, consumer-driven, goal-oriented approach to functional communication therapy described in this chapter. In this section, services that are aimed at the Activity dimension will be described.

A description of Activity-based treatment in which the strengths perspective was used is briefly described. In terms of theoretical background to the treatment, the ICIDH-2 states that the use of personal and nonpersonal aids can be a natural part of performing an activity, hence, treatments at the Activity level might focus on the use of personal and nonpersonal aids. In the example of our client who wanted to take a bus journey, a personal aid might be his wife who assists him with the complex bus schedule. A nonpersonal aid would be a card that would be shown to the bus driver; for example, with the message that he needed time to sit down before the bus moved off. Other strategies such as buying a bus pass instead of using money for fares, are relevant compensatory strategies. Frequently, clients themselves have found solutions to everyday difficulties. It is often a matter of supporting clients through the problem-solving process to encourage them to create their own solutions, to attempt the task, and enjoy the challenge. As proponents of the strengths perspective have often stated, people have an innate capacity to go from strength to strength. Encouraging the individual to participate within a group of people with similar disabilities who have a positive outlook and who have succeeded in some areas is another effective method of facilitating an individual's strengths.

## Social Justice

Within the participation dimension, there is the opportunity not only to focus on the interaction between the individual and society, but also to influence society so that it is more inclusive of individuals with communication disorders generally. For example, in the earlier case example, as an intervention strategy, we could have sought to increase all bus drivers' awareness or understanding of passengers with communication disabilities. This may have not only benefitted our client but also assisted a range of other people with a communication disorder who use buses as a means of transport.

As noted earlier, the social model of disability revolves around the notion that society is not sufficiently inclusive of people with disabilities, that the focus of intervention should be on breaking down barriers to participation at a societal level. In the field of communication and swallowing disorders, achieving equal opportunity in terms of access to appropriate services and resources is a major challenge to achieving optimal participation. Hence, another guiding principle in service provision using a social model is the principle of social justice. Long-held concerns expressed by speech–language pathologists, that people with communication disorders were not sufficiently heard in society, fall under the umbrella of social justice. Activities such as advocacy and publicizing communication disorders are legitimatized in terms of social justice. These professional activities should be thought of as targeting the Participation dimension for clients.

Jordan and Kaiser (1996) note that the low level of understanding about aphasia in society has far-reaching implications. The same could be said about all communication disorders. The implications of this low level of understanding include the poor development of services to people with communication disorders. Poor levels of service provision are often based on inadequate collection of health statistics. Low levels of understanding of communication disorder by people in society also present as barriers to participation by people with communication disorders.

Jordan and Kaiser (1996) describe two situations in the United Kingdom in which barriers to participation were present. In one situation, the barriers were overcome by the speech and language therapist who provided information about aphasia to the professionals involved in a court proceedings (e.g., police, prosecutor, and judge). In particular, the speech and language therapist provided information about how to communicate effectively with the witness who was aphasic following an assault. The second situation did not have such a successful outcome. This was a situation in which a highly articulate person with aphasia was confused by the length and complexity of sentence structure of an interviewer on radio. While the task of raising awareness of communication disorders is most effectively conducted by professional organizations and organizations representing disabled people themselves, individual speech–language pathologists need to involve themselves in activities that raise public awareness of communication disorders. It should be seen as a legitimate part of their role, especially when it is in connection with reducing the barriers faced by individual clients.

Communication-disordered individuals often utilize a range of community resources to participate fully in society. Resources may include self-help groups, community programs, information, or specialist skills. Using a social model approach, speech–language pathologists often link their clients with community resources, if they are indeed available. Hepworth and Larsen (1982) suggest some resource utilization objectives that attempt to facilitate the interaction between individuals and society. These objectives provide speech–language pathologists with a framework for practice when linking communication-disordered individuals to resources in society. The first objective is to help people gain better coping and problem-solving skills. The strengths perspective can be applied here. The second objective is to help people obtain resources. Hence the speech–language pathologist's role is to refer people with communication disorders to existing resources and in the likely event that these are not available, assist in the development of these resources. The third objective is to make organizations responsive to people. Speech–language pathologists need to be aware of discriminatory policies, dehumanizing procedures or inappropriate behaviors and attitudes of others. Another objective is to facilitate interactions between individuals and others in society, as in the court room case described above. This can be accomplished through training of conversational partners (Kagan & Gailey, 1993) or through being the direct link in the chain by acting as a "translator" for the client. Mediating between organizations and influencing policy are further objectives within this framework of practice.

In summary, speech–language pathology services need to encourage social reform, lessen barriers that individual clients face, and support the use of clients' own strengths to seek solutions. The Activity and Participation dimensions can therefore be targeted in therapy.

### Step 4: Postservice Evaluation

Finally, another professional value that guides practice is the need for accountability. There is increasing pressure on clinicians to collect outcomes data as part of their routine clinical practice and Frattali (1998a) states that cost pressures are driving the need for outcomes data. Hesketh and Sage (1999) define a speech–language pathology outcome as the attributable effect of an intervention on a heath state where health is broadly meant to include physical and psychological well-being as well as satisfaction and attitudes to the service. They note that outcome can be measured at three different levels: for individuals, for a service, and for the entire population. Frattali (1998b) suggests that there are three desired outcomes for speech–language pathology clients: modality-specific behaviors, functional abilities, and quality of life.

Enderby (1999) suggests that many clinicians hope to avoid the fashion of outcome measurement by keeping their heads down. Enderby, like others who advocate the use of outcome measures, urges speech–language pathologists to embrace the topic of outcome measurement as a means of improving the quality of our services. Holland (1999) presents another perspective that argues that speech–language pathologists should encourage consumerism in our clients by informing them of the outcome of services. This is consistent with the philosophy of the consumer-driven functional communication approach advocated in this chapter. This approach views outcome measurement as a means whereby clients can be more involved in decisions about service provision. It also encourages consumers to be informed about the outcome of the service that they have received. Hence, accountability to the client is a belief that is embedded in this consumer-driven approach. In practical terms, this means that the therapist's and client's perception of change on stated therapy goals are sought and discussed. A tool for measuring change in performance as a result of therapy is Goal Attainment Scaling, particularly if a goal-orientated approach to therapy has been adopted.

Kiresuk and Sherman (1968) first proposed goal attainment scaling (GAS) as a measure of outcome in community mental health programs. The method gained popularity in the 1970s and then after a decline, its popularity increased again due to the need for quick and simple outcome measures that measure the effect of intervention. In a survey of aphasia therapists in Britain, Hesketh and Hopcutt (1997) reported that some therapists used goal attainment as an outcome measure. The process of GAS is that goals are jointly established with the client and levels of attainment are described. A score of "0" is given to the expected outcome while a score of +2 is given to the most favorable outcome and a score of −2 is given to the least favorable outcome. Intermediate levels (+1 and −1) are also described. Outcome for clients is then measured in relation to whether they reached their goals, while outcome measurement for a given population can be simply the proportion of clients achieving their goals or achieving more than their expected goals. An example of goal attainment scaling for a client is provided in Table 11–2.

One of the major advantages of GAS is that outcome is not based on a prescribed theoretical construct. As can be seen in Table 11–2, goals can be from diverse models of practice targeting different dimensions of disablement. It is therefore particularly suitable for the diverse nature of rehabilitation.

GAS also uses the goals established by the client, therefore the goals are relevant and meaningful to the client. As Dillon et al. (1997) note, a radical approach to developing self-report measures of outcome is to allow clients to develop their own. This ensures that the client and the therapist are not answering a multitude of items that are not relevant to their situation. In addition, the system of precisely describing goals and scaling attainment levels helps the therapist focus on the exact targets of intervention. Goals attainment scaling therefore is a method for measuring outcome regardless of the model of rehabilitation used.

Table 11–2.   An Example of Goal Attainment Scaling for an Adult Client

| | Goal 1:<br>Catching the Bus | Goal 2:<br>Buying a Birthday<br>Gift for His Wife | Goal 3:<br>Participating in<br>Social Functions of<br>Previous Employer |
|---|---|---|---|
| Most favorable outcome (+2) | Able to use the bus without assistance without error all of the time | Able to surprise wife with a gift that he has bought | Client encouraged to attend by former colleagues and interaction enjoyed by all |
| More than expected outcome (+1) | Able to use the bus with the help of his wife without error all of the time | Able to buy gift with minimal help from his wife which does not spoil the surprise | Client encouraged to attend by former colleagues and inter-actions were mostly successful |
| Expected outcome (0) | Able to use the bus with the help of his wife with some errors some of the time | Able to buy gift with wife helping, but trying not to know what the gift is | Invitations to attend were received and accepted but conversations restricted to one or two well-meaning people |
| Less than expected outcome (−1) | Too much help required and too many errors made for continued use of the bus | Attempted to buy gift but wife had to complete the transaction | Invitations received but declined after unsuccessful attempts to interact with former colleagues |
| Least favorable outcome (−2) | Unable to use bus at all | Would not attempt the task | Invitation to attend not received |

GAS ensures that the effectiveness of the consumer-driven, goal-orientated therapy described in this chapter is sufficiently monitored. The principles of GAS fit well with our functional communication approach that emphasizes the setting of individual goals and the monitoring of the outcome of those goals.

## Conclusion

This chapter has described some principles that form the foundation of a model of practice that integrates the Activity and Participation dimensions of the ICIDH-2. The principles of the right of shared decision-making, individualism, social justice, the strengths perspective, and accountability are used to guide professional practice with people with communication disorders.

In practical terms, this means that the first questions that clients are always asked is "Why did you come to this clinic? What do you want to achieve from coming to speech therapy?" Discussion and negotiation about how these needs might be met then follow. Within the discussion, specific goals individual to the client are determined. If the goals are within the Activities dimension, then a menu of possibilities from the Functional Communication Therapy Planner (Worrall, 1999) are discussed with the client and their family. If participation is an issue with the client, then barriers to participation are identified and the client is made aware of community resources that are available. Some clients become aware of the injustices of society toward communication-disordered individuals and become involved in organizations that promote greater community awareness etc. Support of these organizations and individuals is viewed as being an essential part of the speech–language pathologist's role. The strengths perspective focuses clients on their strengths and works to their strengths so that treatment sessions are often problem-solving occasions in which clients are encouraged to initiate their own strategies and develop their own solutions and resources. Strategies that have been used by "successful aphasics" (i.e., those that are living well with aphasia) are suggested by either the speech–language pathologist or other members of the group, if group therapy is part of the service. Finally, ownership of baseline and outcome measures is shared between the clinician and the client. The client's perspective is taken into account and is used to reshape further directions in the client's therapy or reshape the service of the whole facility. This process encourages mutual respect between the therapist and the client and makes "therapy" as unique and exciting for the clinician as for the client.

The profession of speech–language pathology has been encouraged to diversify its scope of practice for some time. New theoretical models (e.g., cognitive neuropsychological models of language processing, or physiological models of speech processing) have encouraged us to be more specific when describing the breakdown at the impairment level and functional approaches and social models have forced many clinicians to take a broader view of the client. Underlying each approach is a set of values.

As a profession, our values should be debated and shared and, if possible, a consensus reached. This chapter has described a set of values used to guide functional communication therapy and has advocated that the profession needs to strive to have clinicians whose values encompass the principles of shared decision-making, individualism, social justice, the strengths perspective and account-ability. However, as Hepworth and Larsen (1982) note, it must be recognized that a profession is made up of individuals and it is the right of individuals to operate from different value perspectives. Speech–language pathologists should accord colleagues who differ on certain value positions, the same respect, dignity, and right to have different perspectives that would be accorded clients. In this con-text, the principles of practice described in this chapter are those of an individual clinician based predominantly on experience of what has made a difference to people's lives.

## Acknowledgment

The author wishes to acknowledge the assistance and contributions of Jenny Egan, a social worker and a speech-language pathologist, to this chapter.

## References

Beukelman, D. R., Yorkston, K. M., & Lossing, C. A. (1984). Functional communication assessment of adults with neurogenic disorders. In A. S. Halpern, M. J. Fuhrer (eds): *Functional assessments in re-habilitation.* Baltimore, MD: Paul H. Brooks.

Biestek, F. P. (1961). *The casework relationship.* London : Allen & Unwin.

Butrym, Z. T. (1976). *The nature of social work.* London: Macmillan.

Charles, C., Gafni, A., & Whelan, T. (1997). Shared decision-making in the medical encounter: What does it mean? (or it takes two to tango). *Social Science and Medicine, 44,* 681–692.

Coulter, A. (1997). Partnerships with patients: The pros and cons of shared decision-making. *Journal of Health Services Research and Policy, 2,* 112–121.

Dillon, H., James, A., & Ginis, J. (1997). Client Orientated Scale of Improvement (COSI) and its rela-tionship to several other measures of benefit and satisfaction provided by hearing aids. *Journal of the American Academy of Audiology, 8,* 27–43.

Enderby, P. (1999). For richer for poorer: Outcome measurement in speech and language therapy: A commentary on Hesketh and Sage. *Advances in Speech–Language Pathology, 1,* 63–65.

Frattali, C. M. (1998a). Outcomes measurement: Definitions, dimensions, and perspectives. In C. M. Frattali (ed): *Measuring outcomes in speech–language pathology* (pp. 1–27). New York: Thieme.

Frattali, C. M. (1998b). Measuring modality-specific behaviours, functional abilities, and quality of life. In C. M. Frattali (ed): *Measuring outcomes in speech–language pathology* (pp. 55–88). New York: Thieme.

Hepworth, D. H., & Larsen, J. A. (1982). *Direct social work practice: Theory and skills.* Homewood, IL: Dorsey Press.

Hesketh, A., & Hopcutt, B. (1997). Outcome measurement for aphasia therapy: It's not what you do, it's the way that you measure it. *European Journal of Disorders of Communication, 32,* 198–203.

Hesketh, A., & Sage, K. (1999). For better, for worse: Outcome measurement in speech and language therapy. *Advances in Speech–Language Pathology, 1,* 37–45.

Holland, A. L. (1980). *Communicative abilities in daily living.* Baltimore, MD: University Park Press.

Holland, A. L. (1999). Consumers and functional outcomes. *Advances in Speech–Language Pathology, 1,* 51–52.

Holland, A. L., & Ross, R. (1999). The power of aphasia groups. In R. Elman (ed): *Group treatment of neurogenic communication disorders: The expert clinician's approach.* Boston: Butterworth-Heinemann.

Hopper, T., & Holland, A. (1998). Situation-specific training for adults with aphasia: An example. *Aphasiology, 12,* 933–944.

Jordan, L., & Kaiser, W. (1996). *Aphasia: A Social Approach.* London: Chapman & Hall.

Kagan, A., & Gailey, G. (1993). Functional is not enough: training conversation partners for aphasic adults. In A. Holland, M. Forbes (eds): *Aphasia treatment: World perspectives.* San Diego: Singular Publishing Group.

Kiresuk, T. J., & Sherman, R. E. (1968). Goal attainment scaling: A general method for evaluating com-prehensive community mental health programs. *Community Mental Health Journal, 4,* 443–453.

Meinhert, R. G., Pardeck, J. T., & Sullivan, W. P. (1994). Issues in social work: A critical analysis. West-port, CT: Auburn House.

Oliver, M. (1996). Forward. In L. Jordan, W. Kaiser (eds): *Aphasia: A social approach*. London: Chapman & Hall.

Saleebey, D. (ed). (1997). *The strengths perspective in social work practice: Second edition*. New York: Longman.

Skinner, C., Wirz, S., Thompson, I., & Davidson, J. (1984). *Edinburgh Functional Communication Profile*. Winslow, Bucks: Winslow Press.

Smith, L. E. (1985). Communicative activities of dysphasic adults: A survey. *British Journal of Disorders of Communication, 20*, 31–44.

Smith-Worrall, L. E., & Burtenshaw, E. J. (1990). Frequency of use and utility of aphasia tests. *Australian Journal of Human Communication Disorders, 18*, 53–67.

Smith, L., & Parr, S. (1986). Therapists' assessment of functional communication in aphasia. *Bulletin of the College of Speech Therapists, 409*, 10–11.

Worrall, L. E. (1995). The functional communication perspective. In D. Muller & C. Code (eds): *Treatment of Aphasia* (pp. 47–69). London: Whurr Publishers.

Worrall, L. E. (1999). *Functional communication therapy planner*. Oxon, UK: Winslow Press.

# 12

## Functional Communication in Cognitive Communication Disorders Following Traumatic Brain Injury

### Brigette M. Larkins
### Linda E. Worrall
### Louise M. H. Hickson

Traditionally, many functional approaches in traumatic brain injury rehabilitation have borrowed heavily from aphasiology. This chapter provides a rationale for the development of a unique functional approach for people with TBI. The attractiveness of the functional approach to payers is also explored from the perspective of the sole insurance agency for head injury in New Zealand. A study of the everyday communicative activities of New Zealanders with TBI describes the impoverished communication that occurs. Functional communication therapy approaches developed for TBI populations are also described.

A functional approach has particular relevance to the rehabilitation of people who have sustained a traumatic brain injury (TBI) for three main reasons. First, the cognitive-communication disorders associated with TBI tend to be long-standing, with the impairment persisting for many years. The chronic nature of the disorder necessitates the introduction of compensatory strategies for reintegration of the individual back into society. Second, the majority of people with TBI are young with many years of living, working and socializing ahead. These young people are frequently only beginning to develop life roles in society when the injury occurs. Hence, there is a particular need for programs that focus on the Participation level of the World Health Organisation's International Classification of Impairments, Activities, and Participation—ICIDH-2 (WHO, 1997; see Chapter 1) for this population.

Finally, the increasing number of individuals with TBI requiring rehabilitation, and the associated costs of such rehabilitation, have highlighted the importance of measuring functional outcomes of intervention with this population. Intervention goals that are functionally based are more meaningful to payers, and functional outcomes justify money invested, by specifying which activity limitations or participation barriers are targeted for improvement.

The first aim of this chapter is to elaborate on the rationale for employing a functional approach in speech-language pathology with this population by presenting the insurer's perspective. The second aim is to describe the influence of the cognitive-communication disorders associated with TBI at the levels of impairment, activity limitation, and participation restriction. This will draw heavily on an observational study of communicative activities of people with TBI in New Zealand. The third aim is to discuss the use of the functional approach in assessment and treatment of individuals with TBI. The lack of a specific functional communication assessment tool for people with TBI is seen as a major challenge in this area. We recommend an everyday observational approach as the key functional communication assessment. From the treatment perspective, a number of broad and specific functional approaches to intervention are described.

## *The Payer Perspective*

Over the last decade, third party payers have increasingly required functional improvement as a basis for reimbursement (Frattali, 1992). New Zealand is no exception. New Zealand, with a total population of approximately 3.75 million, is in the unusual position of having one primary, "no fault" (litigation is denied by law), insurer of its citizens. The Accident Rehabilitation and Compensation Insurance Corporation (ACC) is funded by contributions from every employer and employee, as drawn from road and government taxes. The purpose is to reduce the social, economic, and physical impact of personal injury on individuals and the community. On behalf of the New Zealand Government, the Corporation purchases rehabilitation services. It also provides weekly compensation, set at 80% of the individual's salary, until the individual regains employment. It is therefore crucial for the economic viability of the scheme, that a high proportion of injured individuals successfully return to work or achieve independence.

As a purchaser of functional assessment, ACC clarified its definition of the term functional (ACC/National Health Committee Guidelines for Brain Injury Rehabilitation, 1998). Functional refers to those activities necessary for an individual to participate (function) in his or her own daily living, work/play, social, academic, leisure, or family/community life. In order for a communication outcome (or indeed any outcome) to be considered functional it must pertain to an individual's everyday, real-world activities or behavior.

Functional communication assessment and the consequential functional objectives must therefore include three parameters as discussed below: (1) effectiveness as an outcome rather than technical correctness, (2) relevance to the individual, and (3) integration of the task into the individual's daily life activities.

Effectiveness refers to the way in which a behavior or goal is measured. It signals the importance of achieving successful communication regardless of the technical correctness (i.e., whatever means achieve the end). This coincides with the thinking of Holland (1982), who defined functional as "getting messages across in a variety of ways ranging from fully formed grammatical sentences to appropriate gestures, rather than being limited to the use of grammatically correct utterances" (p. 50). A communication activity would be considered effective therefore even if a device was used to compensate for the impairment. For example, an answering machine, which may be replayed frequently, could be used to compensate for an individual's slowed information processing. The functional outcome for the client is that telephone messages are understood.

Relevance to the individual emphasises the importance of choosing assessment and treatment outcomes that are meaningful to the individual. Determining an appropriate rehabilitation outcome requires considering issues relating to the cultural, social, and personal needs of an individual. From a cultural perspective in New Zealand, increasing eye contact with a speaker would not be a relevant rehabilitation goal for a Maori or Samoan citizen, yet may be appropriate for New Zealanders from other cultures (Metge & Kinloch, 1984). From a social and personal perspective, assessing oral reading would only be appropriate if an individual engages in this activity, and joke-telling would only be relevant to a premorbid raconteur (Elman & Bernstein-Ellis, 1995). Worrall (1995) argues that it cannot be assumed that there is a core set of communication activities in which all people engage and advocates that it is the individual's own communication environment, needs and activities that must be examined.

Integration of the task highlights the notion that activities are not a series of single components but events that interact. Telephoning, for example, is an integrated activity that requires planning, listening, and speaking as well as perhaps reading and writing. Performing a functional activity "involves a complex interaction between the entire cognitive mechanism, personality, and motivational variables, and the environment" (Ylvisaker & Szekeres, 1994, p. 550). While the individual's previous experience may at times provide a structure for regaining skills, when the situation is novel, he or she is unlikely to integrate and generalize the steps in a task without specific therapeutic support. Hagen (1981) reports that an increase in rate, amount, duration, or complexity of task stimuli will negatively influence the performance of individuals with brain injury. It is therefore important that integrated activities are rehearsed for everyday life.

### Cognitive-Communication Impairment Following TBI

The neuropathology of TBI involves injury that may be focal or diffuse. Focal contusions of the anterior and inferior frontal and temporal lobes occur in the majority of trauma cases (Adams et al., 1982; Ommaya & Gennarelli, 1994). The frontal lobes control higher human behavior "executive control" by regulating and integrating cognitive behavioral functioning (Hartley, 1995). Diffuse axonal injury is also a frequent neuropathological finding and results in complex and variable symptomatology. The injury sustained from a TBI therefore can be a mixture of (multiple) focal lesions and diffuse damage, potentially resulting in interruption of any aspect of cognitive and communicative functions. Prigatano et al. (1986) summarize these deficits as impaired ability in attention and concentration, initiation and goal direction, judgement and perception, learning, and memory, speed of information processing, and communication.

Cognitive and physical fatigue also accompany TBI and may be one of the most limiting effects of brain injury, influencing attention, memory, concentration, motivation, and perseverance. Gronwall et al. (1990) note that the individual may be restless, distractable, disorganized or abnormally loquacious. Mood may be exaggerated, with ready laughter or tears. The individual may be swift to argue, difficult to reason with, and may deny fatigue.

The unique sequelae of persons with TBI and their increased survival rates have necessitated the development of specialized brain injury rehabilitation programs in many developed countries of the world (Boake, 1990). Speech-language pathologists have a vital role to play in such programs and their valuable contribution to rehabilitation is becoming increasingly recognized worldwide.

Historically, the importance of speech and language deficits after brain trauma have been minimized and the literature pertaining to TBI has primarily focused on medical management (Groher, 1990). Communication and its role in total rehabilitation were treated in an accessory manner. This occurred because of the lack of accepted terminology to accurately describe the deficits, the paucity of empirical data about treatment efficacy, and the failure to believe that communication deficits secondary to brain trauma deserve special attention as a unique speech and language symptomatology.

Recent advances in the field however have addressed some of these issues. There has been consensus in use of terminology, for example, the commonly used term cognitive-communication impairment (ASHA, 1988). While there has been some, but not enough progress in treatment efficacy research for speech-language pathology following TBI, there remains some controversy about the relationship between language problems following diffuse brain injury and cognitive disruption (Hinchliffe et al., 1998).

Cognitive-communication disorders are prevalent impairments in TBI. Sarno et al. (1986) reported that 100% of 125 consecutive admissions with closed head injury to a rehabilitation facility had some disorder of language efficiency, of which only 37% could be described as aphasia. The characteristic communication profile resulting from TBI has been variously described in the literature. Halpern et al. (1973) reported on the language of confusion; Sarno (1980, 1984), subclinical aphasia; Hagen (1981), cognitive-language disorder; and Prigatano et al. (1986), nonaphasic language disturbances. As noted earlier, in 1988 the American Speech-Language-Hearing Association (ASHA) determined that the combination of characteristics associated with TBI be called cognitive-communication impairment. ASHA (1988) summarized the characteristics as:

- Disorganized, tangential, wandering discourse, including conversational, and monologic discourse (e.g., spoken or written narratives)
- Imprecise language and word retrieval difficulties
- Disinhibited, socially inappropriate language; hyperverbosity; ineffective use of social and contextual cues

or

- Restricted output, lack of initiation
- Difficulty comprehending extended language (spoken or written), especially under time pressure; difficulty detecting main ideas
- Difficulty following rapidly spoken language
- Difficulty communicating in distracting or stressful environments
- Difficulty reading social cues and flexibly adjusting interactive styles to meet situational demands
- Difficulty understanding abstract language, including indirect or implied meaning
- Inefficient verbal learning and verbal reasoning

### Communication at the Activity Level

One of the enigmas about communication following TBI, is that on the surface, the individual's basic language skills may appear intact (Clark, 1994). However, cognitive-communication disorders frequently affect activities that involve communication in a variety of ways (Marsh & Knight, 1991). Social interaction problems occur and may include difficulty initiating conversation, difficulty inhibiting socially inappropriate or impolite language, and difficulty interpreting social cues and roles (Ylvisaker & Urbanczyk, 1990). Wood (1987) describes how disinhibition following TBI leads to over-familiar language and tactlessness.

Using ethnographic methods, Larkins et al. (in press) compared the functional communication activities of 10 individuals who had sustained a TBI with 10 matched controls who had no injury. The types of communication activities, the range and frequency of activities, and the communication environments were investigated. Results obtained from 100 hours of real-life observation (5 hours per participant), communication diaries and participant questionnaires showed that the TBI group engaged in significantly fewer communication activities, had a restricted range of communication activities, and had fewer communication partners, than the control group. The most commonly occurring communication activity for all participants was social chat, defined as a conversation that was interactional rather than transactional, and served a social function associated with pleasure rather than work, that is, the type of communication that can maintain social relationships. Other commonly occurring activities for participants in both groups were telephoning, greeting, giving and receiving instructions, and asking for assistance.

The reasons for the activity limitations were not investigated in the Larkins et al. study, however the ICIDH-2 conceptual framework would suggest that the multitude of impairments associated with TBI such as problems with attention and concentration, initiation and goal direction, judgement and perception, learning and memory, speed of information processing and communication (Prigatano et al., 1986) would contribute significantly to the limitations in communication activity. In addition, giving support to the notion that the ICIDH-2 is not a uni-directional model, it would appear that the participation dimension was having a major impact on the communication activities of TBI participants. Many TBI participants did not have the opportunity to engage in some communication activities because they were not participating in an occupation, or in community or family life. The interaction between the dimensions of the ICIDH-2 provides support for the notion that rehabilitation should consider all dimensions at all times.

## Participation Level

Cognitive-communication disorders also can influence powerfully the success of the individual's social, academic or vocational reintegration or participation in society. Impaired communication interaction may create a negative impression on potential friends or employers, and poor self-awareness and unrealistic expectations may be the primary contributors to poor vocational adjustment.

Larkins et al. (in press) found that participants with TBI were often leading impoverished lives which excluded participation in many life roles. In turn, this influences communication opportunities and ultimately, may have an effect on mental health, well-being, and community integration. The individual's diminished self-awareness and inability to clearly appraise his or her own performance leads to reduced adherence to societal customs and rules, and possible isolation from family and friends. In addition, this lack of awareness means that the ramifications of post-injury changes to life goals are not fully acknowledged, leading to inability to accept assistance and feedback from others (Smith & Godfrey, 1995).

In recent years, the disability movement has gained momentum and there is a greater emphasis on individuals with disability participating in society. For example, wheelchair access to buildings is now mandatory in many countries (Seelman, 1996), and disability groups such as those with spinal cord injury and hearing impairment, lobby government for particular attention. Even within the disability movement however, the TBI survivor is marginalized. The cognitive-linguistic consequences of a brain injury frequently prohibit this group from advocating for themselves. Self-management and autonomy are difficult to attain when the consequences of the injury include reasoning difficulties and disrupted self-monitoring and information processing.

## Assessment Challenges

One of the difficulties facing functional communication assessment, has been the lack of an agreed conceptual understanding of what consititutes functional assessment. Hence, there has been a lack of a theoretical framework to guide the establishment of boundaries as to what is, and what is not, functional communication. There has been debate also as to whether discourse analysis and pragmatic analysis are functional communication assessments (Worrall, 1995). This debate has particular relevance to TBI, as pragmatic behaviors are often affected following TBI.

Functional communication assessments measure the effect of impairment on everyday life; consequently, the nature of that impairment is important. Functional communication assessments however have been devised primarily for aphasic stroke patients. As such, assessment tools have a linguistic emphasis rather than a cognitive-communication emphasis. The language disturbances following TBI are often not aphasia (Murdoch, 1996). While aphasia can occur following TBI, the majority of language disorders exhibited post-TBI differ in their pattern of language breakdown from aphasia (Holland, 1982). The test items in these assessments therefore may not always be relevant, nor sufficiently broad in scope, for use with individuals with TBI.

The more well known functional communication instruments such as the Functional Communication Profile (FCP: Sarno 1969), the Revised Edinburgh Functional Communication Profile (EFCP: Wirz et al., 1990), the Communicative Effectiveness Index (CETI: Lomas et al., 1989), the recently published Communicatiion Activities of Daily Living (CADL–2: Holland et al., 1999) are primarily applicable to adults with aphasia, although test data have often been collected on other populations such as those with TBI. The American Speech-Language-Hearing Association Functional Assessment of Communication Skills for Adults (ASHA FACS: Frattali et al., 1995) was designed to be applicable across a range of communication disorders and was initially standardized on both aphasia and TBI populations. There is however, a recognized need for additional functional communication items that probe critical thinking, problem solving and general higher-level abilities central to the communication concerns of the TBI group. Future research is necessary to determine if a functional communication assessment designed specifically for people with TBI is required. Ethnographic studies such as those undertaken by Larkins et al. (in press), which describe the communicative activities and participation of individuals with TBI, are a way of ensuring that the items in functional communication assessments capture the real-life communication of individuals with TBI.

In the absence of standardized functional communication tools designed specifically for TBI, the speech-language pathologist is advised to develop an individual assessment process that is structured to capture all the information required, yet flexible enough be sensitive to the social, cultural and/or environmental context of the assessment and the individual's communication needs within that context (Groher, 1990). Unlike impairment testing, functional communication assessment can take place anywhere. Functional communication can be evaluated just as easily in an acute care setting, a rehabilitation unit, a community center, the individual's home, at work or at a leisure location. Any standardized testing should be augmented by careful and ongoing observation, family and caregiver reports and an accurate premorbid history (Wilson & Moffit, 1984).

Observation of the individual with TBI in his or her natural contexts identifies the environmental factors influencing communication success or failure. Observation is as important as using standardized tests for assessing executive function (Lezak, in press), and perhaps is the best tool for measuring functional communication (Lomas et al., 1989), particularly in this population. Observation involves watching an individual and his or her interaction with the environment, recording communication behavior and then analyzing and interpreting that behavior. Field observation of functional communication has not been widely reported in the literature. Holland (1982) observed adults with aphasia for a 2-hour period each, to capture a representative sample of natural communication in normal family interactions. Prutting (1982) used 15 minutes of videotaped conversation when investigating the pragmatics of participants with head injury. Milroy (1987) recommends longer periods of observation that not only allow the observer to place the language in its situational context but also desensitises the individual to being watched.

As noted earlier, observation of communication can occur in any environment, but a sample of a variety of communication situations is recommended. A week-long communication diary kept by the client indicating the time, place, topic, and communication partners involved in the interactions will help determine the real-life communication situations that could be observed. Alternatively, an interview could identify the everyday environments within which the individual communicates, and the real-life situations in which communication is an issue. Other important aspects to note are the barriers to communication within the individual's environment, and the participation restrictions that might result from activity limitations or impairments. Once the situations are identified, the client is observed in the real-life situations preferably using a participant observer approach (Spradley, 1980). This approach creates a more natural environment because the observer participates in the activities that are appropriate to maintain natural communication. For example, during a visit to a café, an observer may also eat a meal, or use an exercycle when observing at the participant's gym. The essential features to isolate in any communication situation are the antecedents and consequences within the context of the environment. To identify important communication situations for each individual, observation checklists are available, such as those developed by Hartley (1995) and Worrall (1999). Worrall (1995) suggests that, to determine the relevance of each activity, four main questions need to be answered: (1) was the activity performed premorbidly?, (2) is it performed now?, (3) is the activity missed if it is not performed now?, and (4) why can't the individual perform the activity now? Answering these questions, and thus identifying activity limitations and participation restrictions, should lead to the identification of appropriate functional communication goals for therapy.

## Therapy Approaches

The primary goal of functional communication therapy is to identify and minimize those cognitive-communication factors that interfere with the individual's real-world activities and thus reduce barriers to participation in everyday life. The goal must be to rehabilitate people, not cognition (Ylvisaker & Urbanczyk, 1990). Utilizing regularly occurring everyday activities ensures the individual receives repeated practise, and the natural consequences of success further act to reinforce the relearned skill (Boake, 1990). At the activity and participation levels, the priority is to provide clients with community experiences similar to those they will encounter in everyday life. Therapy integrated into real-life experiences such as shopping, budgeting, workplace practises and social interaction enables individuals with brain injury to succeed at what they most want to do.

Table 12–1 shows the broad and specific approaches to functional communication treatment in TBI stemming from six general models of intervention described by Hartley (1995). Hartley (1995) describes models of intervention that

Table 12–1.   Functional Treatment Approaches in TBI

| General Models of Intervention (Hartley, 1995) | Broad Functional Approaches* (from Hartley, 1995) | Specific Functional Techniques |
|---|---|---|
| Facilitation-stimulation | | |
| Component process training | | |
| Environmental manipulation/ adaption | Environmental adaption | Communication partner training (Ylvisaker et al., 1993) |
| Compensatory strategy training | Compensatory strategy training | Conversational coaching (Ylvisaker & Holland, 1985) |
| Functional skills training Stimulus-response conditioning | Functional skills training | |

*Functional approaches have been identified from Hartley's six models of intervention using the three criteria of effectiveness, rather than technical correctness as an outcome, relevance to the individual, and integration into daily life activities.

target impairments, disability, and handicap. These include facilitation-stimulation, component process retraining, environmental manipulation or adaption, compensatory strategy training, functional skills training, and stimulus-response conditioning. Using the three criteria for functional objectives discussed earlier (i.e., effectiveness rather than technical correctness as an outcome; relevance to the individual; and integration into daily life activities), three of these models of intervention could be said to fall into the category of functional approaches for people with TBI: compensatory strategy training; environmental adaption; and, functional skills training. Using the ICIDH-2 framework, these approaches often overlap, targeting both Activity and Participation level goals. The rationale for these three broad approaches will be briefly described, and then two specific intervention techniques that may be applied in these approaches (communication partner training and conversational coaching) will be described in detail. Both of these specific techniques are described in more detail by Ylvisaker and Holland (1985) and Ylvisaker et al. (1993) and contain many practical suggestions of how a functional approach can be implemented for individuals with TBI. In addition, both techniques combined provide a comprehensive functional approach to intervention, because one technique focuses on the individual while the other focuses on the individual's environment. Therefore, it is recommended that the two techniques be combined for a comprehensive functional approach to TBI intervention.

## Broad Functional Intervention Approaches in TBI

COMPENSATORY STRATEGY TRAINING

Compensatory strategies may take two forms. It may be that the individual is taught compensatory techniques or that the environment is modified to provide compensatory alternatives (Ylvisaker & Holland 1985). Compensatory strategies are either external or internal. External aids may be the same as those utilized by noninjured persons, such as use of a diary. Internal aids range from self-cueing instructions to complex mental associations that may enhance comprehension or retrieval. Compensatory strategies for cognitive-communication disorders may need to be identified and implemented by the therapist initially, as self-derived strategies from individuals with TBI can be inefficient or maladaptive. Key phases in teaching compensatory strategies include the individual with TBI attaining a metacognitive awareness about their performance, valuing a strategic approach, selecting and practicing useful strategies and then applying these strategies in varied situations (Ylvisaker & Szekeres, 1994). As an example, a successful sales manager's oral communication was largely unimpaired following his TBI, however he retained chronic problems with memory, calculation, and written language. He employed a secretary to specifically support these disabilities and he remains in employment.

FUNCTIONAL SKILLS TRAINING

Generalization tend to be particularly difficult for persons with brain injury (Parente & Anderson-Parante, 1990). Wood (1987) emphasized the importance of teaching functional skills within the actual environment in which the skills will be utilized. Scott et al. (1983) detail components of successful generalization training. They recommend training with multiple and/or relevant persons, training significant others to deliver reinforcement, training in multiple settings and scenes, and scheduling regular booster sessions post-treatment. They also suggest that self-initiation of a strategy and self-monitoring are markers for success.

Hartley (1995) states that this approach is based on the assumption that functional skills can be improved through repeated practice and learning in real-life settings. Examples of treatment activities that use this approach are training in making telephone calls, writing checks, and conversing with others (Hartley, 1995).

ENVIRONMENTAL ADAPTION

There are a variety of techniques within this broad approach. An individual's behavior may be dramatically altered simply by environmental change. For example, a vocally aggressive individual in a busy hospital ward may become compliant in a quieter home-like environment. Diller and Gordon (1981) advocate the "engineer's model" of analyzing brain injury problems through observing how the interaction of the individual and the task creates difficulties. Wood (1987) extends this concept to addressing post brain trauma difficulties through investigating the interaction between the environment and individual. Simple removal or alteration of "triggers" can lead to a positive result. Heightening the awareness of triggers and providing management techniques becomes the therapy focus.

Hartley (1995) describes this approach as changing the environment so that the individual can perform adequately despite his or her impairments. The individual with TBI requires no learning, hence this approach is particularly suitable for those individuals with impaired new learning. Examples of specific treatment activities or techniques within this approach are establishing a quiet study area so that the person with attention deficits is not distracted (Hartley, 1995) or training conversational partners within the individual's environment as discussed in more detail later in this chapter (Ylvisaker et al., 1993).

## Specific Functional Techniques for TBI

### CONVERSATIONAL COACHING

Ylvisaker and Holland (1985) used the analogy of "coaching" to support two fundamental theses: that brain injury therapy includes all the elements of effective team coaching and that the most useful therapy outcome is for the clients to learn how to coach themselves. This utilizes the internal compensatory strategies mentioned earlier. This approach emphasizes skill transfer from the rehabilitation profession to the individual with brain injury. The approach focuses on coaching rather than caring because as Willer and Corrigan (1994) note, the medical model that uses caring may foster dependency. An example that contrasts caring with coaching is: after cooking a meal, a caregiver may turn off the appliance for the person with TBI, whereas a coach would ask "what needs to be done now?"

The coaching analogy involves supporting the individual with TBI to rehearse, and gain feedback. It also involves managed risk; allowing the person with TBI to trial independence yet maintaining a "safety net." Increasingly integrative and functional tasks are trialed under increasingly natural conditions. Real-life demands that the TBI survivor must face in his or her vocational, educational, or social life are used as challenges to be overcome.

Coaching, also known as "place and train" or "supported employment" is an established vocational rehabilitation practice in the management of individuals with TBI (Chan et al., 1991). A job coach should be a short-term measure until supports are naturally integrated into the workplace. Abrams and Haffey (1991) advocate employee or peer coaching, flexible schedules, or written/printed cues to guide task performance. They also report that an experienced job coach is a valuable means of breaking down attitudinal barriers in the workplace.

### COMMUNICATION PARTNER TRAINING

Ylvisaker et al. (1993) describe a social-environmental approach to intervention based upon the premise that increasing communication effectiveness of people with TBI is primarily a result of positive interaction with communication partners rather than specific tasks conducted in speech-language pathology sessions. Their functional approach involves targeting the everyday communication partners of people with TBI. They describe a comprehensive approach to communication partner training that extends beyond the traditional hour or two of in-service training. Their program was developed for rehabilitation facilities, however, the principles apply to those individuals receiving rehabilitation outside a specific

TBI rehabilitation facility. First, they maintain that a positive communication culture within the communication environment needs to be established. In this sense, the everyday communication partners of the person with the TBI need to share a set of values that include the notion that communication is central to satisfying interpersonal relationships. In rehabilitation facilities, communicative competence is written into the job descriptions of direct care staff. Once a positive communication culture is fostered, communication training may then involve an in-service lecture followed by interactive sessions with various communication partners. Importantly, situational coaching is offered to those who request it and those who require it. Ylvisaker et al. (1993) therefore provide a real-world perspective and practical suggestions on how to implement a socioenvironmental approach that recognizes the importance of communication partners in recovery from TBI.

In summary, three broad functional approaches to intervention have been described using Hartley's broad framework of intervention approaches in TBI. All approaches simultaneously target both Activity and Participation levels of the ICIDH–2. Two specific techniques have been described by Ylvisaker et al. that encompass all areas of the functional approach, are uniquely suited to clients with TBI, and contain sufficient practical detail for speech-language pathologists to implement in real-life settings.

## *Conclusion*

One of the major issues for individuals who have sustained a TBI is the ability to use language to form and maintain social relationships. The ICIDH–2 is a conceptual approach that assists with the analysis of the consequences of TBI. This framework allows the clinician to clarify and define functional outcomes that are of increasing relevance to payers and other stakeholders in care. Determining functional communication outcomes is an integral component of rehabilitation following TBI. "Functional" involves focusing on communication that is of cultural and social relevance to the individual. Success is marked by the achievement of the desired communication goal regardless of technical skill and, both assessment and therapy are conducted within the context of natural communication environments. This involves a focus away from specific components of linguistic elements toward naturalistic observation of integrated communication activities. In contrast to therapy efforts that focus exclusively on impairment restoration, this chapter has highlighted the importance of therapy that focuses on coaching the individual to communicate effectively in real-life situations and prepare communication partners in order to facilitate functional communication.

Those who survive a TBI face and accept many challenges. Speech-language pathologists must also be challenged by the need to develop and evaluate interventions that make a real difference in people's lives. The functional approach not only has the potential to provide interventions that make a difference, but also seems ideally suited to this population whose very impairments limit their ability to integrate information in the real world.

## *References*

Abrams, D. & Haffey, W. (1991). Blueprint for success in vocational restoration: the work reentry program. In B. McMahon, & L. Shaw (Eds.), *Work Worth Doing: Advances in Brain Injury Rehabilitation*, (pp. 221–244). Florida: Paul M Deutsch Press.

ACC and the National Health Committee. (1998). *Traumatic Brain Injury Rehabilitation Guidelines*, Wellington, New Zealand.

Adams, C., Graham, D., Murray, L. S., & Scott, G. (1982). Diffuse axonal injury due to non-missile head injury in humans: An analysis of 45 cases. *Annals of Neurology, 12*, 557–563.

American Speech-Language-Hearing Association (1988). The role of the speech-language pathologists in the identification, diagnosis, and treatment of individuals with cognitive-communicative impairments. *ASHA, 30*, 79.

Boake, C. (1990). Transitional living centres in head injury rehabilitation. In J. S. Kreutzer & P. Wehman (eds): *Community Integration Following Traumatic Brain Injury*, (p. 115–124). Baltimore: Paul H. Brookes.

Chan, F., Dial, J., Schleser, R., McMahon, B., Shaw, L., Marme, M., & Lam, C. (1991). An ecological approach to vocational evaluation. In B. McMahon, & L. Shaw (Eds.), *Work Worth Doing: Advances in Brain Injury Rehabilitation*, (pp. 117–133). Florida: Paul M. Deutsch Press.

Clark, L. W. (1994). Communication disorders: What to look for and when to refer. *Geriatrics, 49* (June), 51–57.

Diller, L., & Gordon, W. (1981). Interventions for cognitive deficits in brain injured adults. *Journal of Consulting and Clinical Psychology, 49*, 822–834.

Elman, R. J., & Bernstein-Ellis, E. (1995). What is functional? *American Journal of Speech-Language Pathology, 4*, 115–117.

Frattali, C., Thompson, C., Holland, A., Wohl, C., & Ferketic, M. (1995). American Speech-Language Hearing Association Functional Assessment of Communication Skills for Adults. Rockville, MD: ASHA.

Frattali, C. (1992). Functional assessment of communication: Merging public policy with clinical views. *Aphasiology, 6*, 63–83.

Groher, M. (1990). Communication disorders in adults. In M. Rosenthal, E. R. Griffith, M. C. Bond, & J. D. Miller (Eds.), *Rehabilitation of the Adult and Child with Traumatic Brain Injury* (2nd ed., pp. 148–162). Philadelphia: F.A. Davis.

Gronwall, D., Wrightson, P., & Waddell, P. (1990). *Head injury: The facts: A guide for families and caregivers.* Oxford: Oxford University Press.

Hagen, C. (1981). Language disorders secondary to closed head injury: diagnosis and treatment. *Topics in Language Disorders, 1*, 73–87.

Halpern, H., Darley, F. L., & Brown, J. R. (1973). Differential language and neurological characteristics in cerebral involvement. *Journal of Speech and Hearing Disorders, 38*, 162–173.

Hartley, L. (1995). *Cognitive-Communication Abilities Following Brain Injury. A Functional Approach.* San Diego: Singular.

Hinchliffe, F. J. Murdoch, B. E., & Chenery, H. J. (1998). Towards a conceptualisation of language and cognitive impairment in closed-head injury: Use of clinical measures. *Brain Injury, 12*(2), 109–132.

Holland, A. (1982). Observing functional communication of aphasic adults. *Journal of Speech and Hearing Disorders, 47*, 50–56.

Holland, A., Frattali, C., & Fromm, D. (1999). *Communication Activities of Daily Living.* Austin, Texas: Pro-Ed.

Larkins, B., Worrall, L. & Hickson, L. (in press). Everyday communicative activities of individuals with traumatic brain injury living in New Zealand. *Asia Pacific Journal of Speech, Language and Hearing.*

Lezak. M. D. (in press). Nature, applications & limitations of neuropsychological assessment following brain injury. In A. L. Christensen & B. Uzzell, *International Handbook of Neuropsychological Rehabilitation*. New York: Plenum.

Lomas, J., Pickard, L., Bester, S., Elbard, H., Findlayson, A., & Zoghaib, C. (1989). The communicative effectiveness index: development and psychometric evaluation of a functional communication measure for adult aphasia. *Journal of Speech and Hearing Disorders, 54*, 113–124.

Marsh, N. V., & Knight, R. G. (1991). Behavioural assessment of social competence following severe head injury. *Journal of Clinical and Experimental Neuropsychology, 13*, 729–740.

Metge, J. & Kinloch, P. (1984). *Talking Past Each Other, Problems of Cross Cultural Communication.* Wellington: Victoria University Press.

Milroy, L. (1987). *Language and Social Networks.* (2nd ed.). Oxford: Basil Blackwell.

Murdoch, B. (1996) Communication impairments following traumatic brain injury: the neglected sequelae. In J. Ponsford, P. Snow & V. Anderson (Eds.) *International Perspectives in Traumatic Brain In-*

*jury: Proceedings of the 5th conference of the International Association for the Study of Traumatic Brain Injury and 20th Conference of the Australian Society for the Study of Brain Impairment,* (pp. 280–290). Queensland: Australian Academic Press.

Ommaya, A. K., & Gennarelli, T. A. (1994). Cerebral concussion and traumatic unconsciousness. *Brain, 97,* 633–654.

Parente, R., & Anderson-Parante, J. (1990). Vocational memory training. In J.S. Kreutzer & P. Wehman (Eds.), *Community Integration Following Traumatic Brain Injury,* (pp. 157–168). Baltimore: Paul H. Brookes Publishing Co.

Prigatano, G., Roueche, J., & Fordyce, D. (1986). Nonaphasic language disturbances after brain injury. In G. P. Prigatano (Ed.), *Neuropsychological Rehabilitation After Brain Injury,* (pp. 18–28). Baltimore: John Hopkins University Press.

Prutting, C. (1982). Pragmatics as social competence. *Journal of Speech and Hearing Disorders, 47,* 123–133.

Sarno, M. (1969). *The Functional Communication Profile: Manual Of Directions.* New York: Institute of Rehabilitation Medicine.

Sarno, M. T. (1980). The nature of verbal impairment after closed head injury. *Journal of Nervous and Mental Disease, 11,* 685–692.

Sarno, M. T. (1984). Verbal impairment after closed head injury: Report of a replication study. *Journal of Nervous and Mental Disease, 172,* 475–479.

Sarno, M. T. Buonaguro, A., & Levita, E. (1986). Characteristics of verbal impairment after closed head injury. *Archives of Physical Medicine and Rehabilitation, 67,* 400–405.

Scott, R., Himadi, W., & Keane, T. (1983). A review of generalisation in social skills training: suggestions for future research. *Progress in Behaviour Modification, 15,* 114–167.

Seelman, K. (1996). Access. In *Congress Proceedings of the 18th World Congress of Rehabilitation International,* (pp. 89–94). Auckland, New Zealand.

Smith, L. M. & Godfrey, H. P. (1995). *Family Support Programs and Rehabilitation. A Cognitive-Behavioural Approach to TBI.* New York: Plenum.

Spradley, J. P. (1980). *Participant Observation.* New York: Holt, Rinehart & Winston.

Willer, B., & Corrigan, J. D. (1994). Whatever it takes: a model for community based services. *Brain Injury, 8*(7), 647–659.

Wilson, B., & Moffit, N. (1984). (Eds.) *Clinical Management of Memory Problems.* Rockville, MD: Aspen Systems Corp.

Wirz, S., Skinner, C., & Dean, E. (1990). *Revised Edinburgh Functional Communication Profile.* Tucson, Arizona: Communication Skill Builders.

Wood, R. L. (1987). *Brain injury rehabilitation: A neurobehavioural approach.* London: Croom Helm.

WHO (1997). ICIDH-2 International Classification of Impairments, Activities, and Participation. A Manual of Dimensions of Disablement and Functioning.Beta-1 draft for field trials. World Health Organization, Geneva. [http://www.who.ch/programmes/mnh/mnh/ems/icidh/icidh.htm]

Worrall, L. (1995). The functional communication perspective. In C. Code & D. Muller, *Treatment of Aphasia: From Theory to Practice,* (pp. 47–69). London: Whurr.

Worrall, L. (1999). *Functional Communication Therapy Planner.* Winslow Press: Bucks: UK.

Ylvisaker, M., Feeney, T. J., & Urbanczyk, B. (1993). A social-environmental approach to communication and behaviour after traumatic brain injury. *Seminars in Speech and Language, 14*(1), 74–86.

Ylvisaker, M., & Holland, A. L. (1985). Coaching, self coaching and rehabilitation of head injury. In D. F. Johns (Ed.), *Clinical Management of Neurogenic Communicative Disorders,* (pp. 243–257). Boston: Little Brown & Co.

Ylvisaker, M., & Szekeres, S. (1994). Communication disorders associated with closed head injury. In R. Chapey (Ed.), *Language Intervention Strategies in Adult Aphasia,* (4th ed.) (pp. 546–568). Baltimore: Williams & Wilkins.

Ylvisaker, M., & Urbanczyk, B. (1990). The efficacy of speech-language pathology intervention: traumatic brain injury. *Seminars in Speech and Language, 11,* 4, 215–266.

# 13

## A Framework for the Assessment and Treatment of Functional Communication in Dementia

### Rosemary Lubinski
### J. B. Orange

There has been a gradual development of specific communication assessments and interventions for people with dementia. This chapter reviews these approaches and then proposes the Wellness-to-Opportunity framework for a functional communication approach to dementia rehabilitation. A case example describes the practical application of the framework. The chapter concludes with an examination of the obstacles that face speech–language pathologists in implementing a functional approach in dementia.

### Introduction

Several realities face individuals with dementia and their caregivers.[1] First, dementia is a progressive disease that currently has no cure or remission. Declines across cognitive and social domains interfere with independent living and ability to communicate effectively. Second, these declines affect not only the individual, but also

---

[1]The terms "caregiver" and "care provider" are used interchangeably in this chapter and refer to family members or professionals who assume major responsibility for the care of the individual with dementia.

family members or other caregivers. Family members must cope with the incremental challenges of aging and dementia, and for some, the institutionalization of a loved one. These challenges are met by elderly spouses and adult children who come to the caregiving context with competing demands on their coping skills. Care becomes an all-consuming task often relegated to professional caregivers in long-term care settings. Third, maintaining effective communication skills as long as possible must be a priority if individuals with dementia are to receive quality care from family and professional caregivers. Quality care is more probable when individuals with dementia can express their needs and understand their caregivers' verbal and nonverbal communication. It also is more likely to occur when caregivers understand the importance of communication in the care process and are able to call upon a large repertoire of strategies available to facilitate interaction.

These realities translate into distinct challenges for clinicians and researchers interested in evaluating the communication of and providing services to individuals with dementia and their care providers. If the progression of dementia cannot be reversed, slowed, or stopped, what assessment and intervention protocols are appropriate and ethical? What approaches capture the everyday communication difficulties of individuals with dementia, especially in expressing their physical, emotional, and social needs? What approaches capitalize on maintaining and enhancing preserved abilities? What approaches engage care providers and significant others in their interactions with individuals with dementia? Finally, what documentation demonstrates clearly to care providers, researchers, clinicians, and third-party payers that progress (or lack of decline) has been achieved?

In the past 20 years, speech–language pathologists have advanced their understanding of the cognitive and communicative abilities of individuals with dementia. The seminal work of researchers such as Bayles et al. (e.g., 1987, 1992), Bond-Chapman et al. (1998), Ripich et al. (1991), and Ulatowska et al. (1988), and others shows the relationship between cognition and communication. Intervention approaches also have emerged, ranging from adaptations of approaches for individuals with aphasia or traumatic brain injury, indirect approaches that focus on environmental modifications and group programs based on preserved social/communicative skills, to reminiscence based therapies. What is essential is a framework that establishes a theoretically sound basis for assessment and intervention. The model must be functional in that it reflects the everyday needs of individuals with dementia and their communication partners; it must be transparent so that service payers can understand the underlying philosophy, importance, and relevance of assessment and intervention; and it must lend itself to evidence-based practices such that researchers and clinicians can easily and precisely document changes in performance or lack of decline in performance.

This chapter offers one conceptualization of assessment and intervention that is functional, empirically focused, clinician friendly, and evidence based. The chapter begins with a discussion of the nature of dementia and factors affecting assessment and intervention. A brief review of current assessment and intervention approaches to communication and dementia is presented along with a framework to structure assessment and intervention. A case example of how to apply the framework is presented. Finally, future needs of functional communication assessment and intervention approaches to dementia are discussed.

## Nature of Dementia

Dementia is an acquired syndrome characterized by chronic, progressive, and persistent declines in at least three of the following areas: memory, language and communication, visuospatial skills, personality, and cognition (e.g., reasoning, judgment) (Cummings et al., 1980). There are many different types of dementia. The most prevalent form is dementia of the Alzheimer's type (DAT), which accounts for 50 to 65% of all types (Canadian Study of Health and Aging Working Group, 1994; Gorelick & Bozzola, 1991). It is anticipated that the incidence and prevalence rates of DAT will escalate as the percentage of the older adult population increases. Other types of dementia include, but are not limited to, Pick's disease, vascular dementia, frontotemporal lobe dementia, Lewy body disease, semantic dementia, Jacob–Creutzfeldt disease, primary progressive aphasia, dementia associated with motor neuron disease (e.g., Parkinson's disease, Huntington's disease, amyotrophic lateral sclerosis, multiple sclerosis, progressive supranuclear palsy), and dementia associated with HIV infection, among others. Each type of dementia has a distinctive profile of cognitive, language and communication, behavior, personality, medical, and neuromotor features. It is beyond the scope of this chapter to review the language and communication features of each form of dementia. The reader is encouraged to seek more detailed overviews in works by Bayles and Kaszniak (1987), Lubinski (1995), and Ripich (1991).

The language and communication problems associated with dementia are well recognized and are estimated to occur in almost all individuals with dementia (Kempler, 1995). Studies of the experiences of care providers of individuals with dementia show high levels of psychological, emotional, social, and physical stress and burden (Mittelman et al., 1993; Mobily et al., 1992; Schulz & O'Brien, 1994; Wright, 1993). The literature also shows that communication difficulties are perceived by care providers of individuals with dementia to be a primary problem in coping with the disease, and that communication problems increase the risk of early institutionalization (Gurland et al., 1994; Richter et al., 1995; Williamson & Schulz, 1993). Findings also suggest that the negative influence of communication difficulties may be reduced when caregivers possess adequate knowledge of the nature of communication changes over the course of dementia (Clark, 1995). Speech–language pathologists must be prepared to develop and implement communication assessment and intervention programs for individuals with dementia that (a) assess impairment level and functional communication (including discourse and conversational performances); (b) capitalize on communication strengths and problem solving skills of caregivers; (c) target challenging behaviors of individuals with dementia that are communication related and that may contribute to increased levels of caregiver stress and burden; (d) respond to changes in communication over the course of the disease, and to changes in the contexts of care (e.g., home vs. institution; family vs. institutional caregivers; role changes of family caregivers); and (e) make adjustments in physical and psychosocial environments that support communication (Bourgeois, 1997; Clark, 1997; Lubinski, 1995; Tomoeda & Bayles, 1991).

## Review of Current Assessment and Intervention Approaches

Standardized assessments of the linguistic performance of individuals with dementia have been undertaken using traditional tests for aphasia, such as the *Boston Diagnostic Aphasia Examination* (Goodglass & Kaplan, 1983) and the *Western Aphasia Battery* (Kertesz, 1982). Other tests have been used to measure performances in domain-specific areas of language such as expressive and receptive vocabulary (e.g., *Boston Naming Test;* Kaplan et al., 1983; *Peabody Picture Vocabulary Test*–Revised; Dunn & Dunn, 1981) and auditory comprehension (e.g., *Revised Token Test;* McNeil & Prescott, 1978).

A test developed specifically to examine linguistic skills in dementia is the *Arizona Battery for Communication Disorders of Dementia* (ABCD) (Bayles & Tomoeda, 1993). The ABCD is a standardized test designed to profile the linguistic-communicative performance of individuals with early- and middle-stage DAT within the context of a cognitive memory-based model of communication. The ABCD is the current gold standard by which clinicians can differentiate the linguistic-communicative abilities of normal older adults from those who have DAT. The subtests of the ABCD are designed to profile different aspects of expressive and receptive linguistic-communication, along with mental status, declarative episodic memory, and visuospatial construction skills of older adults. The ABCD is standardized on older normal adults and individuals with DAT. It is a popular test among clinicians and researchers, and provides valuable diagnostic information, although it is less helpful for planning, implementing, and monitoring functional communication interventions.

The *Functional Linguistic Communication Inventory* (FLCI) (Bayles & Tomoeda, 1994), on the other hand, is a standardized test designed to document the everyday communicative performance of middle and late-clinical stage individuals with DAT. The FLCI is relatively easy to administer in a short period of time (~30 minutes). It contains 10 components that show older adults' abilities for greeting and naming, answering various types of questions (e.g., open-ended, multiple choice, Yes–No), writing, comprehending signs, matching objects to pictures, reading comprehension, reminiscing, following spoken commands, pantomiming and gesturing, and participating in a topic-directed conversation-like interaction. The test provides a percent correct profile across the 10 domains of functional communication. Normative data enable clinicians to compare performances of individuals with various severity levels of DAT. Moreover, scores can be used to determine strengths and weaknesses of functional communication, plan meaningful, everyday relevant communication interventions, and help guide clinicians in counseling family and professional care providers.

In addition to using measures of functional communication, clinicians should examine the discourse and conversational performances of individuals with dementia in a variety of contexts with several different partners. The current options of discourse protocols include nonstandardized checklists, questionnaires, and surveys that target broad areas of pragmatics, conversation, and discourse including narrative, procedural and expository discourse genres, and pseudo-conversational discourse in the form of extended monologues on topic-specific questions. Clinicians have been reluctant, however, to examine discourse and conversation of individuals with dementia because of the extensive time required to obtain and analyze the data. Recent work by Boles and Bombard (1998) shows that conversational discourse analyses of several measures (e.g., conversation repair, speaking rate, utterance length, speaking efficiency) can be completed quickly in reliable and valid ways using 5- to 10-minutes samples of conversation. Table 13–1 summarizes measures that have been reported in the literature and used to measure pragmatic, discourse, and conversation features of individuals with dementia. A more in-depth discussion of discourse and conversational analyses of older adults, including individuals with dementia, can be found in Bloom et al. (1994); Cherney et al. (1998); and Garcia and Orange (1996). Further, the review by Ripich (1995) provides a comprehensive overview of current communication assessment options for individuals with dementia.

The perceptions of care providers regarding the functional communication and conversation skills of individuals with dementia also must be obtained. Care providers' views provide a base against which clinicians can compare perceived versus tested versus observed performances. The authors of this chapter are in the process of developing such an instrument that examines caregivers' perceptions of the communication difficulties of dementia patients, strategies used to repair the difficulties, and the stress and burden experienced relative to communication difficulties.

Over the past decade, communication intervention for individuals with dementia have focused on strategies to facilitate word-finding skills (Palm & Purves, 1996); improve gestural communication (Hoffman et al., 1988); enhance pragmatic and discourse abilities through participation in socialization groups, activities of daily living, and reminiscence and life review groups (Boczko, 1994; Santo Pietro & Boczko, 1998; Zgola & Coulter, 1988); and reduce anxiety over past emotional crises (i.e., validation therapy) (Morton & Bleathman, 1991). Other approaches such as pet-, art-, massage-, and music-based therapies have been used to promote socialization and stimulate communication.

Communication education and training programs for family and institutional care providers have been developed over the past decade, some of which have been tested empirically. Bourgeois (1991), Clark (1995), and Ripich (1994) support the use of communication-enhancement programs for care providers so that they learn to change their role from an equal partner to a facilitator. They note that training should include learning how to create supportive communication environments and how to modify language use (e.g., using literal, less complex language, and asking fewer open-ended questions). Koury and Lubinski (1995) suggest that the best approach to such training is through role playing of communication scenarios. The reader is directed to more detailed discussions of communication interventions for individuals with dementia and their care providers by Clark (1995), Orange and Colton-Hudson (1998), and Koury and Lubinski (1995).

## A Functional Communication Framework

The information yielded from traditional impairment-based assessment of communication is just one part of the total picture of communication in dementia. Conventional tests do not assess dementia patients' abilities in daily-life situa-

Table 13–1. Summary of Selected Functional Communication Checklists, Questionnaires, and Inventories used for Individuals with Dementia*

| Features | Instruments | | | | | |
|---|---|---|---|---|---|---|
| | FLCI | DAP | PCA | CADS | RSCCD | PAC-D |
| Respondent and population | SLPs and other professionals familiar with dementia score performance of patients with moderate or late-stage dementia | SLPs and other clinicians score performance of individuals with dementia | SLPs rate performance of adults with neurogenic and cognitive-communicative disorders | Individuals self-rate and family caregivers rate aspects of functional communication | SLPs, other clinicians, and family caregivers rate communicative performance of individuals with dementia | SLPs rate pragmatic performance of moderate-severe patients with dementia using 10 common objects |
| Turn-taking | + | + | + | + | + | – |
| Topic | + | + | + | + | + | – |
| Repair | + | + | + | – | + | – |
| Speech acts | + | + | + | + | – | – |
| Linguistic level (cohesion, coherence, etc.) | – | – | – | – | – | – |
| Interactions with others (familiar vs. unfamiliar, groups, etc.) | – | – | – | – | – | – |
| Using and understanding emotions | – | – | – | + | + | – |
| Daily living (greetings, pain, etc.) | + | – | – | – | + | – |
| Using and understanding nonverbal behaviors | + | + | + | – | + | + |
| Using and understanding prosodic features | + | + | + | – | – | – |

Table 13–1. (Continued)

**Instruments**

| Features | FLCI | DAP | PCA | CADS | RSCCD | PAC-D |
|---|---|---|---|---|---|---|
| Respondent and population | SLPs and other professionals familiar with dementia score performance of patients with moderate or late-stage dementia | SLPs and other clinicians score performance of individuals with dementia | SLPs rate performance of adults with neurogenic and cognitive-communicative disorders | Individuals self-rate and family caregivers rate aspects of functional communication | SLPs, other clinicians, and family caregivers rate communicative performance of individuals with dementia | SLPs rate pragmatic performance of moderate-severe patients with dementia using 10 common objects |
| Naming | + | – | + | + | + | + |
| Writing | + | – | – | – | + | – |
| Reading | + | – | – | – | + | |
| Rating/Scoring system | subtest and total percentage scores compared with values from subjects with dementia | rate *present* or *absent* for features in narrative, procedural, and conversation genres; ratings (*excellent, good, adequate, fair, poor*) made for genre, general discourse, and overall performance; discourse profile generated from matrix using number of features present, and general discourse ratings | communicative competence rated on 5-item scale (from *appropriate* to *inappropriate*) for linguistic features in scales (*control of discourse, fluency, and global*) and subscales of interactive features | ratings for 26 items based on 5-point items (*almost always, usually, sometimes, rarely, almost never*); no indication that ratings are quantified | items in verbal and nonverbal domains rated as *normal* or *disordered* (*mild, moderate, severe, absent*); quantitative values assigned to each rating, and verbal and nonverbal subdomain and total ratings calculated | 1 point awarded for spontaneous verbal, functional holding, and gestural responses; 0.5 point awarded for correct response to model; total of 30 possible points |

| Psychometric properties | well-standardized; validity and reliability data published | small samples of normal elderly and early and middle stage Alzheimer's disease; no published validity or reliability data | nonstandardized, no published validity or reliability data | none published | validity, rater agreement, and reliability data published | none |

*Note:*

FLCI—Functional Linguistic Communication Inventory (Bayles & Tomoeda, 1994).

DAP—Discourse Assessment Profile (Terrell & Ripich, 1989).

PCA—Profile of Communicative Appropriateness (Penn, 1985).

CADS—Communication Adequacy in Daily Situations (Clark & Witte, 1991).

RSCCD—Rating Scale of Communication in Cognitive Decline (Bollinger & Hardiman, 1991).

PAC-D—Pragmatic Assessment of Communication—Dementia (England, O'Neill, & Simpson, 1996).

*Adapted from Garcia and Orange (1996).

tions, the strategies they or their communication partners use to maintain everyday communication, nor the impact of the communication difficulties on communication partners. What is needed is a framework for working with individuals with dementia that incorporates an understanding of neuropathological, cognitive, and communicative changes associated with aging and dementia and their relation to physical and social factors that influence communication. This framework should provide clinicians with guidance on how to assess individuals over time, across a variety of cognitive and communicative domains, and within different contexts (e.g., home vs. institutions). It should address the fact that communication is a dyadic process and that communication difficulties experienced by one person affect the other communication partner. The framework should also investigate approaches of evidence-based practice to help document change in performance over time. Finally, the framework should lead to practical suggestions that result in effective communication and improved quality of life for the person with dementia and the care provider.

The framework presented in this chapter makes several assumptions. First, functionality is best achieved when assessment and intervention are viewed as integrated. Assessment must have clear implications for treatment, and treatment must lead to continued assessment as the disease progresses.

Second, the framework focuses on the individual with dementia and his or her communication partners (usually caregivers) who will carry an increasing burden for initiating and maintaining communication.

Third, assessment and intervention are approached from a broad perspective that addresses physical, psychosocial, emotional, and cognitive abilities, and socioeconomic and cultural factors that influence communication.

Fourth, caregivers' perspectives are vital to effective assessment and intervention. Caregivers can provide valuable information regarding communication needs, successful strategies, and actions and environments that contribute to communication problems. For interventions to be effective, caregivers must understand the rationale for intervention, support its philosophy, and participate in the process. It is the caregivers who will be implementing suggestions, modifying them, and providing feedback to clinicians regarding their effectiveness.

Finally, a functional framework must generate numerous occasions and new opportunities for carryover of the various suggested strategies. Although strategies may be generated initially by the speech–language pathologist in consultation with caregivers and significant others, it is essential that caregivers generate new ways of achieving and maintaining communicative effectiveness. Interventions are functional when caregivers approach each communicative event with a positive problem solving attitude.

### "Wellness-to-Opportunity" Framework Requirements

One framework that meets the above requirements is the "Wellness-to-Opportunity" model (Fig. 13–1). It is adapted from earlier work by Lubinski (1988, 1995) on the communication needs of elders and from a model for a comprehensive communication enhancement program for individuals with Alzheimer's disease by Orange et al. (1995). There are four modules to the framework: wellness, skill,

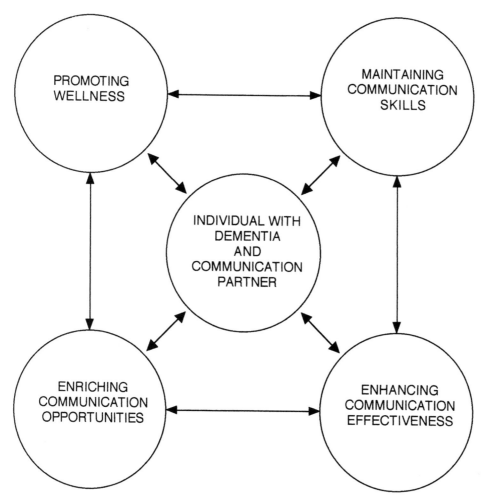

**Figure 13–1.**  Wellness-to-Opportunity framework for functional communication in dementia.

effectiveness, and opportunity. Taken together, they form a functional approach to communicative assessment and intervention for individuals with dementia and their caregivers.

Our framework maintains that assessment and intervention are more functional when the patient and care provider are included and integrated in the process. The framework emphasizes a positive approach in that it focuses on maximizing existing abilities of the individual with dementia and his or her communication partners. Inherent in the framework are opportunities to support communication partners and reinforce their problem-solving abilities. It is comprehensive in that it addresses not only the needs and abilities of the person with dementia and caregiver, but also the physical and social environments in which they communicate. Moreover, the framework considers the maintenance of self-esteem and personhood as a result of individualized assessment and intervention programming. Finally, it is functional in the traditional sense in that the assessments and interventions are relevant to everyday functioning.

Although presented in a linear fashion, the framework is cyclical in design. A dementia patient's needs at any point in time may require integration and repetition of one or more modules of the framework. Note also that the dementia patient and caregiver are at the center of the framework, further emphasizing the necessity to focus on both communication partners.

### Promoting Communication Wellness

In 1981, representatives at the White House Conference on Aging defined health for older individuals as "the ability to live and function effectively in society, to exercise self-reliance and autonomy to the maximum extent feasible, but not necessarily total freedom from disease" (Minkler & Fullarton, 1980, p. 4). This definition is a cornerstone of the wellness approach to health for older persons. It takes a holistic approach that maximizes functional ability, prevents or minimizes disabilities, and maintains dignity toward the end of life (Walker, 1992). Clark (1986) further defined wellness as a process of moving toward greater awareness of and satisfaction from engaging in activities that promote fitness, positive nutrition, positive relationships, stress management, clear life purpose, consistent belief systems, commitment to self-care, and environmental sensitivity/comfort (p. 12). Wellness approaches are based on individuals maintaining healthy lifestyles and relationships through education, self-empowerment, and access to appropriate care.

These same principles can be applied to promoting functional and effective communication between individuals with dementia and their caregivers. Promoting the wellness of the individual with dementia and the caregiver helps create a positive physical and psychological environment where the individual can mobilize personal resources to cope with the challenges of dementia. Individuals who strive to be healthy will want to communicate and work to maintain communication as long as possible.

The first component of the wellness module that can be adapted to promoting functional communication is knowledge about the nature of dementia. Some family members are quite able to describe the communication problems associated with the onset and progression of dementia and acknowledge that these problems contribute to caregiving difficulties (Bayles & Tomoeda, 1991; Orange, 1995; Powell et al., 1995). Family members, however, may not understand the extent of the changes or the link between these changes and cognitive decline. When families are knowledgeable about dementia, they are more likely to assess their relative's needs, be able to provide valuable information to guide clinical assessment, and are more likely to assume responsibility for maintaining communication.

Based on family members' descriptions of recent changes and their perceptions of current behaviors, the clinician might ask a variety of questions that focus on the nature of dementia, the communication problems that are occurring, the strategies that facilitate communication, and the impact of the communication problems on the caregiver and patient. Sample questions are provided in the Appendix for each of the modules of the Wellness-to-Opportunity framework.

Knowledge about dementia is improved via educational programs that combine didactic information with practical problem-solving opportunities. Didactic information might address the nature of dementia, its effects on communication, and the importance of communication in maintaining independence, safety, and socialization. Such information might be supplemented with movie and video presentations and suggested readings. Problem solving is stressed in several types of programs including discussions following video presentations, role-playing sessions, peer discussion sessions, and group focus sessions. Recent work by Ripich et al., (1995), Arkin (1996), Orange and Colton-Hudson (1998), and Santo Pietro and Ostuni (1997) show that education and training programs can enhance overall communication between individuals with dementia and their care providers.

The second element of the wellness model, which has relevance to functional communication, is the promotion of health and fitness. Elders with dementia and their caregivers need to maintain their ability to send and receive messages as competently as possible. This will involve having regular physical examinations with their primary-care physician to identify any potential complicating medical conditions that might compromise communication and therefore warrant treatment. Ramsdell (1990) details the scope of health-care maintenance programs for older individuals.

Communication effectiveness also involves regular hearing and vision screenings to identify and remediate age- and medically related sensory problems. Both senses contribute to cognitive and social stimulation, promote safety, and enhance communicative interaction. Vision and hearing problems are frequently of insidious onset among the elderly and are often overlooked during routine medical visits even though the prevalence of both problems is high. About one in every six persons over the age of 65 years is either blind or has a severe vision impairment. This proportion increases to one in four for those over 85 years (Flax et al., 1993). Hearing loss is the third most prevalent chronic disability among older adults, third only to arthritis and hypertension (Binnie, 1994; Haber, 1994). The prevalence of hearing loss among older adults ranges from 40% to as high as 90% for individuals living in nursing care institutions (Glass, 1990; Schow & Nerbonne, 1980).

Hearing loss among those with dementia is also common and more severe than among age-matched older persons without cognitive decline (Uhlmann et al., 1989; Weinstein & Amsel, 1986). Further, some elders with and without dementia have additional difficulty with central auditory processing that presents particular problems in speech comprehension in normal and degraded listening conditions (Grimes, 1995).

Individuals with dementia, along with their caregivers will be better able to participate in conversations when they can adequately hear and see. A hearing screening involves five components: (a) clinician subjective assessment of difficulties attributable to hearing difficulty; (b) asking the dementia patient and caregiver about their perceived hearing difficulties; (c) performing a pure tone hearing screening; (d) performing impedance testing; and (e) otoscopic examination of the external ear, auditory canal, and tympanic membrane.

The clinician should begin by noting behavioral signs during informal conversation that might indicate a hearing problem. Common symptoms include frequently asking for repetition, mishearing information, carefully watching the speaker's face during interaction, responding inappropriately, and monopolizing turns in conversation. The clinician might also ask the individual with dementia (i.e., primarily individuals in the early clinical stage) or caregiver to complete a self-assessment inventory to identify their perception of any possible hearing problem and its impact on everyday life. Two of the most commonly administered self-assessments are the Hearing Handicap Inventory (Ventry & Weinstein, 1982) and the Self-Assessment of Communication (Schow & Nerbonne, 1982). Both are brief and standardized, although neither is designed specifically for those with dementia. The speech–language pathologist should be prepared to discuss the importance of having a hearing screening performed by a qualified audiologist and to recommend sites where such screenings can be done. The reader is referred to Grimes (1995); Kricos and Lesner (1995); Lichenstein et al. (1991); Pichora-Fuller and Cheesman (1997); and Weinstein (1997) for in-depth discussions of hearing assessment of the elderly and those with dementia.

Speech–language pathologists should also be aware of the possible vision difficulties of elders. Signs and symptoms of potential eye problems include decreased, double, or blurred vision, loss of depth perception, difficulty recognizing colors, vision field changes or neglect, sensitivity to glare, discharge, redness of eye or lids, bulging of eye, headaches, and complaints of eye pain, discomfort, or fatigue. Individuals with diabetes and a family history of eye disease are at particular risk for eye problems. As with hearing problems, elders should be referred to their physician for assessment and appropriate intervention. (See Schumer, 1997 for a more in-depth discussion of vision changes with aging.)

Another aspect of enhancing wellness is to help elders with dementia and their caregivers identify potential activity patterns in their environment. The value of physical exercise for elders is well documented and is considered a critical component to wellness approaches to health maintenance (Walker, 1992). Friedman and Tappen (1991) have suggested that walking has beneficial effects not only on health and physical fitness but also on communication, although their conceptualizations and trial were not well-grounded or controlled (see Orange & Ryan, 1992). Increased mobility will also focus discussion on safety features of the environment. Thus, the clinician might ask the caregiver and dementia patient about their daily living schedules, access to activities of choice, and physical, social, and emotional obstacles that might prevent such access. See Appendix for interview questions that focus on activity patterns.

The fourth component of the wellness framework is rewarding social roles and relationships. Communication is more likely to occur when individuals have meaningful social roles and participate in a variety of activities. Aging in itself is likely to eliminate or change accustomed roles related to work, family life, and leisure. It becomes even more complicated for those with dementia and their family caregivers. For example, some individuals with dementia who want to participate in familiar social activities may be excluded because of perceived incompetence. Others may not have social opportunities available, and this deprivation leads to an increased loss of social skills. Some elders with dementia will have supportive and frequent opportunities for one-on-one and group activities. Finally, the social opportunities of the caregivers may also become restricted as their relative's dementia progresses and caregiving responsibilities increase. Social roles and relationships can be investigated through a series of questions posed to the caregiver and dementia patient. See Appendix for sample questions.

Assessment of social roles and relationships will likely lead to the need for subsequent counseling/education programs. Counseling/educational programs should incorporate information about how to maintain or adapt social roles in the face of declining cognitive abilities and the need for caregivers to replenish their own needs. The speech–language pathologist can host or arrange for such educational programs to be facilitated by social workers, clinical psychologists, geriatricians, geriatric nurses, or other qualified professionals. In some cases, peer counseling programs may also be provided through local Alzheimer's associations, hospitals, adult day programs, long-term care facilities, or senior citizen centers.

Positive mental health is the fifth component to the wellness module. This is not typically a topic addressed by speech–language pathologists; nonetheless, the presence of depression in the individual with dementia or the caregiver will influence their responsiveness to communication intervention. In particular, caregiver depression and stress will influence the availability and sensitivity of the caregiver to communication interchanges with the dementia patient. Caregivers who feel prolonged, unrelieved stress are unlikely to communicate frequently or with enthusiasm or to problem solve difficult communication situations. Speech–language pathologists should be aware of behavioral signs that might indicate stress and depression on the part of the dementia patient or caregiver, including prolonged sadness and crying, feelings of unworthiness, disinterest and social withdrawal, difficulty concentrating, indecisiveness, sleep and appetite changes, and expression of suicidal intent (see reviews in Birren et al., 1992). Four tools to help identify depression are the Beck Depression Inventory (Beck et al., 1961), the Geriatric Depression Scale (Yesavage et al., 1983), the Revised Hamilton Rating Scale for Depression (Warren, 1994), and the Cornell Scale for Depression in Dementia (Alexopoulos et al., 1988). Although diagnosis of depression is a medical responsibility, the speech–language pathologist may be a catalyst in mobilizing caregivers to seek medical help for themselves or their family member and to participate in counseling or respite programs.

## Skills

A functional assessment of communication for individuals with dementia cannot ignore the evaluation of basic receptive, expressive, cognitive, and pragmatic skills. It also provides a baseline against which further skill deterioration can be measured. Identification of communication skills that can be remediated or compensated for will enhance assessment and intervention aimed at communication in everyday contexts.

Communication requires the timely coordination of many skills beginning with cognitive skills that underlie the ability to comprehend and formulate language. An assessment of cognitive skills is crucial in understanding the complete nature of the underlying cognitive deterioration. Although a typical battery involves a comprehensive assessment of intelligence (e.g., Wechsler Adult Intelligence Scale-III; 1997), more typically, assessment will involve administration of a brief mental status examination such as the Mini Mental Status Examination (Folstein et al., 1975), the Mattis Dementia Rating Scale (Mattis, 1976), or the Mental Status Questionnaire (Kahn et al., 1960). In-depth assessments of decline across a variety of domains may have more relevance for functional communication assessment and can be done with instruments such as the Brief Cognitive Rating Scale (Reisberg, 1983), the Clinical Dementia Rating (Hughes et al., 1982), the Functional Assessment Stages (Reisberg et al., 1984), or the Global Deterioration Scale (Reisberg, Ferris et al., 1982).

Other communication skills include the motor aspects of speech, linguistic aspects of communication, pragmatics, and nonverbal communication. Motor speech changes are not manifest usually until late in the progression of the disease, and thus, any difficulties in speech production noticed early in the course of dementia may be of particular clinical significance. Motor speech skills are assessed during administration of cognitive and linguistic tests and through evaluation of conversational speech. Campbell-Taylor (1995) and Garrett and Yorkston (1997) discuss motor speech changes and interventions relative to dementia. The ABCD (Bayles & Tomoeda, 1993) provides skill-based information regarding the communication performance of individuals with dementia while the FLCI (Bayles & Tomoeda, 1994) measures individual's functional communication.

Although there has been an increasing interest in the ability of individuals with dementia to comprehend or use nonverbal communication (e.g., Langhans, 1984; Welland, 1997), there have been no formal, standardized tests developed specifically for this purpose. The ABCD (Bayles & Tomoeda, 1993) has one subtest that assesses pantomime expression. The Pragmatic Assessment of Communication in Dementia (PAC-D) (England et al., 1996) also accepts gestural response as correct or attempts to elicit such responses when dementia patients do not name common items spontaneously. It is likely that there will be more development of methods to assess nonverbal receptive and expressive abilities of individuals with dementia in the near future, particularly at the discourse level.

## Effectiveness

Even when communication skills become seriously compromised, communication between the dementia patient and caregiver still needs to occur. It is the speech–language pathologist's job to identify what strategies caregivers and dementia patients can use to facilitate communication.

One way to identify strategies is to observe the dementia patient and caregiver in natural conversations and document the strategies each person uses to maintain the flow of conversation and repair conversational difficulties. Another approach is to question caregivers regarding the strategies they use. In its final development stage, the Perception of Conversation Index-DAT (Orange et al., 1998) provides the clinician with lists of communication difficulties the dementia patient might have and the strategies that can be used to facilitate communication. For example, the caregiver is asked if specific communicative interactions are difficult for the dementia patient. The caregiver is then asked to indicate the severity of the problem. Finally, the caregiver indicates which items in a list of strategies result in more effective communication. This tool has been empirically designed and at present, represents responses from over 100 family caregivers of individuals with DAT and from over 40 speech–language pathologists with experience with dementia.

Another aspect of effectiveness to evaluate is the availability and use of assistive communication devices. Assistive technologies include those for enhancing vision, hearing, expression, memory, and safety. They range from low-technology aids such as home-made or commercial communication boards and memory reminders to high technology aids such as computers that facilitate reading, digital hearing aids, and personal and environmental computers that assist in independent living and safety. The speech–language pathologist must determine, through observation and from caregivers' comments regarding need for an assistive device, the patient's potential to use a device either independently or with assistance, and the need for referral for comprehensive assistive device evaluation. For those with assistive devices, the speech–language pathologist should ascertain its condition as well as accessibility to, willingness to, and success in using it. In addition, it is useful to determine the caregiver's knowledge of and willingness to use the device, since the caregiver may be the primary person to encourage its use on a daily basis. In some cases, environmental devices, rather than personal assistive devices, will be more suitable. For example, for those dementia patients with hearing loss for whom a hearing aid is inappropriate, F.M. or I.R. room systems may facilitate the reception of sounds, especially when used with compensatory communication behaviors by caregivers. For a more complete discussion of communication technologies for the elderly (see Lubinski & Higginbotham, 1997).

## Opportunity

Perhaps most neglected in traditional assessments of communication of individuals with dementia is their opportunity to communicate. One of the most devastating aspects of dementia is the narrowing of social opportunities to demonstrate communication competencies as physical, social, and mental skills deteriorate. Communication partners naturally limit or avoid situations where communication predicaments present themselves. This attitude compounds other issues that negatively influence communication, such as ageism, institutionalization, depression, and learned helplessness. The speech–language pathologist should determine if the dementia patient resides in a communicatively rich or impoverished environment. In previous publications, Lubinski (e.g., 1995, 1997) suggests that speech–language pathologists assess the physical and social environments to identify factors that either enhance or restrict access to communication opportunities. Lubinski's Communication

Environmental Assessment and Planning Guide (1995) outlines 10 areas for assessment and intervention, each from an environmental and personal perspective.

Communication opportunities can be improved through caregiver education, environmental design or redesign, and modeling of strategies that promote interaction. Family and professional caregivers need to understand that physical and social contexts will affect the presence and quality of communication. Educational programs should focus on simple, easily incorporated suggestions that facilitate communication. For example, caregivers can learn the value of face-to-face seating, adequate lighting and noise reduction, and visual, auditory and physical accessibility to communication partners and activities of choice. In addition, education programs must focus on how families and other caregivers might help individuals with dementia maintain previous social roles or develop new roles. Creative ways to enhance the social environment include increasing intergenerational opportunities such as activities with children of varying ages, adaptive exercise programs (i.e., dancing), and peer visiting programs. Individuals with dementia should be encouraged either to observe or participate in social and cultural events that are appropriate to their age, gender, race or ethnicity, religion, and personal interests.

Finally, as stated previously in the section on wellness, caregivers should be encouraged to satisfy their own physical, social, and emotional needs because healthy caregivers will be more likely to communicate effectively with dementia patients. Caregivers in need of counseling should be referred to appropriate professionals who can provide them with respite resources and other options for caregiving relief.

The following case is presented to illustrate elements of the Wellness-to-Opportunity framework.

## Case Example

BACKGROUND

Mrs. Czarnecki (pseudonym) is a 75-year-old woman who has resided in the Village Woods Adult Care Resident Facility for 4 months. She is a native of Poland, arrived alone in the United States at age 15, married almost immediately, and resided in the same home for nearly 60 years. She worked sporadically as a domestic, had no formal education, but could speak and read English at a functional level. The primary language spoken in the home was Polish. The mother of two married daughters who live nearby and a widow for 12 years, she began having difficulty with managing her home 4 years ago, and reluctantly relocated to her daughter Maya's home on a trial basis about 15 months ago. Maya has twin 13-year-old sons and a 3-year-old daughter. She works as a free lance writer and photographer from her home. Maya's husband had cancer surgery recently and is undergoing chemotherapy. Mrs. Czarnecki's other daughter, Helena, is the vice-president of a national marketing company, has two college-age daughters, and is divorced. Maya and Helena have been estranged as sisters since their father died. The sisters share power of attorney for their mother's affairs and care.

After Mrs. Czarnecki's hospitalization for a mild heart attack and diagnosis of senile-onset diabetes and early–mid-stage Alzheimer's disease 4 months ago, Maya decided that her mother should relocate to an adult-care facility upon hospital discharge. Helena was opposed to this placement as it would deplete their mother's savings and felt that her mother would do better residing with Maya's family. Maya's decision prevailed, and Mrs. Czarnecki was placed in Village Woods Facility.

Mrs. Czarnecki's adaptation to life in the facility has been less than satisfactory. Despite good recovery from her recent heart attack and well-controlled diabetes, she has become increasingly dependent on staff assistance for walking, dressing, and eating. She initiates communication infrequently with staff or residents and responds inconsistently to questions or comments. Although ambulatory, she sits in her room most of the day and participates in few activities. Her daughter Maya makes brief weekly visits, and Helena has visited once since admission. An elderly Polish female friend visits about once a month. Staff have not documented the type or amount of communication that occurs during these visits but have observed that Mrs. Czarnecki seems more animated and compliant afterward.

Mrs. Czarnecki has never had a formal evaluation of her communication, but a hearing screening upon admission to the adult-care facility revealed a mild bilateral high-frequency loss. Dementia was diagnosed by the attending physician during her hospitalization for the recent heart attack. There is no documentation, however, of the type of assessment protocol or tests used to diagnose dementia. Because of her increasing need for skilled nursing care, her inconsistent and limited communication, and the possibility of relocating Mrs. Czarnecki to a skilled nursing facility, the resident planning team has questioned if Mrs. Czarnecki has any communication problems that might be responsive to interventions that could facilitate successful adaptation to life in the present or a new setting. The staff feel that if Mrs. Czarnecki could communicate more effectively, relocation to a nursing home might be forestalled at this time.

## ASSESSMENT

The clinician assigned to this case began a comprehensive, functional assessment by conducting a telephone interview with Mrs. Czarnecki's daughter Maya wherein she explored the following topics: (a) Mrs. Czarnecki's present and past communication skills; (b) her perceptions of her mother's communication difficulties; (c) strategies that facilitate communication with her mother; (d) Mrs. Czarnecki's interests, friendship patterns, present communication needs, and social roles prior to admission to the facility; and (e) questions that Maya had about communication difficulties with her mother. The clinician arranged another phone interview when she would update Maya about the findings from the assessment of her mother's communication. The clinician also spoke with the nurse in charge of the day shift about Mrs. Czarnecki's activity patterns and preferences, difficulties the staff had in communicating with the resident and strategies they used to communicate, the need for a complete hearing evaluation, and the need for a mental health assessment.

Mrs. Czarnecki's communication skills were evaluated using selected subtests of the ABCD, the FLCI, a topic-directed interview following a brief discussion of the purpose of the assessment, and a situational assessment of her communication at mealtime. Scores from the ABCD showed that Mrs. Czarnecki exhibited strong skills repeating anomalous sentences, following single- and multi-step commands, and reading and understanding single words. She exhibited average to poor performance for reading comprehension of paragraphs and understanding comparative questions (e.g., Is supper earlier than breakfast?). Mrs. Czarnecki showed great difficulty on the mental status subtest (5 of possible 13 points), story retelling in immediate and delayed conditions, naming pictured objects, and describing a common object (e.g., nail).

Results from the FLCI showed that Mrs. Czarnecki had strengths in greeting and naming, answering Yes–No and two-choice questions, reading words, reminiscing, and gesturing. She exhibited greater difficulty with answering open-ended and multiple-choice questions, writing, comprehending signs (e.g., rest rooms and enter/exit), demonstrating the use of common objects, and writing.

During a topic-directed interview, Mrs. Czarnecki was asked to tell the clinician about (a) where she grew up, (b) her family, (c) the jobs or work that she did, (d) what she did each day, and (e) her health at present. Mrs. Czarnecki produced few content words in all topics. She used many nonspecific terms (e.g., that, those, someone, thing) and ambiguous referents. It was difficult to follow what she was saying, especially for topics related to recent aspects of her life (what she does each day, her health at present, her family). She did produce more words and was rated by the clinician as being more coherent for topics that tapped her autobiographical memory (e.g., where she was born and raised, jobs she had). Periodically, Mrs. Czarnecki reverted to Polish in answering questions.

A brief assessment of her communication during mealtime revealed that Mrs. Czarnecki initiated no communication with her table mates or the dining room employees. When addressed by another resident, she smiled and responded with affirmative responses that were inconsistently appropriate. Twice she responded with "huh?" that was ignored by her communication partners. The clinician noted that staff never directly faced any of the residents, including Mrs. Czarnecki, when communicating with them nor engaged them in any social communication during meal time.

INTERVENTION

Based on the information collected from Mrs. Czarnecki's daughter Maya, results of standardized testing and discourse in topic-directed interviews and meal time observation, the clinician decided that intervention targeting family and staff would be most beneficial at this time. The clinician met with both daughters to explain how dementia affects communication and their role in creating fulfilling communication opportunities for their mother. During this discussion, it became apparent that both daughters felt distressed when visiting their mother and did not have many strategies to initiate or maintain communication. Neither spoke much Polish, although both felt they could improve their once-fluent levels. This contributed to their own stress and limited visits. They agreed to participate in the Dementia Family Program offered by the social worker and nursing staff at the facility during which the speech–language pathologist offers suggestions for communication enrichment. The daughters agreed to contact their mother's friends and encourage them to visit. The daughters also identified several activities that their mother enjoyed including Polish classical music and gardening. The activities director arranged for Mrs. Czarnecki to attend a community concert of Polish music and participate in the facility's gardening program with her daughters, visiting friends, or volunteers. The activities director also suggested that the daughters become involved as volunteers in one of several programs that might interest their mother and that might promote physical activity such as the planned walking program and bowling. The clinician suggested that the family bring in more of Mrs. Czarnecki's personal items such as photo albums, her collection of madonnas, a box of mementos from previous vacations with her husband, and a church calendar for the wall.

Following assessment, the clinician presented a quarterly inservice program to personal-care aides and dining room staff about how to communicate effectively with individuals with dementia. She highlighted the need to engage residents in social communication during care and meals and to capitalize on long-term memory by reminiscing about personal interests and accomplishments. She discussed simple communication techniques including establishing eye contact, reassuring nonverbal communication, addressing residents by name, speaking in adult-like, well-constructed short, simple, active declarative sentences, and giving one-step commands and limited choice questions. Part of the inservice focused on role-playing difficult communication scenarios involving both cognitive impairment and hearing loss.

The clinician monitored the outcomes of this intervention 1 and 3 months later. Within the first month, Mrs. Czarnecki had a complete hearing assessment. The audiologist recommended a monoaural hearing aid at this time. The speech–language pathologist complemented the initial hearing aid counseling session with follow-up sessions with Mrs. Czarnecki, her personal-care aides, and her daughters. Mrs. Czarnecki's physician referred her to a geriatric psychiatrist who suggested a trial course of medication for depression.

Over the next 2 weeks, the speech–language pathologist noted that Mrs. Czarnecki had had four visits from her daughters and one from two friends. Mrs. Czarnecki had also agreed to attend two activities programs although she did not actively participate. The activities staff arranged for a Polish speaking volunteer to visit Mrs. Czarnecki on a weekly basis. On the advice of the speech–language pathologist, three staff members also agreed to learn several Polish phrases such as "Good day," "How are you?," "Nice to see you," etc. These "social conventions" were intended to create a somewhat linguistically familiar context for Mrs. Czarnecki. Staff members noted that Mrs. Czarnecki appeared to communicate more frequently and with greater enthusiasm in this context than in any other.

Within the next 2 months, both daughters attended the Family Dementia Program held on a Sunday evening. The speech–language pathologist discussed how dementia affects communication and specific strategies that might enhance communication effectiveness. The clinician also offered opportunities to simulate problem communication situations. Helena suggested that her company might be willing to sponsor a community program to make more people aware of dementia and what could be done to help individuals with dementia and their family caregivers.

At the end of 3 months, it was decided that Mrs. Czarnecki would not relocate at this time to a skilled nursing facility. Although still dependent for assistance in dressing, Mr. Czarnecki was attending several activities each week and was initiating more communication with staff and other residents. For example, she spoke spontaneously more often in both English and Polish than had been noted previously. She particularly enjoyed communicating with a recently arrived resident who spoke Polish. She wore her hearing aid every day and appeared more animated with staff, residents, and visitors. A follow-up phone call to Mrs. Czarnecki's daughters revealed that both had been visiting their mother on a weekly basis, felt that they communicated more effectively with her during the visits, and enjoyed participating in the volunteer activities in the facility. Both daughters recognized their mother's recent memory difficulties and focused on reminiscing topics that were familiar to their mother. Maya had become involved in the facility newsletter for residents and families and had brought her children to two family events at the facility. Helena was in the process of building corporate sponsorship for a community dementia awareness program and a video that discussed how to communicate with individuals with dementia.

## Future Needs

Speech–language pathologists face a number of obstacles in implementing a functional communication program for those with dementia simply because improvement in cognitive-linguistic skills is difficult to demonstrate. The problem may be that speech–language pathologists have been counting and documenting the wrong variables. Clinical research is needed to establish evidence-based outcomes for individuals with dementia and their caregivers. For example, outcomes might focus on the improved ability of individuals with dementia to perform activities of daily living with or without assistance, their ability to ambulate safely within the community, home or institutional environment, increased ability to use nonverbal means of communication and assistive communication technologies, and enhanced quality of life. Outcomes that focus on the caregivers also bear investigation including reduction of stress related to communication problems, increased ability to generate strategies to facilitate communication, delay in institutionalization, retention of long-term care personnel, and reduced cost of care. The above outcomes are generally not considered when communication intervention is provided, but they would result in a more functional portrayal of what might be gained through such intervention.

Further, speech–language pathologists need to take a more proactive role in advancing their multiple roles for individuals with dementia and their caregivers. In an era of rapid increase in the absolute and relative number of older adults and the costs associated with their care, payers have demanded clear demonstration of progress for payment. Thus, research needs to focus on the identification of functional criteria of progress and how these criteria can be measured quickly in valid and reliable ways.

To achieve functional goals related to issues such as quality of life, safety, and reduction of caregiver stress, approaches will need to be holistic. This will be accomplished by consultation with other specialists, caregiver training, modeling/demonstrations, and workshops and in-service programs. Traditional individual, biweekly, hourly sessions are not the appropriate venue to achieve changes in the environment and to strengthen caregiver problem-solving abilities.

Most importantly, speech–language pathologists need to move away from their traditional emphasis on improving communication skills to a broader conceptualization of their role and intended outcomes. This can be accomplished by grounding in social theories of aging, concepts such as learned helplessness, and methods for enhancing adult learning. Our focus needs to extend to family and professional caregivers to help them problem solve difficult communication situations and to the environment that provides the physical and social context for communication opportunities. We must stand ready to justify this expanded role with elders with dementia and their caregivers and to determine that this role enhances quality of life and is cost-effective.

## *Appendix*

### Sample Interview Questions Based on the Wellness to Opportunity Framework for Communication in Dementia

PREPARATORY TO INTERVIEW

Remember that the purpose of these questions is to elicit the interviewee's perceptions and encourage insight and problem solving. These questions are only overtures and should be followed through as necessary. Explain to the caregiver why you are asking these questions and why you are focusing on him or her as well as the individual with dementia.

## *Wellness*

### Awareness of Dementia and Impact on Communication

1. What concerns you about your relative's communication?
2. What programs have you participated in that have focused on the nature of dementia or communicating with someone who has dementia?
3. What would you like to know about the changes in communication associated with dementia?

### Health and Sensory Status

1. When did your relative have his/her last physical check-up by the family physician? Have you followed through on his/her suggestions?
2. When did you have your last physical check-up by your family physician? Have you followed through on his/her suggestions?
3. When was your relative's vision last tested? What was the outcome?
4. When was your vision last tested? What was the outcome?

5. Has your relative ever had his/her hearing tested by an audiologist or a hearing doctor? What was the outcome?

6. Have you ever had your hearing tested by an audiologist or a hearing doctor? What was the outcome?

## Activity Patterns and Safety

1. What is a typical day like for your relative?

2. What physical exercise does your relative get each day?

3. What opportunities does your relative have to get around his/her environment independently?

4. What do you do to promote the physical safety of your relative in the home?

## Social Roles and Relationships

1. Describe some favorite interests your relative has had throughout his/her life?

2. What social activities does your relative participate in during a typical week in and out of the home?

3. What activities do you think your relative might like to participate in but does not? Why?

4. What activities do you think generate conversational opportunities for your relative?

5. What responsibilities does your relative have for self-care?

6. Who does your relative communicate with on a typical day?

7. What opportunities do you have to pursue activities of interest?

## Positive Mental Health

1. How frustrated is your relative when he/she has difficulty communicating?

2. How frustrated do you become when you and your relative have difficulty communicating?

3. Do you feel that the difficulty communicating with your relative contributes to your overall stress? Why?

4. What do you do to relieve the frustration or stress you feel because of the communication difficulties with your relative?

5. Have you discussed any symptoms of depression on the part of your relative with your physician? What was the outcome of this discussion?

6. Are you experiencing any depression related to your caregiving role? Have you discussed these symptoms with your physician?

7. What opportunities do you have to pursue your own interests or respite from daily caregiving?

## Skills

1. What difficulties does your relative have in understanding you?

2. What difficulties does your relative have in understanding in group situations?

3. What difficulties does your relative have in expressing himself/herself to you?

4. What difficulties does your relative have in expressing himself/herself to unfamiliar people?

5. Does your relative participate in any reading or writing activities?

6. Does your relative use gesture to compensate for difficulties in expressing himself/herself? How effective are these gestures?

7. What communication skills do you think are best preserved in your relative at this time?

## Effectiveness

1. What do you do to facilitate communication with your relative?

2. What strategies work best to facilitate communication with your relative?

3. What assistive devices do you or your relative use to facilitate communication? (e.g., hearing aid, phone amplifier, calendars, memory dial phones, tape recorders, computers, etc.)

4. How effective are these devices?

5. Are the devices you or your relative use in good working condition?

## Opportunity

1. Where does most communication occur with your relative?

2. Is the lighting adequate in this setting so that your relative can adequately see communication partners?

3. Is this typically a noisy environment that might interfere with your relative hearing what is being said?

4. What social opportunities do you think your relative might like to participate in that would stimulate conversations?

5. Do you feel that others in the environment understand the special communication needs of your relative?

## *References*

Alexopoulos, G. S., Abrams, R. C., Young, R. C., & Shamoian, C. A. (1988). Cornell scale for depression in dementia. *Biology of Psychiatry, 23,* 271–284.

Arkin, S. M. (1996). Volunteers in partnership: An Alzheimer's rehabilitation program delivered by students. *American Journal of Alzheimer's Disease, 11,* 12–22.

Bayles, K. A., & Kaszniak, A. (1987). *Communication and cognition in normal aging and dementia.* Boston: College Hill Press.

Bayles, K. A., & Tomoeda, C. K. (1991). Caregiver report of prevalence and appearance order of linguistic symptoms in Alzheimer's patients. *The Gerontologist, 31,* 210–216.

Bayles, K. A., & Tomoeda, C. K. (1993). *Arizona battery for communication disorders of dementia.* Tucson, AZ: Canyonlands Publishing.

Bayles, K. A., & Tomoeda, C. K. (1994). *Functional linguistic communication inventory.* Tucson, AZ: Canyonlands Publishing.

Bayles, K. A., Tomoeda, C. K., & Trosset, W. (1992). Relation of linguistic communication abilities of Alzheimer's patients to stage of disease. *Brain and Language, 42,* 454–472.

Beck, A. T., Ward, C. H., Mendelson, M., & Erbough. (1961). An inventory for measuring depression. *Archives of General Psychiatry, 4,* 561–571.

Binnie, C. A. (1994). The future of audiological rehabilitation: Overview and forecast. *Journal of the Academy of Rehabilitative Audiology Monographs, 27,* 13–24.

Birren, J. E., Sloane, R. B., & Cohen, G. D. (eds.)(1992). *Handbook of mental health and aging* (2nd ed.). San Diego, CA: Academic Press.

Bloom, R. L., Obler, L. K., de Santi, S., & Ehrlich, J. S. (eds). (1994). *Discourse analysis and applications: Studies in adult clinical populations.* Hillsdale, NJ: Lawrence Erlbaum Publishers.

Boles, L., & Bombard, T. (1998). Conversational discourse analysis: Appropriate and useful sample sizes. *Aphasiology, 12,* 547–560.

Bollinger, R., & Hardiman, C. J. (1991). *Rating scale of communication in cognitive decline.* Buffalo, NY: United Educational Services.

Bond-Chapman, S., Peterson-Highly, A., & Thompson, J. L. (1998). Discourse in fluent aphasia and Alzheimer's disease: Linguistic and pragmatic considerations. *Journal of Neurolinguistics, 11,* 55–78.

Bourgeois, M. (1991). Communication treatment for adults with dementia. *Journal of Speech and Hearing Research, 34,* 831–844.

Bourgeois, M. (1997). Families caring for elders at home: Caregiver training. In B. B. Shadden, M. A. Toner (eds): *Aging and communication: For clinicians by clinicians* (pp. 227–249). Austin, TX: ProEd.

Boczko, F. (1994). The Breakfast Club: A multi-modal language stimulation program for stimulation program for nursing home residents with Alzheimer's disease. *American Journal of Alzheimer's Care Related Disorders and Research, 9,* 35–38.

Campbell-Taylor, I. (1995). Motor speech changes. In R. Lubinski (ed): *Dementia and communication* (pp. 70–83). San Diego: Singular Publishing Co.

Canadian Study of Health and Aging Working Group. (1994). Canadian study of health and ageing: Study methods and prevalence of dementia. *Canadian Medical Association Journal, 150,* 899–913.

Cherney, L. R., Shadden, B. B., & Coelho, C. A. (1998). *Analyzing discourse in communicatively impaired adults.* Gaithersburg, MD: Aspen Publishers.

Clark, C. (1986). *Wellness nursing: Concepts, theory, research and practice.* New York: Springer.

Clark, L. W. (1995). Interventions for persons with Alzheimer's disease: Strategies for maintaining and enhancing communicative success. *Topics in Language Disorders, 15,* 47–66.

Clark, L. W. (1997). Communication intervention for family caregivers and professional health providers. In B. B. Shadden, M. A. Toner (eds): *Aging and communication: For clinicians by clinicians* (pp. 251–274). Austin, TX: ProEd.

Clark, L. W., & Witte, K. (1995). Nature and efficacy of communication management in Alzheimer's disease. In R. Lubinski (ed): *Dementia and communication* (pp. 238–256). San Diego: Singular Publishing.

Cummings, J. L., Benson, D. F., & LoVerme, S. (1980). Reversible dementia. *Journal of the American Medical Association, 243,* 2434–2439.

Dunn, L. M., & Dunn, L. M. (1981). *Peabody Picture Vocabulary Test—Revised.* Circle Pines, MN: American Guidance Service.

England, J. E., O'Neill, J. J., & Simpson, R. K. (1996). Pragmatic assessment of communication in dementia (PAC-D). *American Journal of Alzheimer's Disease, 11,* 7–10.

Flax, M. N., Golembiewski, D., & McCaulley, B. (1993). *Coping with low vision.* San Diego: Singular Publishing Group.

Friedman, R., & Tappen, R. M. (1991). The effect of planned walking on communication in Alzheimer's disease. *Journal of the American Geriatrics Society, 39,* 650–654.

Folstein, M. F., Folstein, S. E., & McHugh, P. R. (1975). Mini mental state: A practical method for grading the cognitive state of patients for the clinician. *Journal of Psychiatric Research, 12,* 189–198.

Garcia, L., & Orange, J. B. (1996). The analysis of conversational skills of older adults: Current research and clinical approaches. *Journal of Speech–Language Pathology and Audiology, 20,* 123–135.

Garrett, K., & Yorkston, K. (1997). Assistive communication technology for elders with cognitive and language disabilities. In R. Lubinski, D. J. Higginbotham (eds): *Communication technologies for the elderly: Vision, hearing, and speech* (pp. 203–234). San Diego: Singular Publishing Group, Inc.

Glass, L. (1990). Hearing impairment in geriatrics. *Geriatric rehabilitation.* Boston: College-Hill Press.

Goodglass, H., & Kaplan, E. (1983). *Boston Diagnostic Aphasia Examination.* Philadelphia: Lea & Febiger.

Gorelick, P. B., & Bozzola, F. G. (1991). Alzheimer's disease: Clues to the cause. *Postgraduate Medicine, 89,* 1157–1158.

Grimes, A. (1995). Auditory changes. In R. Lubinski (ed): *Dementia and communication* (pp. 47–69). San Diego: Singular Publishing Group.

Gurland, B., Toner, J., Wilder, D., Chen, J., & Lantigua, R. (1994). Impairment of communication and adaptive functioning in community-residing elderly with advanced dementia. *Alzheimer's Disease and Associated Disorders, 8,* 230–241.

Haber, D. (1994). *Health promotion and aging.* New York: Springer-Verlag Publishing.

Hoffman, S., Platt, C., & Barry, K. (1988). Comforting the confused: The importance of nonverbal communication in the care of people with Alzheimer's disease. *American Journal of Alzheimer's Care and Related Disorders Research, 3,* 25–30.

Hughes, C. P., Berg, L., Danzinger, Cohen, & Martin. (1982). A new clinical scale for staging of dementia. *British Journal of Psychiatry, 140,* 566–572.

Kahn, R., Goldfarb, A., Pollack, M., et al. (1960). Brief objective measures for the determination of mental status of the aged. *American Journal of Psychiatry, 117,* 326–328.

Kaplan, E., Goodglass, H., & Weintraub, S. (1983). *Boston Naming Test.* Philadelphia: Lea & Febiger.

Kempler, D. (1995). Language changes in dementia of the Alzheimer type. In R. Lubinski (ed): *Dementia and communication* (pp. 98–114). San Diego: Singular Publishing Group.

Kertesz, A. (1982). *Western Aphasia Battery.* New York: Grune & Stratton.

Kricos, P., & Lesner, S. (1995). *Hearing care for the older adult: Audiologic rehabilitation.* Boston: Butterworth-Heinemann.

Koury, L., & Lubinski, R. (1995). Effective in-service training for staff working with communication-impaired patients. In R. Lubinski (ed): *Communication and dementia* (pp. 279–291). San Diego: Singular Publishing Group.

Langhans, J. J. (1984). Pantomime recognition and pantomime expression in persons with Alzheimer's disease. Unpublished doctoral dissertation, University of Arizona.

Lubinski, R. (1995). Environmental considerations for elderly patients. In R. Lubinski (ed): *Communication and dementia* (pp. 257–278). San Diego: Singular Publishing Group.

Lubinski, R. (1997). Perspectives on aging and communication. In R. Lubinski, D. J. Higginbotham (eds): *Communication technologies for the elderly: Vision, hearing and speech* (pp. 1–22). San Diego: Singular Publishing Group.

Lubinski, R., & Higginbotham, D. J. (eds). (1997). *Communication technologies for the elderly: Vision, hearing and speech.* San Diego: Singular Publishing Group.

Mattis, S. (1976). Mental status examination for organic mental syndrome in the elderly patient. In L. Bellak & T. B. Karasu (eds): *Geriatric Psychiatry.* New York: Grune & Stratton.

McNeil, M., & Prescott, T. E. (1978). *Revised Token Test.* San Diego: Psychological Corporation.

Minkler, M., & Fullarton, J. (1980). *Health Promotion, Health Maintenance and Disease Prevention for the Elderly.* Unpublished background paper for the 1981 White House conference on aging, prepared for the Office of Health Information, Health Promotion, Physical Fitness and Sports Medicine, Washington, DC.

Mittelman, M., Ferris, S., Steinberg, G., Shulman, E., Mackell, J., Ambinder, A., & Cohen, J. (1993). An intervention that delays institutionalization of Alzheimer's disease patients: Treatment of spouse-caregivers. *The Gerontologist, 33,* 730–740.

Mobily, P., Mass, M., Buckwalter, K., & Kelley, L. (1992). Geriatric mental health: Staff stress on an Alzheimer's unit. *Journal of Psychosocial Nursing, 10,* 25–31.

Morton, I., & Bleathman, C. (1991). The effectiveness of validation therapy in dementia: A pilot study. *International Geriatric Psychiatry, 6,* 327–330.

Orange, J. B. (1995). Perspectives of family members regarding communication changes. In R. Lubinski (ed): *Dementia and communication* (pp. 168–186). San Diego: Singular Publishing Group.

Orange, J. B., & Colton-Hudson, A. (1998). Enhancing communication in dementia of the Alzheimer's type. *Topics in Geriatric Rehabilitation, 14,* 56–75.

Orange, J. B., Lubinski, R., Ryan, S., Dvorsky, A., & Harkness, D. (1998). The Perception of Conversation Index—Dementia of the Alzheimer type. Unpublished manuscript.

Orange, J. B., & Ryan, E. B. (1992). The effect of planned walking on communication. Response to Friedman and Tappen. *Journal of American Geriatrics Society, 40,* 296.

Orange, J. B., Ryan, E., Meredith, S., & MacLean. (1995). Application of the communication enhancement model for long-term care residents with Alzheimer's disease. *Topics in Language Disorders, 15,* 20–35.

Palm, S., & Purves, B. (1996). Management of a word-finding deficit in discourse: A case example. *Journal of Speech–Language Pathology and Audiology, 20,* 155–166.

Penn, C. (1985). The Profile of Communicative Appropriateness: A clinical tool for the assessment of pragmatics. *The South African Journal of Communication Disorders, 32,* 18–23.

Pichora-Fuller, M. K., & Cheesman, M. F. (1997). Special issue on hearing and aging. *Journal of Speech–Language Pathology and Audiology, 21,* 75–142.

Powell, A. L., Hale, M. A., & Bayer, A. J. (1995). Symptoms of communication breakdown in dementia. Carer's perceptions. *European Journal of Disorders of Communication, 30,* 65–75.

Ramsdell, J. (1990). A rehabilitation orientation in the workup of general medical problems. In B. Kemp, K. Brummel-Smith, J. Ramsdell (eds): *Geriatric rehabilitation* (pp. 23–40). Boston: College Hill Press.

Reisberg, B. (1983). *Alzheimer's disease: The standard reference.* New York: Three Free Press.

Reisberg, B., Ferris, S. H., Anand, R., et al. (1984). Functional staging of dementia of the Alzheimer's type. *Annals of NY Academy of Science, 435,* 481–486.

Reisberg, B., Ferris, S. H., DeLeon, M. J., & Crook. (1982). The global deterioration scale for assessment of primary degenerative dementia. *American Journal of Psychiatry, 139,* 1136–1139.

Richter, J. M., Roberto, K. A., & Bottenberg, D. J. (1995). Communicating with persons with Alzheimer's disease: experiences of family and formal caregivers. *Archives of Psychiatric Nursing, 9,* 279–285.

Ripich, D. N. (1991). *Handbook of geriatric communication disorders.* Austin, TX: Pro-Ed.

Ripich, D. N. (1994). Functional communication with AD patients: A caregiver training program. *Alzheimer Disease and Associated Disorders, 8,* 95–109.

Ripich, D. N. (1995). Differential diagnosis and assessment. In R. Lubinski (ed): *Communication and dementia* (pp. 188–222). San Diego: Singular Publishing Group.

Ripich, D., Vertes, D., Whitehouse, P., Fulton, S., & Ekelman, B. (1991). Turn-taking and speech act patterns in the discourse of senile dementia of the Alzheimer's type patients. *Brain and Language, 40,* 330–343.

Ripich, D. N., Wykle, M., & Niles, S. (1995). Alzheimer's disease caregivers: the FOCUSED program. *Geriatric Nursing, 16,* 15–19.

Santo Pietro, M. J., & Ostuni, E. (1997). *Successful communication with Alzheimer's disease patients: An inservice manual.* Boston: Butterworth-Heinemann.

Santo Pietro, M. J., & Boczko, F. (1998). The Breakfast Club: Results of a study examining the effectiveness of a multi-modality group communication treatment. *American Journal of Alzheimer's Disease, 13,* 146–158.

Schow, R. L., & Nerbonne, M. (1980). Hearing levels among elderly nursing home residents. *Journal of Speech and Hearing Disorders, 45,* 124–132.

Schow, R. L., & Nerbonne, M. (1982). Communication screening profile uses with elderly clients. *Ear and Hearing, 3,* 133–147.

Schulz, R., & O'Brien, A. T. (1994). Alzheimer's disease caregiving: An overview. *Seminars in Speech and Language, 15,* 185–194.

Schumer, R. (1997). Changes in vision and aging. In R. Lubinski, J. Higginbotham (eds): *Communication technologies for the elderly: Vision, hearing, and speech* (pp. 41–70). San Diego: Singular Publishing Group.

Terrell, B., & Ripich, D. N. (1989). Discourse competence as a variable in intervention. *Seminars in Speech and Language Disorders, 10,* 282–297.

Tomoeda, C. K., & Bayles, K. A. (1991). The efficacy of speech–language pathology intervention: Dementia. *Seminars in Speech and Language, 11,* 311–319.

Uhlmann, R., Rees, T., Psaty, B., & Duckert, L. (1989). Validity and reliability of auditory screening tests in demented and non-demented older adults. *Journal of General Internal Medicine, 4,* 90–96.

Ulatowska, H. K., Allard, L., Donnell, A., Bristow, J., Haynes, S. M., Flower, A., & North, A. (1988). Discourse performance in subjects with dementia of the Alzheimer type. In H. Whitaker (ed): *Neuropsychological studies in nonfocal brain damage* (pp. 108–131). New York: Springer-Verlag.

Ventry, I., & Weinstein, B. (1982). The hearing handicap inventory for the elderly: A new tool. *Ear and Hearing, 3,* 128–133.

Walker, S. (1992). Wellness for elders. *Holistic Nurse Practitioner, 7,* 38–45.

Warren, D. (1994). *Revised Hamilton rating scale for depression.* Los Angeles: Western Psychological Services.

Webster Ross, G., Cummings, J. L., & Benson, D. F. (1990). Speech and language alterations in dementia syndrome: Characteristics and treatment. *Aphasiology, 4,* 339–352.

Wechsler, D. (1997). Wechsler Adult Intelligence Scale-III. San Antonio, TX: Psychological Corporation.

Weinstein, B. (1997). Hearing aids and older adults. In R. Lubinski, D. J. Higginbotham (eds): *Communication technologies for the elderly: Vision, hearing, and speech* (pp. 129–160). San Diego: Singular Publishing Group, Inc.

Weinstein, B., & Amsel, L. (1986). Hearing loss and senile dementia in the institutionalized elderly. *Clinical Gerontologist, 4,* 3–15.

Welland, R. J. (1997). Face-to-face with dementia: Recent perspectives on verbal and nonverbal communication. Miniseminar presented at the Annual New York State Speech–Language–Hearing Association Convention, Buffalo, NY, April.

Williamson, G. M., & Schulz, R. (1993). Coping with specific stressors in Alzheimer's disease caregiving. *The Gerontologist, 33,* 747–755.

Wright, L. K. (1993). *Alzheimer's disease and marriage.* Newbury Park: Sage Publications.

Yesavage, H., Brink, T., Rose, T., et al. (1983). Development and validation of a geriatric depression screening. A preliminary report. *Journal of Psychiatric Research, 17,* 37–49.

Zgola, J. M., & Coulter, L. G. (1988). I can tell you about that: A therapeutic group program for cognitively impaired persons. *American Journal of Alzheimer's Care Related Disorders and Research, 3,* 17–22.

# 14

# Assessment and Treatment of Functional Communication in Dysarthria

## Pamela M. Enderby

**Dysarthria treatment has evolved from narrow, specific interventions to more holistic interventions that include a functional approach. The chapter reviews the many speaker and listener variables that influence a dysarthric speaker's communicative effectiveness. The importance of assessing impairments, disabilities and handicaps is illustrated by describing dysarthria outcome data using the Therapy Outcome Measures developed in the United Kingdom. Differences in outcomes with different populations suggest that measurement and intervention at all levels must be included.**

## Introduction

The term dysarthria has been used over the last 100 years to define a disorder of speech resulting from lesions within the nervous system (Arnold, 1965). However, the concepts relating to dysarthria have become more comprehensive and refined, and this term is now generally used to encompass disorders beyond that of articulation alone. For example, Darley et al. (1975) state that "Dysarthria comprises a group of speech disorders resulting from disturbances in muscular control due to impairment of any of the basic motor processes involved in the execution of speech." Thus, the present use of the term is still restricted to neurogenic speech dysfunctions resulting from impairment of the central or peripheral nervous system, but it includes disruptions of speech related to neuromotor, respiratory, and phonatory disorders. Frequently the term "motor speech disorder" is used synonymously with dysarthria, however, the definition of dysarthria usually excludes speech disorders of structural, psychological, or motor planning origin. This chapter primarily considers the narrower context of dysarthria.

Dysarthria can range in severity from a disorder that is so mild that it is only noticeable during rapid speech or the variation is only perceived by the speaker, to a disorder so severe that no functional speech is present. Frequently the latter is termed anarthria.

While it is generally accepted that dysarthria is the most common of the acquired speech disorders, the specific figures related to its incidence and prevalence cannot generally be relied upon. Many studies relating to specific neurological diseases (e.g., multiple sclerosis) have reported the incidence of different symptoms, but the precision in collecting data on dysarthria may not have been particularly sensitive, causing an under-reporting. Despite this, it is reported that dysarthria is present in approximately 33% of all patients with brain injuries (Sarno et al., 1986); 8% of individuals with cerebral palsy (Worster-Drought, 1974); and varies from 19 to 100% in individuals with degenerative neurological diseases. The lower figure is indicated for the population of those with multiple sclerosis. Whereas studies indicate that in the later stages of Parkinson's disease and motor neurone disease nearly all those affected have moderate to severe dysarthria (Darley, 1978; Darley et al., 1972; Logemann & Fisher, 1981).

## History of Speech Therapy for Dysarthria

Dysarthria often results in an abnormal quality of speech and reduced intelligibility. However, the main emphasis on the role of the speech and language therapist in the treatment of dysarthria in the 1950s and 1960s was to analyze the dysfunctions contributing to the speech disorder to assist with classifying the dysarthria as part of the diagnostic process. Additionally, those working with dysarthria at that time found that this was an avenue for exploring the neurophysiological underpinning of the speech system and much work was conducted to improve the understanding of normal speech processes.

Despite being the most common of the acquired expressive communication disorders, dysarthria has attracted relatively little attention in the literature. There are far fewer texts and research papers related to the physiological and acoustic bases, methods of assessment, and treatment or the evaluation of the effectiveness of treatments of dysarthria than other speech or language disorders (Enderby & Emerson, 1995; Yorkston, 1996). This may be related to the fact that acquired dysarthria is frequently associated with either severe brain damage or with progressive neurological disease and there has, in the past, been a negative attitude to the role of therapy in these areas.

More recently there has been a change in emphasis in to the role of rehabilitation for patients with acquired disorders with a better understanding of the importance of addressing issues related to disability and handicap along with those associated with the impairment. These changes in the context of rehabilitation have permeated into the speech therapy of dysarthria and it is now possible to plot the evolution of dysarthria therapy in the following way:

- Early physiological approaches to the impaired speech mechanism (proprioceptive neuromuscular facilitation, sensory training, muscle strengthening, emphasis on diagnostic and classification procedures).
- Therapy for basic motor speech processes, such as articulation, resonance, prosody and phonation, etc.
- Applications of instrumentation, including intra-oral appliances, amplification, and biofeedback.
- Facilitation of intelligibility by enhancing oral speech, supplementing speech with gestural systems, etc., or replacing oral communication with communication aids/systems.
- Integrated rehabilitation of dysarthria, including consideration of the psychosocial aspects and implications of oral motor disorders (e.g., development of support groups, counselling, adaptive techniques).

While speech therapy has progressed from narrow specific interventions to more holistic approaches, this should not result in diffuse unfocused programmes of treatment (Yorkston & Beukelman, 1994).


### Treatment of Dysarthric Impairment, Disability, and Handicap

The professional literature on dysarthria has tended to dwell upon the treatment of the impairment, that is, the disorder itself. The disruption of speech caused by damage to neural pathways and cortical regions may give rise to patterns of speech related to lower motor neurone involvement, upper motor neurone involvement, cerebellar disorders, extrapyramidal disorders, and mixed system disorders. Some therapeutic approaches have suggested the importance of identifying the underlying nature of the dysarthria in planning a treatment to attend to the specific deficit. Furthermore, it is recommended that the contributing factors to the dysarthria in terms of the speech processes involved, be they respiratory, velopharyngeal, laryngeal, or related to the movements of the oral mechanism such as the tongue and the lips are analyzed (Netsell, 1998). The therapist's work on the impairment is informed by knowledge as to whether the disordered speech process is dysfunctional due to inadequate range, timing, or fluency of movement along with knowledge of the associated deficits secondary to the primary dysfunction. For example, the therapist would determine whether the person's inability to produce the phoneme /p/ is due to inadequate lip closure or due to poor intra-oral pressure unrelated to lip closure but related to either respiratory or velopharyngeal problems.

While the treatment of dysarthric speech is important and should not be dismissed, there needs to be a redressing of the balance so that rehabilitation programs fully consider the purpose of speech, that is, for communication. The outcome of regaining effective communication should underpin all goals in a cohesive therapy package. This may require changing emphasis of treatment, for example, reconsidering the proportions of time given within therapy in treating pervading disorders rather than addressing alternative or supplementary methods of communication. There are many pressures on therapists to follow an im-balanced course in their treatment of impairment and disability. First, our train-ing leads us to have a greater understanding about the treatments involved with specific impairments, and we are inadequately prepared in the areas of treating communication disorders in their broader context. Furthermore, patients with ac-quired disorders frequently wish to address the speech deficit itself in an attempt to overcome it so that life can return to as it was, rather than seeking compensa-tory approaches, which indicate an acceptance of the more permanent nature of the disabling condition.

In some circumstances working on the dysarthric impairment may lead to a pat-tern of activities and exercises converse to those required for the disability (e.g., in-telligibility). A good example would be in the area of speed of speech. With many dysarthric patients, the intelligibility and communicative effectiveness is im-proved by reducing the speaking speed to below that of normal. However, if the goal of treatment was to reduce the impairment so that speaking functions were more in line with the norm, the emphasis of treatment might be on increasing the speed of speech, which could in turn compromise communicative effectiveness. It is important for the therapist to have a clear understanding of the route treatment is taking by identifying goals in terms of the final outcome. It should go without saying that those goals cannot be owned by the therapist alone. Rather, the em-phasis of treatment and an understanding of its direction should be shared by the patient and the therapist along with caregivers who hopefully will be extending and supporting the therapeutic program (Sims, 1998).

## Communicative Effectiveness

This chapter now concentrates upon the disability/activity features of dysarthria by considering the many factors that affect intelligibility and communicative ef-fectiveness. Whereas treating the speech impairment may well be an isolated ac-tivity, treating intelligibility immediately moves the emphasis of consideration to include the speaker and the listener as encoding and decoding are involved in the concept of intelligible messages. Evidently more complexity is implied when con-sidering intelligibility than is suggested by the use of the related terminology, such as articulation, recognizability, identifiability and discriminability, which are important features but only part of the interaction in communication.

Communicative effectiveness is determined by numerous factors; including so-cial context, message content, the stimulus signal, and the medium used for sig-nal transmission along with the speaker and the speaker's speech mechanism. This is further compounded by the many characteristics of the listener and the environment.

Chial (1984) has argued that while there is a need to examine the individual components of "operational intelligibility," there is also a need to study less structured communication with vocabularies, listeners, messages and signals, which collectively contribute to intelligibility and impact on communicative ef-fectiveness. However, even this apparently inclusive list has omitted aspects such as the environment and other paralinguistic features of communication and the contribution of nonverbal facets of the communication process.

The concept of operational intelligibility suggests that basic phonetic intelligibility is conditioned by physical, pragmatic, and linguistic contexts. The physical context includes extraneous noise and vibration produced by the system as well as other environmental influences. Elements of the pragmatic context include the ongoing event, influences of past and present events, and social constraints filtered through the listeners' knowledge and experience regarding communication. Linguistic context is provided by the listeners' and speakers' knowledge of the probability within linguistic coding. Thus, speech comprehension is the end product (the output) of this complex communication channel, which is originally stimulated by the message conceived by the speaker. For the purposes of this chapter, I separate the listener and speaker variables although this split is obviously artificial as communication is entirely interactive. For example, the speaker will often adjust a message if it is apparent that the listener is having difficulty (Verdolini et al., 1985).

## Listener Variables

The manner in which listeners receive messages varies a great deal and is affected by such aspects as processing time, familiarity, experience, hearing, age, tolerance (physical and psychological), and environment.

Aspects of speech such as prosody and other paralinguistic features, such as pausing and stress, also have a measurable effect on speech intelligibility. These features not only convey separate information that add to the core information so that nuances of meaning can be conveyed, but also these specific aspects of the acoustic signal assist the listener in planning or systematizing decoding, thereby aiding this decoding. For example, decoding is aided by temporal pauses, in that content information is highlighted above redundant information (Gold, 1980; Osberger & McGarr, 1982; Maassen, 1984). Dysarthric patients who have difficulty in phrasing are placing the listener at a disadvantage by reducing his/her ability to decode and omitting cues that highlight to the listener the pertinent issues in the message.

There is strong research evidence that perceived speech quality and intelligibility are particularly related to the listener's view of prosody and pitch evenness (Hawkins & Warren, 1994). Monotonous pitch, or pitch breaks can have a noticeably disruptive effect upon the listener's ability to interact appropriately with the speaker. In this context, it has been found that, within certain parameters, articulation has less of a negative affect on the listener than errors of prosody. Despite this, many clinicians will spend their time working on improving phonemic accuracy rather than considering the features that cause a greater disruption to overall communication. More than two decades ago Wingfield and Klein (1971) and Wingfield (1975) compared prosodically anomalous with normal sentences with accelerated presentation and found a greater deterioration of intelligibility for the former than the latter. This finding was confirmed by Huggins (1978) whose experiments indicated that intelligibility decreased considerably when intonation and temporal structures of sentences were distorted. Studies examining the effect of fundamental frequency corrections of deaf speech showed that corrections yielded a small but sufficient improvement in intelligibility but overuse of intonation resulted in a deleterious effect (Maasen & Povel, 1984).

Breath control is important for maintaining continuity and integrity of an utterance and can thus be related to overall speech rate and division of the utterance into coherent chunks of information (Crystal, 1987). The absence of appropriate "chunking" has been found to lead to reduced intelligibility. Maasen (1986) found that by adding pauses to identify word boundaries, intelligibility of sentences was measurably improved. A control feature in this study also indicated that this increase was not merely due to the general deceleration of the speaking rate. Thus, it appears that this manipulation of segmental and supra-segmental aspects could help the listener play an active role in the communication process.

Words spoken in context are more easily understood by the listener than words heard out of a meaningful context (Punzi & Kraat, 1985). To a certain extent this can be explained by predictability and redundancy of the environment of the sentence (Lieberman, 1963). The predictability of the sentence may affect the accuracy of articulation by the speaker as well as having an effect upon the listener's attitude. For example, if a speaker is placing an unpredictable word within a sentence, he/she will increase the duration and be more precise with the articulation to assist the listener in identifying the anomaly. Dysarthric speakers would have greater difficulty in being able to assist the listener in this way, therefore methods of coping with unfamiliar or unpredictable material should be incorporated into treatment. For example, it may be necessary for a dysarthric speaker to use extra visual clues or spelling clues in these circumstances (Crow & Enderby, 1989).

Sentences and phrases offer linguistic cues and aid the listener in narrowing the pool of possible words that could follow. Other research has shown that context may assist the listener in a broader way by helping the listener to "tune in," giving acoustic information that allows decode parameters associated with an individual speaker to be established. Studies of persons with unfamiliar accents have shown that listeners "tune in" and can decode what is said with increasing ease as the person speaks and that this is not necessarily related to becoming familiar with the context. The implications of these research findings to the treatment of persons with dysarthria or those using speech synthesis are obvious. To help the listener, it is important that any information carrying words are embedded within a context that allows the person to focus and to tune in. Beukleman and Yorkston (1979, 1980) have reported several studies in a program of research related to listener's judgements of dysarthric speech. One of many important findings was that judgements of clarity for the moderately disordered speech were improved by naive judges with increasing passage familiarity and exposure, suggesting that listeners were overlooking the specific acoustic parameters as they were able to predict and became more familiar with the speaking style.

When speech is less clear, listeners use different strategies to help to maintain the conversation. Different listeners use different strategies but the more strategies used lead to greater success. Conversational analysis has shown that some listeners are more flexible and varied in the approaches they take to maintaining conversational flow. Some of these strategies involve prediction, but it would appear that predicting syntax is more important for the listener than conforming semantics. Therefore, if a speaker is having difficulty getting a message across the listener will interpret a sentence to conform to grammatical rules even when it does not make sense semantically. Because of the effort of speaking with dysarthria, many individuals will alter their language structure to simplify the message and to save effort. Unfortunately this secondary effect of dysarthria may have a disruptive influence on the listener. Speech and language therapists interested in improving conversational interaction must be aware that placing emphasis on language structure may be appropriate even in the absence of a language impairment.

The concept of listener effort and attention is interesting. Obviously there are some conditions that encourage attention, including the cocktail party scenario, that is, if a listener's name is used his attention will increase. When a listener is having difficulty understanding, as may occur with unamplified abnormal speech in moderate background noise, he/she may tend to pay more attention than when he/she is in a more favorable environment (Verdolini et al., 1985). This increased attention may recruit the listener being more attentive to lip reading, nonverbal signals, and paralinguistic clues. While this ability to attend may be difficult to sustain, it may well be that the listener's subconscious efforts to attend can be used to the dysarthric person's benefit. It is possible that some dysarthric persons with quiet speech may be more effective in gaining and maintaining attention without a speech amplifier than with one. The natural adjustment of volume and clarity, to combat natural noise, can be used in speech and language therapy to increase a small amount of stress upon the dysarthric person's system to assess the maximum achievement possible by the individual. Frequently speech and language therapists will suggest that persons with dysarthria talk in a quiet environment, and while this may be appropriate, it may also be of therapeutic benefit to practice in noisy environments to improve stamina and attention.

Background noise is one environmental factor affecting intelligibility. Others include the physical characteristics of the environment. Cox et al. (1987) found that there were significant intelligibility differences observed between speakers in different environments, such as living rooms, classroom, and social event room. One subject in their trial demonstrated that some voices are particularly susceptible to degradation due to reverberation in different environments and the perception of intelligibility by listeners seemed to show that individual speakers could naturally accommodate to the different acoustic parameters of different environments in different ways.

### Speaker Variables

This chapter is emphasizing the aspects of disability/activity by dwelling upon methods of improving communicative effectiveness. Factors, primarily from a listener viewpoint, have been considered, but now attention is given to variables related to the speaker, which can be manipulated to improve the success of an interaction. The many features related to the dysarthric impairment and specific approaches to treatment of them will not be addressed. These are well covered in Dworkin (1991) and Duffy (1995).

Clarity of articulation, appropriacy of phonation, resonance, and volume are all essential components in conveying information that can be understood by a listener. There are many features other than the neuromotor impairment that affect precision, force, and accuracy of articulation, some of these are linguistic, psychological, and environmental. The link between linguistic structure and articulation is recognized (Crystal, 1987; McGarr, 1981), but not clearly understood. Leiberman (1963) showed that words isolated from unpredictable sentences were more intelligible than words isolated from predictable ones, possibly a result of the subconscious recognition by the speaker that the listener will need extra assistance resulting in effort at articulatory accuracy. Similarly, speakers frequently adjust their speech if they perceive that the message is not being received. For example, sudden noises or other distractions may lead the speaker to change vocal output by pausing, changing the rate of speech, increasing the amplitude or even repeating or adding information (Lane & Traud, 1971; Verdolini et al., 1985) in an attempt to maintain intelligible communication. The perception by the speaker that a listener is uncertain has a direct effect upon the speaker's articulatory consistency. Research has demonstrated that children with phonological problems adjust their speech by producing better phonetic productions, when talking to someone who was clearly not understanding them, than when the listener gave the appearance that they were understanding (Weiner & Ostrowski, 1979). Thus, it appears that the recognition of communication failure affects the speech production. Speech and language therapists and others will frequently falsely affect comprehension of a dysarthric client to maintain conversational flow, to avoid embarrassment, or in an effort to gain further clues to assist in interpretation. This common "therapeutic" ploy may not be appropriate and may well be disadvantageous to the speaker by not facilitating them to make adjustments to their disordered speech in order to assist the listener.

The range of what is viewed as normal (acceptable, intelligible) speech is broad. Individual variability of phonological production, personal patterns of stress, and prosody along with the subject's usual pitch and volume adjustments, all lead to identifiable patterns of speech that make it easy for a listener to identify one speaker from another without being in visual contact. These communication "finger prints" make it difficult to specify what the norm is; therefore, it is probably easier to look at those that fall beyond these parameters which can be more easily identified as abnormal.

There are many persons who are not dysarthric, but who are not as communicatively competent as others and do not repair or maintain the flow of conversation with alacrity.

Teaching strategies for communication repair to persons with disordered speech is more necessary with some clients than with others. However, probably all dysarthric persons require some attention to ensure that they take some degree of control and responsibility for assisting the listener to participate within the communicative interaction. It is unlikely that we will be able to change the culture which at present disadvantages people with speech disorders and leads to discrimination. Thus, virtually all dysarthric patients will, on occasions, meet individuals or groups of people who do not react in ways that are either appropriate, empowering, or respectful; they will meet prejudice and hostility so, as therapists, we should endeavor to ensure that the dysarthric person is equipped to be resilient and resourceful to assist those who have concerns, fears, or prejudices to react more appropriately. Rehearsing introductory sentences, or having notes that clearly identify how a listener should react to dysarthric speech or a communication aid can defuse anxiety as well as placing the conversation control in the speech impaired person's hands.

## Assessment of Dysarthric Impairment, Disability, and Handicap

This chapter has drawn attention to the needs of the dysarthric patient beyond that related to the treatment of impairment alone. There is an increasing awareness in the discipline of speech and language therapy that attention to the immediate deficit is inadequate for rehabilitating a patient. Generally, there is an acceptance that it is important that functional communication and the well-being of the client should receive consideration and attention, not only in the treatment but also in monitoring progress (See Hustad et al., 1998). The Therapy Outcome Measure (TOM) (Enderby & John, 1997) is one available measure that was developed to provide speech and language therapists with a broader approach to the monitoring of the communication disorder, allowing identification of the speech or language impairment in the context of what the person can achieve communicatively, how he/she is coping socially and considering the level of distress or well-being. The development of the TOM followed analysis of the approaches undertaken by therapists in the treatment of a broad range of different speech and language disorders. While traditionally we have several tools to assist us with clarifying the degree of the impairment, the study concluded that we are not well equipped to reflect the general needs of the patient and whether treatment had an impact on these broader issues. TOM comprises four dimensions; Impairment, Disability/Activity, Handicap/Participation, and Well-being. The first three of these are based upon the dimensions of the World Health Organization (WHO) International Classification (Usten, 1997) and the fourth represents the area in which therapists are commonly involved in trying to facilitate. The outcome measure has an 11-point ordinal scale. The integers (0 to 5) are defined with descriptors of symptoms and behaviors, making distinctions between each whole point on the scale. A half point (0.5) is used to reflect the judgement that a patient's presentation is between the two descriptors. The scale provides category ratings on each of the single dimensions reflecting the severity of the difficulties. A categorical ordinal scale can be considered as having some integral properties. Each numerical rating of the core scale has an attached descriptor specifically developed for a client group (e.g., learning disability, laryngectomy, hearing disorders, dysfluency, dysphasia, dysphonia, developmental disorders, and dysarthria). These descriptors help the therapist to identify the "best fit" of a scale point (See Appendix).

The motivation behind the development of this measure was the need for a simple, standardized, and objective measure to reflect the status of the individual across the different dimensions of health that commonly concern a speech and language therapist and to redress the balance from an impairment emphasis to that recognizing the functional, social, and emotional consequences of a disorder. The measure is used by the therapist at the start of an episode of care and again at the end. This allows the patient, as well as the therapist, to review the goals of treatment and to monitor effectiveness. Attention to the psychometric properties has resulted in several publications, however, we acknowledge there is still room for further work (Enderby & John, 1997; Enderby et al. 1998; Enderby & John, in press). The scales have been found to have face and content validity from the perspective of the therapist. The results of many reliability studies based mainly on multiple assessors viewing videos of patients, or being presented with composite case histories indicate adequate inter-rater reliability with Kappa values of between 0. 43 to 0.91 showing moderate to excellent reliability. Details on all pyschometric studies are reported in the technical manual of the TOMs (Enderby & John, 1997).

Table 14–1 compares the outcomes of patients with dysarthria associated with four common conditions; stroke (15 subjects), head injury (six subjects), Parkinson's disease (eight subjects), and cerebral palsied adult (nine subjects). These adult patients were all referred as new candidates to speech and language therapy within a 6-month period and had received at least one episode of care. An episode of care is usually defined as a period of therapy when the major goals are static. When goals change a new episode of care is begun. Within this study most episodes were between 6 and 8 weeks in length. The percentage change reflects the start score by using the calculation

$$\frac{end - start}{start} \times 100.$$

Inspection of the data indicates that, unsurprisingly, the greatest gains with regard to dysarthric impairment were related to stroke and head injury patients, whereas those with the progressive neurological disease (Parkinson's disease) made a smaller incremental improvement in this domain and those with long-standing cerebral palsy showed no gains in this area.

Despite the lack of improvement in the area of impairment, the cerebral palsy group made a remarkable gain of 38% in the area of disability. Patients with head injury showed gains of 58% in this domain. Changes to disability rather than impairment scores are expected in populations with long-standing disorders, especially when therapy is targeted at the disability level.

While those patients with stroke and head injury showed improvements in the area of handicap/participation (25%, 33%, respectively) those with Parkinson's disease and cerebral palsy showed less gain. The persons with cerebral palsy already had high start scores in this domain as compared to the other four groups. They also showed high start scores related to well-being. The persons with head injury, while showing the lowest start score in the well-being domain, made gains of 29% by the end of the episode of care. Stroke patients made the largest improvement in this area, but did not achieve the high scores indicated by the adult cerebral palsy at the end of the episode of care.

These results show, albeit crudely, that the dysarthrias associated with the different underlying conditions have disproportionate effects upon the areas of impairment, disability, handicap, and well-being and that therapy may impact on

Table 14–1.  Therapy Outcome Measures Mean Start, End, and Change Scores and Overall Percentage Gain. Comparison of Outcomes of Four Client Groups With Dysarthria

| | Impairment | | | Disability/Activity | | | Handicap/Participation | | | Well-being | | |
| --- | --- | --- | --- | --- | --- | --- | --- | --- | --- | --- | --- | --- |
| | Start | Change | End | Start | Change | End | Start | Change | End | Start | Change | End |
| Stroke<br>n = 15 | 1.7 | 0.9<br>53% | 2.6 | 2.35 | 0.8<br>36% | 3.2 | 2.6 | 0.7<br>27% | 3.3 | 2.45 | 1.1<br>45% | 3.55 |
| Head Injury<br>n = 6 | 2.1 | 0.9<br>42.8% | 3.0 | 1.9 | 1.1<br>58% | 3.0 | 2.4 | 0.8<br>33% | 3.2 | 1.7 | 0.5<br>29% | 2.2 |
| Parkinson's Disease<br>n = 8 | 1.7 | 0.05<br>2.9% | 1.75 | 2.65 | 0.3<br>11.3% | 2.95 | 2.55 | 0.1<br>4% | 2.7 | 3.05 | 0.35<br>11.5% | 3.4 |
| Adult Cerebral Palsy<br>n = 9 | 3.00 | 0.00<br>0% | 3.00 | 2.65 | 1.0<br>38% | 3.65 | 3.65 | 0.5<br>13.7% | 3.70 | 4.1 | 0.2<br>4.9% | 4.3 |

these in different ways. It is likely that the approach taken by the speech and language therapist, along with the impact on the individual with dysarthria, will affect the outcomes in different areas. Identifying the level of difficulty in the different domains at the beginning and during treatment can help the speech and language therapist and the client achieve an appropriate balance in therapy that can be individually tailored and monitored.

## Conclusion

There have been many disciplines that have contributed to our knowledge of what helps disordered speech become intelligible. The diverse sources of research that we can apply range from studies related to the interference of slap from helicopter blades to the distortion of the sound signal made by environmental substances. Furthermore, we are learning more about what assists a listener in abstracting messages that may be sent in adverse circumstances. Speech and language therapists can use a range of techniques beyond that of improving the acoustics and phonology to ensure that their clients can be more effective communicators. It is important to view the impaired speech within the general context of rehabilitation, not only in planning the treatment program, but also in considering the most appropriate way of measuring and monitoring the interventions aimed at exploiting every possible factor to improving communicative success and the well-being of the client.

## Appendix

### Dysarthria

Identify descriptor that is "best fit." The patient does not have to have each feature mentioned. Use 0.5 to indicate if patient is slightly better or worse than a descriptor.

**Impairment** (as appropriate to age)

0   **Severe dysarthria:** severe persistent articulatory/prosodic impairment. Inability to produce any distinguishable speech sounds. No oral motor control. No respiratory support for speech.

1   **Severe/moderate dysarthria** with consistent articulatory/prosodic impairment. Mostly open vowels with some consonant approximations/severe festinaton of speech. Extremely effortful or slow speech, only 1 or 2 words per breath. Severely limited motor control.

2   **Moderate dysarthria** with frequent episodes of articulatory/prosodic impairment. Most consonants attempted, but poorly represented acoustically/moderate festination. Very slow speech, manages up to 4 words per breath. Moderate limitation oral motor control.

3   **Moderate/mild dysarthria:** consistent omission/articulation of consonants. Variability of speed. Mild limitation of oral motor control or prosodic impairment.

4   **Mild dysarthria:** slight or occasional omission/mispronunciation of consonants. Slight or occasional difficulty with oral motor control/prosody or respiratory support.

5   **No impairment.**

### Disability (as appropriate to age)

0   Unable to communicate in any way. No effective communication. No interaction.

1   Occasionally able to make basic needs known with familiar persons or trained listeners in familiar contexts. Minimal communication with maximal assistance.

2   Limited functional communication. Consistently able to make basic needs/conversation understood, but is heavily dependent on cues and context. Communicates better with trained listener or family members or in familiar settings. Frequent repetition required. Maintains meaningful interaction related to here and now.

3   Consistently able to make needs known, but can sometimes convey more information than this. Some inconsistency in unfamiliar settings. Is less dependent for intelligibility on cues and context. Occasional repetition required. Communicates beyond here/now with familiar persons, needs some cues and prompting.

4   Can be understood most of the time by any listener despite communication irregularities. Holds conversation, required some special consideration, particularly with a wider range of people.

5   Communicates effectively in all situations.

### Handicap (as appropriate to age)

0   Unable to fulfill any social/educational/family role. Not involved in decision making/no autonomy/no control over environment. No social integration.

1   Low self-confidence/poor self-esteem/limited social integration/socially isolated/ contributes to some basic and limited decisions. Cannot achieve potential in any situation.

2   Some self-confidence/some social integration/makes some decisions and influences control in familiar situations.

3   Some self-confidence, autonomy emerging. Makes decisions and has control of some aspects of life. Able to achieve some limited social integration/educational activities. Diffident over control over life. Needs encouragement to achieve potential.

4   Mostly confident, occasional difficulties integrating or in fulfilling social/role activity. Participating in all appropriate decisions. May have difficulty in achieving potential in some situations occasionally.

5   Achieving potential, autonomous and unrestricted. Able to fulfill social, educational, and family role.

**Well-being/Distress** (as appropriate to age)

0 **Severe constant:**
upset/frustration/anger/distress/embarrassment/concern/withdrawal

1 **Frequently severely:**
upset/frustration/anger/distress/embarrassment/concern/withdrawal

2 **Moderate consistent:**
upset/frustration/anger/distress/embarrassment/concern/withdrawal

3 **Moderate frequent:**
upset/frustration/anger/distress/embarrassment/concern/withdrawal

4 **Mild occasional:**
upset/frustration/anger/distress/embarrassment/concern/withdrawal

5 **No inappropriate:**
upset/frustration/anger/distress/embarrassment/concern/withdrawal

## *References*

Arnold, G. E. (1965). Central nervous disorders of speaking: Dysarthria. In R. Luchsinger, G. E. Arnold (eds): *Voice, Speech, Language*. Belmont: Wadsworth.

Beukelman, D., & Yorkston, K. (1979). The relationship between information transfer and speech intelligibility of dysartic speakers. *Journal of Communicable Diseases, 13*, 189–196.

Beukelman, D., & Yorkston, K. (1980). Influence of passage familiarity on intelligibility estimates of dysartic speech. *Journal of Communicable Diseases, 13*, 33–41.

Chial, M. (1984). Evaluation microcomputer hardware. In A. J. Schwartz (ed): *Handbook of microcomputer applications in communication disorders*. San Diego: College Hill Press.

Cox, R., Alexander, C., & Gilmore (1987). Intelligibility of average talkers in typical listening environments. *Journal of the Acoustical Society of America, 81*, 1598–1608.

Crow, E., & Enderby, P. (1989). The effects of an alphabet chart on the speaking rate and intelligibility of speakers with dysarthria. In K. M. Yorkston, D. R. Beukelman (eds): *Recent advances in clinical dysarthria* (pp. 99–108). Austin, TX.

Crystal, J. (1987). Towards a bucket 'theory' of language disability: Taking account of interaction between linguistic levels. *Clinical Linguistics and Phonetics, 1*, 7–22.

Darley, F. L. (1978). Differential diagnosis of acquired motor speech disorders. In F. L. Darley, D. C. Spriestersbach (eds): *Diagnostic methods in speech pathology* (2nd ed.). New York: Harper and Row.

Darley, F. L., Aronson, A. E., & Brown, J. R. (1975). *Motor speech disorders*. Philadelphia, PA: W. B. Saunders.

Darley, F. L., Brown, J. R., & Goldstein, N. P. (1972). Dysarthria in multiple sclerosis. *Journal of Speech and Hearing Research, 15*, 229–245.

Duffy, J. R. (1995). *Motor speech disorders: Substrates, differential diagnosis and management*. Baltimore: MD: Mosby.

Dworkin, J. (1991). *Motor speech disorders: A treatment guide*. Mosby: St Louis.

Enderby, P., & Emerson, J. (1995). *Does speech and language therapy work: A review of the literature*. London: Whurr Publishers.

Enderby, P., & John, A. (in press). Therapy outcome measures in speech and language therapy: Comparing performance between providers. *International Journal of Language and Communication Disorders*.

Enderby, P., & John, A. (1997). Therapy outcome measures (speech and language therapy). London: Singular Publications.

Enderby, P., John, A., & Petheram, B. (1998). Therapy outcome measure: Physiotherapy, occupational therapy and rehabilitation nursing. London: Singular Publishing Group, Inc.

Gold, T. (1980). Speech production in hearing impaired children. *Journal of Communicable Diseases, 13*, 397–418.

Hawkins, S., & Warren, P. (1994). Phonetic influences on the intelligibility of conversational speech. *Journal of Phonetics, 22*, 493–511.

Huggins, A. W. F. (1978). Speech timing and intelligibility. In J. Requin (ed): *Attention and performance VIII* (pp. 279–297). Hillsdale, NJ: Erbaum.

Hustad, K. C., Beukelman, D. R., & Yorkston, K. M. (1998). Functional outcome assessment in dysarthria. *Seminars in Speech and Language, 19*, 291–302.

Lane, H., & Traud, B. (1971). The Lombard sign and the role of hearing in speech. *Journal of Speech and Hearing Research, 14,* 677–709.

Lieberman, P. (1963). Some effects of semantic and grammatical context on the production and perception of speech. *Language and Speech, 6,* 172–187.

Logemann, J. A., & Fisher, H. B. (1981). Vocal tract control in Parkinson's disease: Phonetic feature analysis of mis-articulations. *Journal of Speech and Hearing Disorders, 46,* 248–352.

Maasen, B. (1986). The role of temporal structure and information in deaf speech. In C. Johns Lewis (ed): *Intonation in discourse.* London: Croom Helm.

Maasen, B., & Povel, D. (1984). The effect of correcting fundamental frequency on the intelligibility of deaf speech and its interaction with temporal aspects. *Journal of the Acoustical Society of America, 76,* 1673–1681.

McGarr, N. (1981). The effect of context on the intelligibility of hearing and deaf children's speech. *Language and Speech, 24,* 255–264.

Netsell, R. W. (1998). Speech rehabilitation for individuals with unintelligible speech and dysarthria: The respiratory and velopharyngeal systems. *Journal of Medical Speech–Language Pathology, 6,* 107–110.

Osberger, M. J., & McGarr, N. S. (1982). *Speech production characteristics of the hearing impaired in speech and language: Advances in basic research and practice,* vol. 8. New York: Lass Academic.

Punzi, L. M., & Kraat, A. (1985). The effect of context on preschool children's understanding of synthetic speech—A pilot study. *Working Papers in Speech Language Pathology, 13,* 84–106.

Sims, J. (1998). Respect for autonomy: Issues in neurological rehabilitation. *Clinical Rehabilitation, 12,* 3–10.

Sarno, M. T., Buonagura, A., & Levita, E. (1986). Characteristics of verbal impairment in closed head injured patients. *Archives of Physical Medicine and Rehabilitation, 67,* 400–405.

Usten, B. (1997). News on the ICIDH. Centre for standisation of Informatics in Health Care; *Newsletter* 4, pp. 2–7.

Verdolini, K., Skinner, M., & Patton, T. (1985). Effect of amplification on the intelligibility of speech produced with an electrolarynx. *Laryngoscope, 95,* 720–726.

Weiner, F., & Ostrowski, A. (1979). Effects of listener uncertainty on articulatory inconsistency. *Journal of Speech and Hearing Disorders, 44,* 487–493.

Wingfield, A. (1975). The intonation and syntax interaction: Prosadic features in perceptual processing of speech. In A. Cohen, S. Nooteboom (eds): *Structure and process in speech perception* (pp. 146–160) New York: Springer Verlag.

Wingfield, A., & Klein, J. D. (1971). Syntactic structure and acoustic patterns in speech perception. *Perceptual Psychophysiology, 9,* 23–25.

Worster-Drought, C. (1974). Suprabulbar paresis: Congenital suprabulbar paresis and its differential diagnosis with special reference to acquired suprabulbar paresis. *Developmental Medicine & Child Neurology, 16*(Suppl. 30), 1–33.

Yorkston, K. (1996). Treatment efficacy: Dysarthria. *Journal of Speech and Hearing Research, 39,* 546–557.

Yorkston, K. M., & Beukelman, D. R. (Eds). (1994). Motor speech disorders: Advances in assessment and treatment. In (pp. 103–118). Baltimore: Paul H. Brookes Publishing.

# 15

# Assessment and Treatment of Functional Swallowing in Dysphagia

## Barbara C. Sonies

**The dominance of dysphagia rehabilitation within speech–language pathology in the health-care sector has spawned a number of dysphagia assessment scales. This chapter reviews a broad range of scales within the context of the World Health Organization's ICIDH-2. The review concludes that there is still a need for broad-based functional measures of dysphagia that assess swallowing in natural contexts and have sufficient reliability and validity to monitor change.**

## Introduction

Since the early 1990s, the majority of clinical practice referrals for speech–language pathologists in many health-care settings in the United States has been to request service for individuals with dysphagia or disordered swallowing. A similar increase in referrals for dysphagia treatment is occurring throughout the European community. This increase has produced an emphasis on accountability and ability to chart progress. More than charting progress, it is essential to be able to determine whether the individual has received benefit from services provided in dysphagia to increase function and reduce handicap. When examining the ability to ingest a normal meal, the functional components imply that the individual can eat most foods safely and comfortably in a natural environment despite the swallowing impairment.

### Functional Eating Behavior

The definition of functional communication, as stated in Chapter 1 (p. 3) "ability to receive or convey a message, regardless of the mode, to communicate effectively and independently in a given environment" (ASHA, 1990, p. 2) can be easily modified for eating. Therefore, for the purposes of this chapter, I define *functional eating behavior* as the "ability to eat a meal effectively and independently in a given environment so as to sustain adequate nutrition for a healthy life style." There is a need to measure the meal-time ability of the dysphagic individual to determine whether functional eating behavior has been achieved.

To date, there is no standard or accepted scale to measure or monitor whether functional independence in eating has been achieved. Anecdotal evidence exists from patient interviews to suggest that some individuals, who have learned to compensate for swallowing impairments by using postural changes and other swallowing maneuvers, are not satisfied with the outcome. This creates an interesting gap between reduction of swallowing impairment, improvement of eating safety, and the person's expectations of their level to return to function. Many persons cannot accept less than premorbid ability to eat as a positive functional outcome. This creates a challenge for those who are designing and validating dysphagia outcome measures.

It is the intent of this chapter to report on a representative sample of swallowing functional outcome scales and to describe them in relationship to the assessment domains they include. Later segments of this chapter will review some of the existing nonstandardized dysphagia outcome measures, categorize them using the ICIDH-2 model, and discuss the future from the perspective of integration of swallowing disorders into this model, driving outcomes research.

## *Handicap (Participation Restriction) Versus Disability (Activities Limitation)*

There are several scales that have been used to describe function in dysphagia that will be discussed in a later section. The majority of these scales focus on understanding the impairment caused by a specific physiological or biomechanical event (i.e., duration of motion of the hyoid bone, opening of the upper esophageal sphincter, pharyngeal transit time, relation of structure motion to bolus flow). An example of a scale that focuses on a biomechanical outcome is the *Penetration-Aspiration Scale* (Rosenbek et al., 1996). This tool includes an 8-point scale dealing exclusively with the location of material entering the airway and whether attempts are made to expel the material from the airway. Although, this scale is clinically helpful, it does not focus on how moving from one level to the next level on the scale affects the patient's ability to improve eating function. There has been a push to examine dysphagia in relation to the effect of impairment on feeding activity and to attempt to better understand how a disadvantage impacts on the individual. However, these few measures are in their infancy and are usually being developed by a single facility [i.e., SWAL-QOL under development at University of Wisconsin, Madison, WI (Wisconsin Speech–Language and Hearing Association, 1996); and the Dysphagic Disability Index, Henry Ford Hospital, Detroit, MI (Silbergleit et al., in press)].

To determine whether the current measures that exist for dysphagia are relevant to the model proposed in Chapter 1, it is necessary to place them into categories that might not have been intended when they were originally constructed. Few, if any, scales were developed to fit neatly into the ICIDH-2 classification scheme. Many of the existing scales used to evaluate swallowing disorders examine only the impairment(s) that can be determined from an instrumental swallowing examination (i.e., videofluorography, ultrasound, nasoendoscopy, electromyography, manometry, scintigraphy, auscultation, electroglotography) (Sonies, 1994; Sonies & Frattali, 1997). Because most dysphagia scales have not been designed to evaluate disability or handicap, they conform to a medical model in which the diagnostic signs signaling a treatment approach are identified. Most outcome scales have been developed by individual health-care facilities and are used only within that particular program. Few are widely shared and few have been standardized or tested to determine their psychometric properties.

### Continuum of Care

To be effective in achieving independence, dysphagia management requires a continual and ongoing process as the patient progresses from the levels of acute care, subacute care, to long-term care, and to home care (Sonies & Frattali, 1997). At each level, an outcome measure can be introduced to evaluate current and predict future activity levels. A system describing the responsibilities of the speech–language pathologist managing neurological communication disorders at the acute, subacute, inpatient rehabilitation, home care, and outpatient rehabilitation levels of care is described by Coelho (1998). It is possible that a person with a stroke could enter an acute care facility and after 3 to 5 days be discharged as a fully independent eater. It is hoped that an outcome scale would be able to predict the prognosis. In the continuum of care model an outcome measure could be used at entry into each level of care. For example, by using the "Critical-Clinical Pathway Outcome Scale" (Sonies & Frattali, 1997), which is part of the Beaumont Outcome Software System (BOSS) (Merson et al., 1995), patients in an acute care setting who received only consultative services or were screened (but not treated) for dysphagia could be tracked during their acute hospitalization. This scale examines entry points along the continuum of care rather than behavioral outcomes associated with treatment. For example, on this measure, the highest scale value is: "The evaluation and treatment have been completed, and the medical staff has been apprised of patient's swallowing status. The discharge plan has been completed and patient is ready for the next phase of rehabilitation. All medical forms and referrals have been completed" (Sonies & Frattali, 1997, p. 22). This type of outcome measure has not typically been included in outcomes data.

### Functional Scales for Examining Ability to Eat, Drink, and Swallow

#### Components of Dysphagia Scales and Outcomes Measures

In reviewing the existing outcome measures, a general scheme emerged in which measures either focused on a narrow spectrum of items (e.g., saliva management, aspiration, oral/nonoral feeding) or tried to include as many types of items as possible that were deemed pertinent to the functional assessment of swallowing (e.g., response delay + aspiration + supervision + independence + diet modifications + bolus size). Many of these scales depend on a combination of instrumental test results and subjective behavioral observations during eating to assign scores. The components usually included in part, or in various combinations, in these measures are as follows: aspiration, risk for aspiration, pulmonary complications, bolus transfer, swallow delay or timing, functional eating ability, secretion management, compensations, type of diet, oral or nonoral feeding, dependence/supervision, food consistency, amount eaten orally and nutrition/hydration.

## Population-Specific Measures

Most of the scales that have been developed for dysphagia use a numerical point scale or a severity rating scale (normal, mild, mild/moderate, moderate, moderate/severe, severe, profound) and contain items pertaining to impairment and disability; rarely do they examine handicap. The scales that have been developed often focus on a specific population or age group. For example, there are functional outcome scales that are being developed for Secretion Management, Pediatric Swallowing, Birth to Kindergarten, Developmentally Disabled Adults, and Adult Dysphagics by task forces of the American Speech–Language Hearing Association (e.g., ASHA Special Interest Division 13, Task Force on Functional Outcomes, 1997). These measures will be discussed later as to how they fit into the categorical descriptions of function.

An example of a population-specific outcome measure is found in a study by Logemann et al. (1992). They evaluated the percentage of head and neck cancer patients who achieved normal eating and drinking function after laryngectomy. Outcomes examined were the time to achieve oral intake, time to return to a preoperative diet, duration of tube feeding placement, and time to achieve a normal swallow. The major measures were time and mode of eating. No rating or hierarchical scales were developed and the outcomes were stated in percentages.

Assessment of health-related quality of life for head and neck cancer patients includes, in large part, their ability to eat in the most natural setting (List et al., 1990). A set of outcome measures was developed and tested on 50 adult patients from 3 months to 6 years after having had major surgery for head and neck cancer (D'Antonio et al., 1996). The scale relates disease-specific measures to functional status in the scope of the quality of life experienced by the patient. Measures of quality of life and functional status were rated in three areas, *Eating in Public, Understandability of Speech,* and *Normalcy of Diet,* with a score of 100 indicating normalcy or no restrictions in each area. *Eating in public* appears to be a scale of handicap as it queries where and how individuals eat in normal environments. Normalcy of diet is a scale of disability as it gives a numerical score to various types of foods that the person is able to eat without restriction. Two additional measures of quality of life and functional status were included in the study: Functional Assessment of Cancer Therapy—FACT (Cella et al., 1994) and University of Washington Quality of Life Questionnaire (UW-QOL). Both of these measures contain categories or items that evaluate ability to eat and swallow. The

FACT focuses more on general items of physical and social/emotional well-being and includes eating issues in a category called additional concerns. The UW-QOL has a category for eating including chewing and swallowing where the individual rates how "well they can perform." Correlations were determined between these measures and disease-specific measures. Cella et al. (1994) found that general and disease-specific instruments each contributed differing degrees of information regarding how individuals perceived quality-of-life functions. These measures could easily be applied to other groups of individuals to objectively assess the implications of dysphagia as a handicap.

An Amytrophic Lateral Sclerosis (ALS) Severity Scale was developed to deal with this specific neurologically impaired adult population (Hillel et al., 1989; Yorkston et al., 1993). This 10-point scale (with "10" indicating normalcy) is subdivided into five discrete categories in order of severity: Normal Eating Habits, Early Eating Problems, Dietary Consistency Changes, Tube Feeding, and Nonoral Feeding. Biomechanical, durational, and instrumental measures are not necessary for assignment of ratings on the ALS Severity Scale. This measure is geared toward the level of disability and the handicap imposed on the individual by the observed and self-reported changes in eating ability. It examines how the patient handles food and liquids and whether nutrition can be maintained through oral methods.

Waxman et al. (1990) have developed a Dysphagia Severity Rating Scale for Parkinson's Disease to attempt to examine the progression of dysphagia in relation to the progression of the condition. It contains a 7-point rating scale ranging from severe dysphagia to normal swallowing. In this scale the results of a videofluorographic swallowing study are used to determine aspiration, duration of the swallow, and benefit of therapeutic strategies for several of the levels. In this scale the patient's self-report as well as their need to vary consistency of diet is threaded throughout the levels. This scale focuses on levels of disability.

The Functional Communication Measure: Pediatrics (ASHA, National Treatment Outcome Data Collection Project, Field Test Edition, 1995–1996) is a 7-point rating scale with an added zero (0) included if the behavior could not be tested. This scale intertwines impairment with disability in all of the levels but does not address handicap until Level 7 "normal feeding to meet nutritional needs with an appropriate diet in all situations." The lowest level of function, Level 1, Profound impairment, and Level 2, Severe impairment, are measures of physiology (i.e., "protective reflexes, gagging, and coughing, lack of secretion management, hypersensitivity") of a severity to preclude or limit feeding. Levels 3 and 4, Severe to Moderate impairment, address functional eating and need for diet modifications and supervision. Levels 5 and 6, Moderate to Mild impairment, again focus on functional eating and lessening of diet modifications or compensations with minimal or no supervision.

The ASHA Functional Communication Measure: Birth to Kindergarten Feeding and Swallowing Scale (ASHA, Field Test Edition, 1995–1996) is another 7-point scale that is a simpler scale with a primary focus on whether feeding is nonoral or oral and whether supervision is needed. This scale is oriented toward feeding expectations at different chronological ages. A similar 7-point scale was developed and field tested in 1997 to examine saliva management in this same group of children from birth to kindergarten. Its singular focus is drooling, and saliva management including the need for oral suctioning. These measures are currently undergoing reliability and validity testing. There are no requirements for objective quantification using instrumental procedures in any of these measures as they depend on clinical/behavioral observations.

A swallowing scale for Developmentally Disabled Adults has been developed as part of the ASHA Functional Outcomes Project (ASHA Field Test Edition, 1996–1997). Adults with developmental disabilities are often institutionalized and differ from adults who develop dysphagia as a result of disease, injury, or treatment of diseases. This group has primary difficulty with secretion management and may require assistance in feeding. This 7-point scale focuses on secretion symptoms and management and oral hygiene, components of an underlying impairment.

### General Measures of Dysphagia for Adults

Cherney et al. (1986) developed a Functional Severity Level scale, which ranges from Severe (nonfunctional), Moderately Severe (interferes with function), Mild and Minimal (adequate but reduced), to Normal (adequate). The authors describe the severity levels to be goal directed to develop treatment plans and monitor progress. This scale is focused on the manner in which the individual is nourished and the amount of supervision required in the more severe stages, and progresses to focus on what type of diet the individual eats in the milder stages. The focus is on disability with some discussion of handicap.

Another general scale of swallowing function is a 7-point scale developed by the ASHA Task Force. The Ability to Swallow Scale (ASHA, FOMS, 1997) does not describe what "functional" actually means but uses the term "functional to meet nutritional needs" throughout the scale. This scale is an attempt to use observational criteria of a general, nonspecific nature to indicate whether the individual is handicapped or disabled.

Salassa (1997) described the rationale for the Functional Outcome Swallowing Scale (FOSS). From this physician's perspective, a "successful swallowing scale should be meaningful, clinically relevant, simple, limited and uses readily available parameters that are straightforward." This scale has five stages with criteria in each that specify various impairments or medically observable characteristics. For example, at the first or highest level, the presence of episodic or daily symptoms of dysphagia such as reflux, globus (sensation in the throat), odynophagia (painful swallow), and throat-clearing are included as within normal functioning. The second level is "stable but with abnormal function" determined by barium swallow or fiberoptic evaluation. Weight loss and presence of reflexes, neurological signs, and aspiration are used as criteria for instability or abnormality at the subsequent three levels leading to the recommendation of nonoral feeding in patients who experience "complete swallowing failures."

Marianjoy Rehabilitation Hospital and Clinics in Wheaton, IL has developed a scale called PECS© (1998), which includes an Ability to Swallow Measure based on videofluoroscopic studies and a Functional Swallow Scale using a 7-point severity rating scale. The amount of assistance/dependence required at each of the seven levels of severity is included in the rating. The Ability to Swallow is a measure of impairment and the Functional Swallow measures disability. A recent study of 900 patients using PECS Functional Swallow Scale assessed the impact of dysphagia on the disposition of patients at discharge from acute rehabilitation to a skilled nursing facility (SNF) or an extended care facility (ECF) (Hutchins et al., 1998). The authors reported that patients recovering from a stroke who were dependent for feeding were discharged to a SNF or an ECF more frequently than patients who were independent for feeding and those who did not have dysphagia. When examining frequency of discharge to home with family supervision, persons who had dysphagia and were dependent for feeding were discharged less frequently than persons without dysphagia. This survey gives a nice rationale for the use of outcome measures and has practical applications for care.

A tool used in Australia called the Royal Brisbane Hospital Outcome Measure for Swallowing (RBHOMS) was developed to be used to meet the needs of patients with a broad range of etiologies in acute care facilities, rehabilitation settings, and within the community (Thompson-Ward & Morton, 1998). It was designed to measure change in swallowing function over time as a result of speech pathology intervention and is described as a measure of swallowing disability. The psychometric properties of the RHBOMS have been studied in 285 patients by examination of inpatient speech pathology files at the Royal Brisbane Hospital. This is one of the few measures that has been subjected to psychometric analysis. The psychometric analysis indicated that there was high inter-rater reliability ($r = 99$), content validity, and discriminatory power. The measure has four stages of oral intake from Nil by mouth (e.g., NPO, nothing per oral) to Maintaining Oral Intake and contains a 10-point ordinal rating scale with details of specific clinical characteristics that may or may not be present at each of these levels. Case examples and practice samples to rate are included in the assessment procedures to assist the rater in making a decision as to the stage and level that best fits the patient with dysphagia. This measure appears to be promising for assessment of functional outcomes in dysphagia.

The Guidelines for Functional Outcome Assessment Measurement of Swallowing FOAMS, developed by the Wisconsin Speech–Language and Hearing Association (1996), is also a 7-point scale in which a level 7 is functional and level 1 is profound impairment. It focuses on duration of the swallow and the types of diet consistency and compensatory swallowing strategies that are used to accomplish feeding. This outcome measure is primarily a disability index with some components of impairment.

The NOVA Scale for Swallow Function and Pneumonia Risk Prediction (Lonegan et al., 1997) uses a 7-point scale with 1 indicating "total assistance" and 7 "complete independence." It was developed to demonstrate whether the patient had gained functional independence as a result of dysphagia intervention. This scale was modeled after the Functional Independence Measure (FIM) and uses concepts of levels of assistance required to ensure safe swallow patterns or to justify nonoral feeding. Risk for aspiration and aspiration pneumonia are included.

It is intended for use in nursing facility settings and is intended to be used at admission and discharge. This scale is primarily a scale of disability with some components of impairment included.

The ASHA Dysphagia Special Interest Division 13, Task Force on Functional Outcomes for Dysphagia, was charged with developing an Adult Outcomes Scale at a working meeting held in 1996 in Ann Arbor, MI. Table 15–1 displays the matrix developed by Sonies et al. (ASHA, 1997). The matrix is a 7-point scale with seven categories that contain measures based on physiology of swallowing usually gleaned from instrumental studies as well as functional or behavioral measures (Table 15–1). This scale has not been validated to date, as is common with many of the measures described in this chapter. Because it has attempted to simplify and categorize outcomes into seven categories (supervision, assistance, ability to eat, social eating, response delay, bolus transfer, airway protection, and risk of aspiration), it may be easier to use than measures that do not separate out these areas. This scale, intended for adults with any etiology causing dysphagia, combines the concepts of impairment, disability and handicap and can be used at any point along the continuum of care.

Another general outcome measure of swallowing for adults, National Outcomes Measurement System (NOMS), was circulated after field testing by ASHA (1998). This measure of swallowing is a 7-point scale where level 7 indicates that the individual can eat independently even if they need to use compensatory strategies to ensure that swallowing is safe for all consistencies. It therefore focuses on safety and efficiency when eating, and does not penalize individuals if they have an impairment that they can compensate for by using therapeutic maneuvers.

Dietary level is the primary domain of this swallowing measure. In fact, the instructions specify that if all the criteria in the intermediate levels are not met, dietary level should be used to assign the rating. Dietary levels and restrictions are defined for solids and liquids and rated whether there are minimum, moderate, or maximum restrictions at each of three reduced levels. For example, maximum restriction is defined as follows: "diet is two or more levels below a regular diet status in solid and liquid consistency." A level-2 reduction in solids occurs if "meats are chopped or ground, vegetables are of one consistency or mashed with a fork." A level three reduction on this scale in swallowing solid food is "when meats and vegetables are pureed." Thus, this scale uses an overall 7-point rating and an accompanying scale to determine the rating for dietary levels and restrictions. There is no mention of the satisfaction level or social consequence of dysphagia.

## *Adult Measures of Handicap (or Participation)*

The SWAL-QOL, being developed at the University of Wisconsin Hospital and William S. Middleton VA Hospital in Madison, WI (McHorney et al., 1998), is an outcome measurement tool that appears to meet the criteria of a test that does focus on participation of the patient. It measures functional quality of care from the patients' perspective and is now being standardized. Because it does focus on the patient's perspective, questions included relate to how long it takes to eat and how dysphagia isolates the patient from friends and family.

Table 15–1. Dysphagia Functional Outcomes—Adult Scale-Summary Matrix

| Level | Supervision Assistance | Ability to Eat | Social Eating Ability | Response Delay | Bolus Transfer Motility | Airway Protection | Risk of Aspiration |
|---|---|---|---|---|---|---|---|
| 0 | unable to evaluate | NPO | unable to evaluate | unable to evaluate | unable to evaluate | poor | constant |
| 1 | 1 : 1 physical assistance | NPO | no oral eating | >10 sec all bolus | unable to transfer, no swallow | no clearing of secretions, wet gurgling, no cough | aspiration on all attempts |
| 2 | 1 : 1 physical or supervisory assistance | Oral intake <10%, tube primary, tastes only | therapeutic tasting in a controlled environment | <10 sec all bolus | attempts to transfer often unsuccessful | responses delayed or weak, intermittent airway clearance, wet gurgly, cough does not clear | present on >90% occurrence, cannot use compensations, laryngeal penetration |
| 3 | 1 : 1 physical or supervisory assistance intermittent | partial oral 10–50%, bolus restrictions one type | therapeutic feeding in limited settings (SNF dining room w/aide) | <5 sec 2 or more bolus types | uncontrolled flow to pharynx | uses compensations, laryngeal penetration, protective responses intermittent, cough clears on request, intermittent wet gurgly | compensations unreliable, secretions cleared by cough or expectorating, aspiration 50–90% |
| 4 | constant group supervision with 1 : 1 cueing | >50% oral, tube only as supplement for one bolus type | eats with familiar person in limited settings (e.g., home or institution) | <5 sec 1, 2.5–5.0 sec for remaining types, pharyngeal swallow response | piecemeal, able to transfer with multiple swallows | spontaneous cough clears effectively, wet gurgling only with bolus swallow | aspiration 10–50%, uses compensation, intermittent penetration |
| 5 | general group supervision, cueing | 100% oral, limits in bolus size, viscosity, or texture | eats in wider social setting or restaurant with familiar persons | 2.0–2.5 sec all types | transfer is uncoordinated | pharynx clears with swallow or spontaneous cough | aspiration <10%, uses compensations, infrequent penetration |
| 6 | infrequent group supervision or cueing | 100% oral, modified dysphagia diet | eats in all social settings with familiar person present | 1.5–2.0 sec for most, 2.0–2.5 for one type | residue clears with swallow | adequate, normal cough | none with compensations, no penetration |
| 7 | none related to dysphagia | no dietary restrictions related to dysphagia | independent appropriate eating in all social contexts | 1.5–2.0 sec, normal duration | no unusual oral residue | adequate, normal cough | none |

ASHA Task force Nov. 1997—Draft.

Another measure geared toward quality of life is the Dysphagia Disability In-dex under development at the Henry Ford Hospital, Division of Speech–Lan-guage Sciences and Disorders in Detroit, MI (Silbergleit et al., in press). This is a 25-item scale with three subscales (physical, functional, and emotional) that uses a 5-point critical difference measure to demonstrate actual changes over several administrations. It was standardized on a variety of patient groups with dyspha-gia. Included among the items are "I eat less because of my swallowing problem" and "I don't enjoy eating as much as I used to." This scale indicates how the pa-tient perceives their disability and handicap.

## Discussion

Specialists in dysphagia have focused their efforts on selection of appropriate di-agnostic techniques to identify biomechanical components of dysphagia and on the management of dysphagia impairment. Specific measures of how dysphagia management impacted on patients' level of functioning when eating were not stressed until the 1990s when the health-care system began to modify its payment practices. Assessment of outcomes has been recognized recently as a necessary component of case management and fiscal responsibility. The conceptual frame-work defined by the World Health Organization (WHO) (ICHDH & ICIDH-2) is becoming the standard terminology to describe outcome measures in dysphagia. Although there are other interpretations of impairment, disability, and handicap used by dysphagia specialists, the trend is for developing new terminology based on this framework. Outcome measures that focus on the severity of the impair-ment caused by dysphagia are most commonly used to rate swallowing disorders as they can use biomechanical and instrumental measures. Impairment scales usually require a clinical examination to assess abnormality and an instrumental procedure (e.g., videofluorography, fiberoptic examination, and ultrasound imaging) to assess physiology and timing of the swallow. Swallowing outcome measures that address disability levels are coming of age and new measures may include the limitations on diet, oral intake, airway protection, or safety when eat-ing. The inclusion of the restrictions faced by individuals in their natural eating environment has been largely overlooked until the last few years. Participation restrictions imposed on the individual when eating in public and the need for su-pervision are included in the 1997 ASHA Task Force Matrix (see Table 15–2). In-clusion of this type of item is not pervasive and is clearly absent in most scales.

There is a need to develop functional measures in dysphagia, which are broad-based, use natural situations, and have sufficient reliability or validity to track functional eating changes in real-life situations to ensure that the individual can eat independently. Most of the functional swallowing measures that currently ex-ist are unidimensional, therefore narrow in focus. A single focus measure, such as one that only evaluates aspiration/penetration or response delay, may have va-lidity in projecting the consequences of a specific disease, but it reveals little re-garding the individual's success when eating. Few measures of function in dys-phagia have a behavioral component and the majority are focused on severity of performance, rather than level of success, independence, or ability to attain a healthy life-style.

Table 15–2.  Summary of 17 Dysphagia Functional Outcome Scales

| Title/Abbreviation | Author/Year | Scoring Scale | Assessment Domains | WHO Classification Component |
|---|---|---|---|---|
| FOAMS | Wisconsin-Speech-Language–Hearing Association | 7-point | Duration of swallow, Consistency of diet, Compensations | Impairment, Disability |
| PECS | Hutchins B et al. (1998) RFI Wheaton, Illinois | 7-point, 2 scales | Instrumental assessment, Assistance/dependence | Impairment, Disability |
| FOSS | Sallassa (1997) | 5 stages | Physiology, Medical conditions | Impairment |
| NOVA | Nova Care, Lonegan et al. (1997) | 7-point | Nursing home, Levels of assistance, Risk for aspiration | Impairment, Disability |
| FCM—Birth to Kindergarten | ASHA, NOMS (1995–1996) | 7-point | Oral nonoral feeding, Supervision levels | Disability |
| FCM—Pediatrics | ASHA, NOMS (1995–1996) | 7-point | Physiology, Dietary Modifications | Impairment, Disability |
| ASHA Functional Outcomes Task Force Matrix | ASHA Special Interest Division 13 working group (1997) | 7-point, 7-areas | Physiology, Duration, Airway, Ability to eat, Social eating | Impairment, Disability, Handicap |
| FCM—Secretion Management | ASHA, NOMS (1995–1996) | 7-point | Oral Secretions | Impairment |
| ASHA—Swallowing | ASHA, NOMS (1995–1997) | 7-point | Dietary Level | Disability, Activity Limitation |

| Measure | Reference | Scale | Parameters | Classification |
|---|---|---|---|---|
| FCM—Developmentally Delayed Adults | ASHA, NOMS (1996–1997) | 7-point | Secretion management<br>Oral hygiene | Impairment |
| Dysphagia Severity Rating Parkinson's Disease | Waxman et al. (1990) | 7-point | Aspiration<br>Duration<br>Diet and treatment | Disability |
| FCM—Ability to Swallow | ASHA, NOMS (1996) | 7-point | Observational<br>Meets nutritional needs | Disability |
| Functional Severity | Cherney et al. (1986) | Severity Levels | Type of diet supervision | Disability |
| ALS Severity Scale | Hillel et al. (1989)<br>Yorkston et al. (1993) | 10-point | Eating Habits<br>Eating Problems<br>Diet Consistency | Disability<br>Handicap |
| RBHOMS | Thompson-Ward, Moton (1998)<br>Queensland, Australia | 4 stages<br>10 levels | Oral intake | Disability |
| Head & Neck Cancer FACT | Cella et al. (1993) | 100 points | Dietary Modifications<br>Physical and social well-being | Disability<br>Handicap |
| Head & Neck Cancer Quality of Life UW-QOL | University of Washington<br>D'Antonio et al. (1996) | 100 points | Eating in public<br>Eating performance | Activity<br>Disability<br>Handicap |

The majority of the current scales do not address the limitations in social situations imposed by swallowing disorders and do not emphasize the sociocultural or physical environment. Rarely are the limitations in roles of family, work, or recreation addressed by the component scales or categories considered in the outcome measures for dysphagia.

This chapter has served to identify that new directions are needed in functional outcome assessment to assure that individuals with swallowing disorders are able to be reintegrated into their social environments. It is apparent that most of the measures in use do not address the issue of *functional eating behavior* described at the beginning of this chapter.

Swallowing outcome measures should assess the domains of eating that can be used effectively to chart the progress of the individual, determine if swallowing therapy is effective, and to address the roles of the person with the disability in their social setting. For example, it is suggested that the swallowing problem be viewed in relationship to how dysphagia affects the emotional stability, happiness, socialization, friendships, and satisfaction with life of the person with the impairment. Once we have an indication of which measures are most influential for patient function and well-being, the most critical elements of an assessment can be used to focus on dysphagia treatment. Many of the measures mentioned in this chapter may provide the basis for these decisions in the future.

## References

ASHA (1997). Task Force on Functional Outcomes Working Group Draft. Rockville, MD: Author.

ASHA (1998). National Outcomes Measurement System (NOMS) for Speech–Language Pathology and Audiology, Adult Care Component. Rockville, MD: Author.

Cella, DF. (1994). *Manual for the Functional Assessment of Cancer Therapy (FACT) Scales* and the *Functional Assessment of HIV (FAH) Scale* (Vers. 3). Chicago, IL: Rush-Presbyterian-St. Lukes Medical Center.

Cella, D. R., Tulsky, D. S., Gray, G., et al. (1993). The Functional Assessment of Cancer Therapy Scale: Development and validation of the general measure. *Journal of Clinical Oncology, 11,* 570–579.

Cherney, L. R., Cantieri, C. A., & Pannell, J. J. (1986). *Clinical evaluation of dysphagia.* Gaithersburg, MD: Aspen Publishers.

Coehlo, C. (1998). Post-acute clinical management: Rehabilitation of the patient with neurological communication disorders. In A. F. Johnson, B. H. Jacobson (eds): *Medical speech–language pathology: A practitioner's guide* (pp. 390–408). New York: Thieme.

D'Antonio, L., Zimmerman, G. J., Cella, D. F., & Long, S. A. (1996). Quality of life and functional status measures in patients with head and neck cancer. *Archives of Otolaryngology Head and Neck Surgery, 122,* 482–487.

Hillel, A. D., Miller, R. M., Yorkston, K. M., McDonald, E., Norris, F. H., & Konikow, N. (1989). Amyotrophic Lateral Sclerosis Severity Scale. *Neuroepidemiology, 8,* 142–150.

Hutchins, B., Hildner, C. D., & Fuss, K. (1998). Recommended discharge placement patterns of patients dependent in dysphagia. Presented at ASHA, San Antonio, TX.

List, M. A., Ritter-Sterr, C., & Lansky, S. B. (1990). A performance status scale for head and neck cancer patients. *Cancer, 66,* 564–569.

Logemann, J. A., Pauloski, B. R., Rademaker, A., Cook, B., et al. (1992). Impact of the diagnostic procedure on outcome measures of swallowing rehabilitation in head and neck cancer patients. *Dysphagia, 7,* 179–186.

Lonegan, C., Smith, S., & Huehn, A. M. (1997). NovaScale for Swallow Function and Pneumonia Risk Prediction. Woodbury, MN: Nova Care Contract Rehabilitation Division.

McHorney, C. A., & Rosenbek, J. C. (1998). Functional outcome assessment of adults with oropharyngeal dysphagia. *Seminars in Speech and Language, 19,* 235–246.

PECS©. (1998). The rehabilitation outcome reporting systems: Manual for clinicians version 3.0. Aurora, IL: PECS, Inc.

Rosenbeck, J. C., Robbins, J., Roecker, E. B., Coyle, J. A., & Wood, J. L. A. (1996). A penetration-aspiration scale. *Dysphagia, 11,* 93–98.

Salassa, J. R. (1997). A Functional Outcomes Swallowing Scale (FOSS) for staging dysphagia. Paper presented at the 39th Meeting of the American Society for Head and Neck Surgery, Scottsdale, AZ.

Silbergleit, A. K., Jacobson, B. H., & Sumlin, T. (in press). Dysphagia Disability Index. Patient self-assessment of swallowing. Division of Speech–Language Sciences and Disorders. Detroit, MI: Henry Ford Hospital.

Sonies, B. C. (1994). Dysphagia: A model for differential diagnosis for adults and children. In L. R. Cherney (ed): *Clinical management of dysphagia in adults and children.* Gaithersburg, MD: Aspen Publishers.

Sonies, B. C., & Frattali, C. F. (1997). Critical decisions regarding service delivery across the health care continuum. In B.C. Sonies (ed): *Dysphagia: A continuum of care.* Gaithersburg, MD: Aspen Publishers.

Thompson-Ward, E.C., & Morton, A. L. (1998). Psychometric evaluation of the Royal Brisbane Outcome Measure for Swallowing: Validity, reliability and responsivity data. Paper presented at the 2nd Australasian Dysphagia Conference, Melbourne, Australia.

Waxman, M. J., Durfee, D., Moore, M., Morantz, R. A., & Koller, W. (1990). Nutritional aspects and swallowing function of patients with Parkinson's disease. *Nutrition in Clinical Practice, 5,* 196–199.

Wisconsin Speech–Language and Hearing Association (1996). FOAMS: Functional Outcome Measure of Swallowing Ability, Madison, WI.

Yorkston, K. M., Strand, E., Miller, R., Hillel, A. D., & Smith, K. (1993). Speech deterioration in amyotrophic lateral sclerosis: Implications for the timing of intervention. *Journal of Medical Speech–Language Pathology, 1,* 35–46.

# 16

# Assessment and Treatment of Functional Communication Following Right Hemisphere Damage

## LEORA R. CHERNEY
## ANITA S. HALPER

**The functional approach for people with right hemisphere damage is based upon the premise that the underlying cognitive-communication impairment impacts the activity limitation and participation restrictions in this population. Current assessments for right hemisphere damage are reviewed and three criteria for characterizing functional treatment are proposed. These are that the expected outcomes are defined in functional terms, treatment materials are meaningful to the individual patient, and treatment activities are oriented toward generalization to the patient's natural environment. Examples of treatment activities that contain these characteristics are described.**

## Introduction

The management of patients with right hemisphere damage (RHD) is challenging to speech-language pathologists. Damage to the right hemisphere results in a cluster of cognitive deficits that reduces the patient's effective and efficient use of communication skills. Such cognitively based disorders of communication have been referred to as cognitive-communicative impairments (American Speech–Language–Hearing Association, 1987).

This chapter describes the characteristics of right hemisphere cognitive-communicative disorders at the World Health Organization (1997) levels of impairment and activity. We take the point of view that functional communication is within the realm of activity, but recognize that its consequences may extend into the participation level. However, because most speech–language pathologists do not typically focus their treatment at the level of participation, we address primarily the impairment and activity levels. We include a discussion of current evaluation tools, implications for development of long- and short-term goals, and components of functional communication activities.

## Characteristics

As the term *cognitive-communicative* implies, the two major areas of impairment are cognition and communication. The cognitive areas that are impaired include the processes of attention, perception, memory, organization, reasoning, and problem-solving. The major area of communicative impairment is pragmatics. Figure 16–1 is a schematic representation of these impairments and their interrelationships. These impairments may limit effective communication skills at the activity level, and ultimately impact on quality of life (Cherney & Halper, 1996). This conceptual framework has grown from our clinical experience of more than 20 years with this population. It is not intended to be a theoretical model of brain organization and function, but a clinical guide for selecting appropriate evaluation and treatment materials. The premise of the framework is that the performance of any functional communicative behavior or activity is dependent on the underlying cognitive and pragmatic processes. When communication breaks down in a specific task, the underlying reason or impairment needs to be identified so that interventions can be applied. Because each of these underlying cognitive impairments are complex and have been described differently by various authors, our definitions of these processes are reviewed below. A brief discussion of pragmatic impairments follows.

### Impairment Level: Cognition

Attention disturbances are exhibited in the following areas: directing attention to specific sensory stimuli (focused attention); maintaining attention to the stimuli over a period of time (sustained attention); focusing attention on specific stimuli while ignoring irrelevant stimuli (selective attention); shifting attention from one task to another (divided attention); and focusing and sustaining attention on more than one task simultaneously (divided attention) (Sohlberg & Mateer, 1989). The most clinically significant disorder of attention that occurs in patients with right hemisphere damage is left-side neglect. The individual is unaware and does not respond to stimuli in the left hemispace. Neglect is more common in the visual modality, but may occur in the auditory, olfactory, or tactile modalities (Mesulam, 1985a).

Similar to attention, memory is a complex process. An individual with right hemisphere damage may demonstrate impairment in any of the operations of memory, namely, encoding, storage, and retrieval. Encoding or memorizing is the process by which the representation of an event is formed and constructed (Sig-

# Communication Enhancement Model

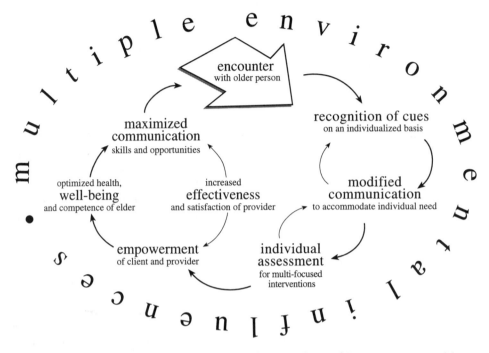

**Figure 16–1.** Schematic representation of interrelationships among cognitive–communicative processes. (Reproduced with permission from Cherney, L. R. & Halper, A. S., 1996.)

noret, 1985). Storage is the process of transferring a transient memory into permanent storage. Retrieval occurs when the memory traces in permanent storage are activated and made available for use. Our own research with word list recall indicates that the encoding process is most difficult for these patients (Cherney et al., 1995; Halper et al., 1996).

Individuals structure their environment by integrating sensory stimuli into meaningful units; this process is referred to as perception (Lezak, 1983). Patients with right hemisphere damage often experience perceptual difficulties that may occur in the auditory and visual modalities. Visual perceptual deficits include problems with figure-ground perception, color recognition, and visual–spatial relationships. Auditory perceptual deficits include problems with perception of music and prosody.

The higher level cognitive processes of organization, reasoning, and problem solving may be impaired in the right hemisphere population. Organization is the ability to sort, categorize, sequence, and prioritize information. Reasoning is the ability to think abstractly and draw inferences and conclusions based on supposed information. Problem-solving is a multicomponent process and involves the following steps: recognizing and analyzing a problem, developing alternate solutions for solving the problem, evaluating the solution, selecting the most appropriate solution, and evaluating its effectiveness (Luria, 1966; Szekeres et al., 1987). Judgment is an integral part of problem-solving and involves forming an opinion or estimate and predicting the consequences of an action based on known information. An aspect of judgment is social judgment in which the individual knows what is appropriate and inappropriate and can apply reasoning to social situations (Sohlberg & Mateer, 1989). Pragmatic deficits in patients with right hemisphere damage further affect problems in social judgment.

## Impairment Level: Pragmatics

Pragmatics is central to any discussion of cognitive-communicative problems in right hemisphere damage. For the purpose of this chapter, we are borrowing terminology from Davis (1986), who defines pragmatics as comprising three contexts—extralinguistic, paralinguistic, and linguistic. Deficits in these contexts coincide with the impairment level.

According to Davis (1986), the extralinguistic context exists apart from the utterance itself. It includes external factors such as the setting and participants, and internal factors such as emotional state, and knowledge of the participants. The extralinguistic context may be reflected by nonverbal behaviors such as gestures, body posture and position, eye contact, and facial expression.

The paralinguistic context includes the suprasegmental features of intonation and prosody that are used to convey emotions or to signal semantic interpretation or syntactic analysis. Raising pitch to indicate a question or changing stress patterns of word (e.g., re'cord or rec'ord) are examples of the use of prosody. The linguistic context refers to verbal behavior or discourse, a string of connected speech units. These three contexts interrelate in different ways depending on the communication task at the activity level.

The Pragmatic Communication Skills Rating Scale of the Rehabilitation Institute of Chicago Evaluation of Communication Problems in Right Hemisphere Dysfunction—Revised (RICE-R) (Halper et al., 1996) offers a tool for identifying pragmatic impairments. It lists nonverbal (extralinguistic and paralinguistic) and verbal (linguistic) characteristics of pragmatics that include intonation, facial expression, eye contact, gestures/proxemics, conversation initiation, turn taking, topic maintenance, response length, presuppostion, and referencing skills.

## Activity Level: Pragmatics

There are different kinds of communication tasks including narrative, procedural, and conversational discourse. These communication activities are dependent on intact skills at the impairment level and are essential for communication in everyday life contexts (e.g., interacting with a friend, making a telephone call to gain information). Narrative discourse is the generation of a series of events usually recounted in the first or third person (e.g., telling a memorable experience or retelling a story). Procedural discourse refers to describing the steps involved in completing a task (e.g., how to make a sandwich). In narrative and procedural discourse, the speaker must provide complete on-topic information without producing irrelevant or tangential information.

Conversational discourse refers to a cooperative exchange of information between two or more persons. Skills required for effective conversation include the appropriate initiation of a conversation, introduction of a new topic, maintenance of a topic, and turn-taking skills. Effective conversation also relies heavily on the adequate comprehension and production of nonverbal behaviors. For example, a speaker uses eye contact to evaluate the listener's interest in the topic, to establish role dominance, and as a turn-taking signal.

Table 16–1.   Underlying Impairments of Pragmatics

| Activity | Overt Characteristics of the Impairments | Underlying Impairments |
|---|---|---|
| Narrative Discourse | Off-topic information, irrelevancies, errors in cohesive ties, incomplete information | Pragmatics—linguistic context |
| | Flat, monotonous prosody | Pragmatics—paralinguistic context |
| | Too much/little information because of incorrect presupposition, limited/inappropriate facial expression | Pragmatics—extra-linguistic context |
| Procedural Discourse | Off-topic information, irrelevancies, errors in cohesive ties, incomplete information | Pragmatics—linguistic context |
| | Flat, monotonous prosody | Pragmatics—paralinguistic context |
| | Too much/little information because of incorrect presupposition, inappropriate/absent gestures | Pragmatics—extra-linguistic context |
| Conversational Discourse | Inappropriate turn-taking, inappropriate/absent topic initiation and shifting, inappropriate/reduced eye contact, errors in cohesive ties | Pragmatics—linguistic context |
| | Flat, monotonous prosody | Pragmatics—paralinguistic context |
| | Limited or inappropriate facial expression, inappropriate use of body posture and gestures, maintains a distance that is too close or too far from the conversational partner, provides too much/too little information because of incorrect presupposition | Pragmatics—extra-linguistic context |

An important aspect of discourse production that crosses all communication tasks is the use of cohesive ties that allows for a smooth and logical flow of information (Halliday & Hasan, 1976). There are several types of cohesive ties such as reference, substitution, ellipsis, conjunction, and lexical cohesion. The most common of these is reference, which is the use of pronouns, demonstratives (this/that), or comparatives to refer to previously mentioned items. Cohesive ties facilitate discourse that is more organized so that information is ordered logically (e.g., temporally or procedurally around a main theme).

### Relationship Between Impairment and Activity Levels

Table 16–1 illustrates how the extralinguistic, paralinguistic, and linguistic contexts and the RICE-R pragmatic characteristics mesh with each other and the WHO (1997) terminology. Similarly, Table 16–2 provides examples that illustrate how the different underlying cognitive and pragmatic impairments and their overt characteristics might contribute to problems at the activity level.

## Assessment

Comprehensive evaluation of patients with RHD must include assessment at the impairment and activity levels. Because a functional treatment program can focus on either of these levels, it is essential that both be addressed during the evaluation. Therefore, the clinician identifies the primary cognitive and/or pragmatic impairments, which contributes to a performance deficit at the activity level.

In addition, it is important to consider how the impairment and activity limitations restrict participation. For example, a patient who has impairments in organization and pragmatics may have difficulty relating experiences/events in a

Table 16–2.    Underlying Impairments of Communication Activities

| Activity | Overt Characteristics of the Impairments | Underlying Impairments |
|---|---|---|
| Retelling a joke | Irrelevancies, repetitions, literal interpretation (missing the punchline), missing details | Pragmatics (see Table 16–1), Memory, Reasoning |
| Reading a story aloud | Omission of words on the left side of the page, misreading words, monotone delivery | Attention (left-side neglect), Visual Perception, Pragmatics (see Table 16–1) |
| Writing a thank you note | Perseveration of strokes, omission of strokes, ignoring the left side of the paper | Visual Perception, Attention (left-side neglect) |
| Balancing a check book | Perseveration of strokes, omission of strokes, ignoring the left side of the paper, unable to keep columns straight, addition and subtraction errors | Visual Perception, Attention (left-side neglect), Memory |

meaningful, organized, and concise manner. As a result, conversations (activity level) fail because the patient tends to be verbose, tangential, and disorganized (overt characteristics of the impairment level). This in turn restricts the patient's social interactions and could lead to social withdrawal, isolation, and loneliness (participation level).

Knowledge of the effects of impairments on activities and participation is essential to appropriate identification and prioritization of treatment goals. Depending on the patient's unique needs and circumstances, the impact of the impairment on the activities and participation may be different. Therefore, in developing a treatment plan, clinicians need to collect information relevant to the patient's potential degree of participation in community life.

Currently, there are three tests of communication skills that have been developed primarily for individuals with RBD. Table 16–3 lists their major subtests and identifies the impairment level and associated functional communication behaviors addressed at the activity level. The Mini Inventory of Right Brain Injury (Pimental & Kingsbury, 1989) is a 27-item screening tool that was standardized on 30 patients with right hemisphere damage and 30 normal controls. It provides a cutoff score that differentiates normal subjects from patients with RHD. The RIC Evaluation of Communication Problems in Right Hemisphere Dysfunction-Revised (RICE-R) (Halper et al., 1996) screens areas of deficits typically found in this population and clinically important to the rehabilitative process. It was standardized on 40 patients with right hemisphere stroke and 36 normal subjects. Cutoff scores for differentiating normal subjects from patients with right hemisphere damage are given (Cherney et al., 1996). In addition, guidelines for severity levels (mild, moderate, and severe) are provided for each subtest. The Right Hemisphere Language Battery—2nd ed. (RHLD) (Bryan, 1994) according to its author, was designed primarily to identify the presence of language disorders in patients with RHD. It was standardized on 30 neurologically normal subjects, 40 patients with RHD, and 40 subjects with aphasia. The raw scores for each subtest can be converted to T-scores that allow comparison of performance across subtests.

The tests described above assess some aspect of the impairment level. Some subtests, such as conversation on the RHLD and RICE-R and writing on the RICE-R address the activity level. None of these tests address the participation level. The clinician often can infer the potential problems at the activity and participation levels from those deficits identified at the impairment level. In the interest of time and limited reimbursement, it is not always possible to perform a comprehensive functional assessment. For example, the clinician can infer that the patient will have problems with reading when the patients demonstrates left neglect on the visual scanning task of the RICE-R.

There are other tests available that are applicable to this population. Again, none of these assessment tools evaluate at the participation level. Rather, they target specific areas of impairment such as memory, attention and left neglect, and pragmatics. Table 16–4 lists some of these tests and the area of impairment assessed (Baddeley et al., 1995; Brookshire & Nichols, 1993; Delis et al., 1987; Mesulam, 1985b; Prutting & Kirschner, 1987; Robertson et al., 1994; Terrell & Ripich, 1989; Wilson et al., 1987). In addition, some of these tests attempt to evaluate performance in more functional tasks and these are indicated. Each clinician should

Table 16–3.  Tests for Patients with Right Hemisphere Damage

| Test/Tasks | Impairment | Activity/Functional Communication Behavior |
|---|---|---|
| **Mini-Inventory of Right Brain Injury (Pimental & Kingsbury, 1989)** | | |
| Visual Processing | Visual Perception, Attention (including left side neglect) | Reading Drawing Writing |
| Language Processing | Reasoning, Prosody | Understanding and expressing humor and other types of abstract language |
| Emotion and Affect Processing | Pragmatic | Communicating emotions |
| General Behavior and Psychic Integrity | Attention | Maintaining participation in communication activities |
| **RIC Evaluation of Right Hemisphere Dysfunction-Revised (Halper, Cherney, Burns, & Mogil, 1996)** | | |
| Behavioral Observation Profile | Orientation, Attention, Memory | Telling time, day, date, and season Finding your way around the environment Remembering important daily events |
| Pragmatic Communication Skills Rating | Pragmatics | Participation in a conversation Telling a story |
| Visual Scanning and Tracking | Visual Perception, Attention (left-side neglect) | Reading |
| Assessment and Analysis of Writing | Visual Perception, Attention (left-side neglect) | Writing |
| Metaphorical Language | Reasoning | Understanding abstract language in communication activities |
| **The Right Hemisphere Language Battery-Second Edition (Bryan, 1995)** | | |
| Metaphor Picture Test | Reasoning | Understanding abstract language in communication activities |
| Written Metaphor Test | Reasoning | Understanding abstract material during reading |
| Comprehension of Inferred Meaning | Reasoning | Understanding inferential information during communication activities |
| Appreciation of Humor | Reasoning | Understanding humor |
| Lexical-Semantic Test | Semantics | Recognizing words in communication activities |
| Production of Emphatic Stress | Pragmatics | Conversing with vocal inflection |
| Discourse Analysis | Pragmatics | Participating in a conversation |

review those tests that are available and determine which ones are appropriate for any given patient. Even tasks that are not an everyday functional activity such as listening to a paragraph and answering questions may provide important information. Such a task allows the clinician to infer that the patient may have difficulty in such everyday activities as listening to the news or a lecture.

Two measures have been developed to assess communication skills at the activity level. The American Speech–Language–Hearing Association Functional Assessment of Communication Skills for Adults (ASHA-FACS) (Frattali et al.,

Table 16–4.   Impairment-Specific Tests for Patients with Right Hemisphere Damage

| Test | Impairment | Functional Tasks Included | Examples of Functional Tasks |
|---|---|---|---|
| Behavioural Inattention Test (Wilson, Cockburn, & Halligan, 1987) | Left neglect | Yes | Telling time Reading a menu |
| California Verbal Learning Task (Delis, Kramer, Kaplan, & Ober, 1987) | Memory | No | |
| Discourse Abilities Profile (Terrell & Ripich, 1989) | Pragmatics | Yes | Having a conversation |
| Discourse Comprehension Test (Brookshire & Nicholas, 1993) | Reasoning | No | |
| Doors and People (Baddeley, Emslie, & Nimmo-Smith, 1995) | Memory | No | |
| Pragmatic Protocol (Prutting & Kirchner, 1987) | Pragmatics | Yes | Having a conversation |
| Rivermead Behavioural Memory Test (Wilson, Cockburn, & Baddeley, 1991) | Memory | Yes | Remembering an appointment Remembering a short route |
| Test of Everyday Attention (Robertson, Ward, Ridgeway, & Nimmo-Smith, 1994) | Attention | Yes | Map reading Using a telephone book |
| Verbal and Non-Verbal Cancellation Test (Mesulam, 1985) | Left neglect | No | |

1995) assesses the four domains of social communication, communication of basic needs, daily planning, and reading, writing, and number concepts. These domains are appropriate to assess regardless of the type and severity of the communication disorder. The ASHA-FACS has quantitative and qualitative scoring. The qualitative scoring dimensions of adequacy, appropriateness, promptness, and communication sharing can capture the functional deficits associated with cognitive-communicative disorders of patients with RHD. Field testing to validate the use of this test for this population is underway. The Communication Activities in Daily Living-2 (CADL-2) (Holland et al., 1998) was recently revised and the updated norming sample includes patients with right hemisphere stroke. This test assesses communication activities in the following seven areas: reading, writing, and using numbers; social interaction; divergent communication; contextual communication; nonverbal communication; sequential relationships; and humor/metaphor/absurdity.

The above tests focus on assessment at the impairment and activity levels. To assess at the participation level, it is necessary to use tools that are designed to measure the quality of life. There are several aspects of quality of life, such as life satisfaction, well-being and morale, functional ability, and social interaction as well as stress and psychiatric disturbance. As a result, there are a variety of measures associated with each of these aspects of quality of life. While a review of these scales is beyond the scope of this chapter, the interested reader is referred to Measuring Health: A Review of Quality of Life Measurement Scales (Bowling, 1997), which is a guide to many of these scales. Because impairments and activity limitations have an impact on participation, it is important that quality-of-life measurements be included in any comprehensive evaluation.

## A Functional Approach to Treatment

We take the point of view that there are several ingredients necessary to characterize treatment as functional. Each of the following aspects is discussed in detail: expected outcomes defined in functional terms; treatment materials that are meaningful to the individual patient; and treatment activities oriented toward generalization to the patient's natural environment. We have adopted a broad definition of functional treatment and consider treatment to be functional if these three ingredients are present.

Outcomes are changes in status that result from an intervention. Outcomes, if they are to be functional, must be appropriate and relevant to the individual patient. Therefore, the clinician must take into consideration several factors that are patient-specific. These include: patient/caregiver goals; patient needs/preferences; premorbid educational background; vocational background and plans; avocational interests; cultural variations; and anticipated discharge placement. For example, consider the patient who has visual perceptual problems that interfere with reading. This is a problem that needs to be addressed for the retired patient who was an avid reader, spent much of his premorbid leisure time reading, and plans to live alone. However, it is not a problem that needs to be addressed for the retired patient who did not like to read, spent his leisure hours gardening and listening to music, and plans to go home with his spouse.

In addition, the clinician must consider the type and severity of the underlying impairments when determining functional outcomes in patients with RHD. For example, if a patient does not exhibit impairment in pragmatics, a functional outcome related to participation in conversation may not be an appropriate target of treatment. For a patient who has a moderate impairment in pragmatics, the functional outcome might be participation in a group conversation. On the other hand, the patient with severe impairments in pragmatics might have a functional outcome of appropriate initiation of questions related to basic needs.

In patients with RHD, the major problem is the *use of language* that impacts on skills needed for social interactions, work, and recreational activities. There have been two approaches to addressing functional outcomes. One approach is to focus on communication functions in the context of daily life activities, such as using the telephone, participating in a conversation, listening to television or radio, and following instructions for homework assignments. Formal outcome measures such as the ASHA-FACS (Frattali et al., 1995) and informal observations of patient performance of these functional activities provide information about the patient's progress toward a specific goal.

The second approach is to categorize the use of language according to the language modalities of auditory comprehension, oral expression, reading, and writing. Frattali (1998) considers these modality-specific outcome measures to be skills underlying communication rather than functional communication. However, in clinical practice we have found this modality-specific approach to be useful for functional goal delineation and assessment of progress. We use the Rehabilitation Institute of Chicago Functional Assessment Scale (RIC-FAS V; 1998) to facilitate the determination of functional outcomes. The RIC-FAS V is a 7-point scale that rates medical management, health maintenance, self-care, mobility, communication, cognitive status, psychosocial status, community integration, and vocational areas. The communication areas include auditory comprehension,

Table 16–5.   RIC Functional Assessment Scale: Money Management

**Domain:**   Community Integration
**Item Name:**   Money Management
**Definition:**   Handling money, making change (includes evaluating correct amount of change) and balancing a checkbook. Premorbid money management skills should be considered when rating this modality.

**Scale Points**

| | |
|---|---|
| 7 = Normal | Normal ability to manage money. A subject may receive this rating if money management is functional with no assistance required and is at premorbid level. |
| 6 = Minimal Impairment | In most situations, subjects complete monetary transactions readily or with only mild difficulty. Self-monitors and self-corrects transactions and self-initiates compensatory strategies as needed. |
| 5 = Mild Impairment | Completes monetary transactions with more than 90% accuracy. Cues may be required to facilitate accuracy less than 10% of the time. |
| 4 = Mild to Moderate Impairment | Subject can pay out correct amount of money and make change. Can inconsistently (more than 50% of the time) complete other monetary transactions (e.g., balancing a checkbook, figuring out tips); requires assistance for these tasks. |
| 3 = Moderate Impairment | Subjects can pay out correct amount of money and make change for daily purchases more than 50% of the time. Moderate cueing may be required. Unable to perform any other monetary transactions. |
| 2 = Moderate to Severe Impairment | Subject can pay out correct amount of money and make change for simple, small transactions (e.g., $1.00, $5.00) 25% of the time. Requires maximal cues. Unable to perform any other monetary transactions. |
| 1 = Severe Impairment | May not perform any monetary transactions or may perform simple transactions (e.g., counting money, making simple change) less than 255 of the time. |
| 0 = Not applicable (e.g., premorbidly illiterate, decreased visual acuity) | |

*Source:* Rehabilitation Institute of Chicago Functional Assessment Scale Manual Version IV. (1996). Chicago: Rehabilitation Institute of Chicago.

oral expression, reading comprehension, written expression and pragmatics as well as other areas (e.g., motor speech disorders) that usually are not affected by the cognitive-communicative deficits of RHD. In addition, money management skills that may be impaired are included under the domain of community integration.

The RIC-FAS V (1998) severity levels and descriptors are used to assist in determining functional outcomes. To illustrate its use, we will focus on the money management scale. Money management includes such activities as handling money, making change, and balancing a checkbook (see Table 16–5). During the initial evaluation of the patient, impairments are assessed, problem areas such as money management are identified, and the patient's level of functional skills is estimated according to the severity levels described in Table 16–5. The functional outcome anticipated at the time of discharge is similarly rated taking into consideration individual factors and the severity of impairment. Appropriate interventions are selected based on the patient's impairments, his/her current functional status in this modality, and the anticipated functional outcome. Then, at discharge, the patient's functional status is again rated and compared with initial status to determine functional gain.

A functional orientation to treatment requires task-specific materials that are meaningful to the patient. The clinician can use items or simulate activities from the patient's home, work, and other environments. While this seems obvious, we have seen clinicians select materials that are convenient and readily available (e.g., workbooks) rather than carefully considering the relevance of the materials to specific patients. Table 16–6, for example, lists functional everyday materials for visual scanning and tracking (Halper et al., 1996). Clinicians need to remem-

Table 16–6.   Functional Materials for Visual Scanning and Tracking

Bus, train, or airline schedule
Catalogs
Dictionary
Directions on food packages
Grocery lists
Local magazines or newspaper listing of activities (e.g., movies, restaurants, and
   museums)
Maps
Menus
Newspaper ads
Newspaper headlines
Newspaper listings of national and foreign weather information
Nutritional information on food products
Phone book
Racing form
Recipes
Table of contents
TV guide
Vending machines

Source: Halper, A. S., Cherney, L. R., & Burns, M. S. (1996). Treatment of cognitive-communicative skills in patients with right hemisphere damage. In A. S. Halper, L. R. Cherney, M. S. Burns (eds.): *Clinical management of right hemisphere dysfunction,* 2nd ed. (pp. 57–96). Gaithersburg, MD: Aspen Publishers, Inc.

ber that even though these materials are functional in nature, they are not relevant to all patients. For example, if a patient has never used public transportation and does not intend to do so at discharge, bus and train schedules would not be appropriate. Reading menus may be appropriate for the patient going to a nursing home where opportunities for menu selection are provided as well as for the patient who is going home and enjoys eating out.

To provide functional treatment, it is essential that it be delivered in areas other than the clinic room. While treatment may begin inside the clinic doors, it is important to do as many activities as possible in more natural environments. Clinicians can simulate natural environments by introducing visual or auditory distractions such as noise and people, or by conducting treatment on the nursing unit, in the cafeteria, in the gift shop, or other locations outside the treatment facility. For example, the use of a functional paper-and-pencil treatment activity for visual scanning may not be as effective as allowing the patient to scan and select items in the vending machine in the cafeteria. Another way to facilitate generalization is through the use of group treatment. It provides opportunities for patients to practice their communication skills with other individuals while receiving clinician and peer support. Group therapy provides an excellent transition from the therapeutic environment to the patient's natural environment.

Our approach to functional treatment includes outcomes defined in functional terms, materials meaningful to the patient, and generalization to natural environments built into the treatment program. The treatment methods selected can be either impairment or activity based, or can be a combination of the two, but always with the goal of improving functional performance in the patient's natural environments. For example, consider the patient who can inconsistently read sentence-level material (moderate to severe impairment according to the RIC-FAS-V; 1998) as a result of visual perceptual and left-side neglect problems. Our projected outcome from the RIC-FAS-V is that the patient will be able to read one to two paragraphs (moderate impairment). The clinician may choose to work at the level of impairment on the left neglect itself via visual scanning and tracking of words using functional materials such as menus and newspaper ads. Alternatively, the clinician may choose to work at the level of activity by having the patient read paragraphs from the newspaper using compensatory strategies, such as a red line down the left side of the paragraph and verbal cues. We consider both of these treatment approaches functional.

Table 16–7 provides examples of functional outcomes, impairments, and interventions for oral expression, reading, and writing. The interventions suggested are generic in nature and can be adapted to a specific patient's impairment and anticipated functional outcome based on unique needs and preferences.

## Conclusion

This chapter has reviewed the cognitive-communicative characteristics of right hemisphere damage, assessment tools, and a functional communication treatment approach as they relate to the WHO levels of impairment, activity, and participation. While we are moving in a direction that emphasizes level of participation, there are many gaps in our knowledge and practice that affect assessment,

Table 16–7. Sample Interventions for Patients with Right Hemisphere Damage

| Problem | Activity/Functional Outcome | Impairment | Interventions |
|---|---|---|---|
| Difficulty with oral expression | Will retell a personal experience | Deficits in nonverbal pragmatics (eye contact, facial expression, intonation, gestures and proxemics) | Practicing appropriate intonation, facial expression, and gestures while relating a story (read or spontaneous) with clinician modeling and providing cues and feedback |
| | | Deficits in verbal pragmatics (topic maintenance, referencing) | Listening for relevant components of the story prior to retelling it; Practicing retelling a personal event or story focusing on using appropriate references (e.g., pronouns, deictic terms) |
| | | Deficits in organization | Sequencing the relevant components of the story |
| Difficulty with oral expression | Will participate appropriately in a conversation | Deficits in nonverbal pragmatics (eye contact, facial expression, intonation, gestures and proxemics) | Identifying instances of nonverbal and verbal pragmatic impairments from a videotape, audiotape, or script of a conversation |
| | | Deficits in verbal pragmatics (conversational initiation, turn-taking, topic maintenance, referencing) | Engaging patient in a conversation and have patients use specified pragmatic skills appropriately and provide cues as needed |
| Difficulty reading | Will use functional, everyday materials pertinent to patient needs (e.g., TV guide, phone book, address book, bus/train/plane schedules) | Attention/left neglect Perception/visuospatial disorganization | Scanning and tracking exercises—horizontally and vertically using functional materials (symbols, numbers, words, times, channels, names, phone numbers) and using appropriate compensatory strategies (e.g., red line, Velcro) |
| Difficulty reading | Will read the newspaper | Perception/visuospatial disorganization | Identifying key components of the newspaper (e.g., name of newspaper, date of paper, page number) to determine that it is oriented correctly (not upside down) |
| | | Attention/left neglect | Scanning and tracking exercises—letters, words, phrases using compensatory strategies (e.g., pointing, red line Velcro) |

Table 16–7. (Continued)

| Problem | Activity/ Functional Outcome | Impairment | Interventions |
|---|---|---|---|
| | | Memory | Oral reading of components of newspaper (e.g., headlines, picture captions, articles) using compensatory strategies (e.g., pointing, red line Velcro) |
| | | | Directing the patient to look for specific information prior to reading (e.g., the "who, what, where, when, how" of the story) |
| | | | Explaining the humor in the story |
| | | Reasoning | Drawing conclusions based on known information in the article |
| | | | Predicting the end of the article after reading only a part of it |
| Difficulty writing | Will write a personal letter/article | Attention/left neglect and Perception/visuo-spatial disorganization | Scanning and tracking exercises—words and Writing a brief note using compensatory strategies (e.g., red line velcro, raised or highlighted horizontal lines) |
| | | Pragmatic disturbances/topic maintenance and informational content | Identifying relevant information Outlining and sequencing key points to be included in the letter |
| | | Organization problems | Grouping key points for meaningful paragraphs |

treatment, and measures of functional outcomes (Tompkins et al., 1998). In particular, there is a paucity of research on the effect of cognitive-communicative problems on the level of participation, including such dimensions as quality of life of individuals with right hemisphere damage. However, patients, family members, and caregivers have provided anecdotal evidence of problems in life satisfaction generally and social interactions specifically. While our ultimate goal is to improve the patient's participation in life activities, our skills as speech–language pathologists allow us to have the most effect at the impairment and activity levels. Efficacious treatment provided at these levels will also improve the overall quality of life of our patients.

## References

American Speech–Language–Hearing Association. (1987). The role of speech–language pathologists in the habilitation and rehabilitation of cognitively impaired adults: A report of the subcommittee on language. *ASHA 29*, 53–55.

Baddeley, A., Emslie, H., & Nimmo-Smith, I. (1995). *Doors and people.* Suffolk, England: Thames Valley Test Company.

Bowling, A. (1997). *Measuring health: A Review of quality of life measurement scales,* 2nd ed. Bristol, PA: Open University Press.

Brookshire, R. H., & Nicholas, L. E. (1993). Discourse Comprehension Test. Tucson: Communication Skill Builders.

Bryan, K. L. (1994). The Right Hemisphere Language Battery, 2nd ed. London: Whurr Publishers, Ltd.

Cherney, L., & Halper, A. S. (1996). A conceptual framework for the evaluation and treatment of communication problems associated with right hemisphere damage. In A. S. Halper, L. R. Cherney, M. S. Burns (eds): *Clinical management of right hemisphere damage,* 2nd ed. (pp. 21–29). Gaithersburg, MD: Aspen Publishers, Inc.

Cherney, L. R., Halper, A. S., & Drimmer, D. P. (1995). Word list recall and recognition by subjects with right hemisphere stroke. *Brain and Language, 51,* 51–53.

Cherney, L. R., Halper, A. S., Heinemann, A. W., & Semik, P. (1996). RIC evaluation of communication problems in right hemisphere dysfunction-Revised (RICE-R): Statistical background. In A. S. Halper, L. R. Cherney, M. S. Burns (eds): *Clinical management of right hemisphere damage,* 2nd ed. (pp. 31–40). Gaithersburg, MD: Aspen Publishers, Inc.

Davis, G. A. (1986). Pragmatics and treatment. In R. Chapey (ed): *Language intervention strategies in adult aphasia,* 2nd ed. Baltimore: Williams & Wilkins.

Delis, D. C., Kramer, J. H., Kaplan, E., & Ober, B. A. (1987). California Verbal Learning Test. San Antonio: The Psychological Corporation.

Frattali, C., Thompson, C., Holland, A., Wohl, C., & Ferketic, M. (1995). American Speech–Language–Hearing Association Functional Assessment of Communication Skills for Adults. Rockville, MD: ASHA.

Frattali, C. M. (1998). Measuring modality-specific behaviors, functional abilities, and quality of life. In C. M. Frattali (ed): *Measuring outcomes in speech–language pathology* (pp. 55–88). New York: Thieme.

Halliday, M. A. K., & Hasan, R. (1976). *Cohesion in English.* London: Longman.

Halper, A. S., Cherney, L. R., & Burns, M. S. (1996). Treatment of cognitive-communicative skills in patients with right hemisphere damage. In A. S. Halper, L. R. Cherney, M. S. Burns (eds): *Clinical management of right hemisphere dysfunction,* 2nd ed. (pp. 57–96). Gaithersburg, MD: Aspen Publishers, Inc.

Halper, A. S., Cherney, L. R., Burns, M. S., & Mogil, S. I. (1996). RIC evaluation of communication problems in right hemisphere dysfunction-revised (RICE-R). In A. S. Halper, L. R. Cherney, M. S. Burns (eds): *Clinical management of right hemisphere damage,* 2nd ed. (pp. 99–132). Gaithersburg, MD: Aspen Publishers, Inc.

Halper, A. S., Cherney, L. R., Drimmer, D. P., & Chang, O. (1996). Right hemisphere stroke: Performance trends on word list recall and recognition. *Archives of Physical Medicine and Rehabilitation, 77,* 837.

Holland, A. L., Frattali, C. M., & Fromm, D. (1998). *Communication activities of daily living,* 2nd ed. Austin, TX: Pro-Ed.

Lezak, M. (1983). *Neuropsychological assessment,* 2nd ed. New York: Oxford University Press.

Luria, A. R. (1966). *Human brain and psychological processes.* New York: Harper & Row.

Mesulam, M. M. (1985a). Attention, confusional states and neglect. In M. M. Mesulam (ed): *Principles of behavioral neurology* (pp. 125–169). Philadelphia, PA: FA Davis, Co.

Mesulam, M. M. (1985b). Verbal and Visual Cancellation Test. Philadelphia: F.A. Davis.

Pimental, P. A., & Kingsbury, N. A. (1989). Mini Inventory of Right Brain Injury. Austin: Pro-Ed.

Prutting, C. A., & Kirchner, D. M. (1987). A critical appraisal of the pragmatic aspects of language. *JSHD, 52,* 105–119.

Rehabilitation Institute of Chicago Functional Assessment Scale Manual, vers. V. (1998). Chicago: Author.

Robertson, I., Ward, T., Ridgeway, V., & Nimmo-Smith, I. (1994). Test of Everyday Attention. Suffolk, England: Thames Valley Test Company.

Signoret, J. L. (1985). Memory and amnesia. In M. M. Mesulam (ed): *Principles of behavioral neurology* (pp. 169–192). Philadelphia, PA: F.A. Davis Co.

Sohlberg, M. M., & Mateer, C. (1989). *Introduction to cognitive rehabilitation.* New York: Guilford Press.

Szekeres, S. F., Ylvisaker, M., & Cohen, S. B. (1987). A framework for cognitive rehabilitation. In M. Ylvisaker, E. M. R. Gobble (eds): *Community re-entry for head injured adults* (pp. 87–136). Boston: College Hill Press.

Terrell, B., & Ripich, D. (1989). Discourse competence as a variable in interventions. *Seminars in Speech and Language, 10,* 282–297.

Tompkins, C. A., Lehman, M. T., Wyatt, A. D., & Schulz, R. (1998). Functional outcome assessment of adults with right hemisphere brain damage. *Seminars in Speech and Language, 19,* 303–323.

World Health Organization (1997). ICICH-2 International Classification of Impairments, Activities and Participation. Geneva: Author.

Wilson, B., Cockburn, J., & Halligan, P. (1987). Behavioural Inattention Test. Suffolk, England: Thames Valley Test Company.

Wilson, B., Cockburn, J., & Baddeley, A. (1991). The Rivermead Behavioural Memory Test. Suffolk, England: Thames Valley Test Company.

# SECTION 4

# *Assessment and Treatment of Functional Communication in Different Settings*

# 17

# A Socioenvironmental Approach to Functional Communication in Hospital In-Patients

## ROBYN T. MCCOOEY
## DEBORAH TOFFOLO
## CHRIS CODE

**This chapter describes the many barriers to effective communication in hospitals. These include patient-related difficulties such as sensory loss and speech and language disorders, staff-related communication difficulties such as the lack of time hospital staff have to communicate with patients, and environment-related communication difficulties such as continuous background noise. A new functional approach for hospital in-patients that links communication disadvantage to quality improvement is described. The approach is being trialed in an Australian acute care hospital that emphasizes the role of communication in client satisfaction. The development of an Australian assessment procedure is also presented.**

## Introduction

Speech–language pathology practice in acute care hospitals has changed dramatically over the last decade. Health-care systems worldwide have undergone major restructuring to improve efficiency and restrain expenditure, resulting in shorter lengths of patient stay (Katz et al., 1998). The speech–language pathologist's caseload in acute care hospitals has also changed. Ninety-five percent of certified speech–language pathologists in U.S. hospitals now regularly manage patients with dysphagia (American Speech–Language–Hearing Association,

1997). Larger and more varied caseloads, the priority of patients with dysphagia over other patients, and shorter lengths of stay, have resulted in less time for assessment and management of patients with acquired communication disorders.

Although speech–language pathologists have less time for in-patients with acquired communication disorders, they continue to use traditional approaches when in-patients are seen. A recent international survey of 165 clinicians working in acute care settings found that the most popular tests in the United States, Canada, and Australia for assessment and management of aphasia were the Boston Diagnostic Aphasia Examination (BDAE) (Goodglass & Kaplan, 1972), The Western Aphasia Battery (WAB) (Kertesz, 1982), and the Boston Naming Test (BNT) (Kaplan et al., 1984; Katz et al., 1998). In the United Kingdom, the most frequently used tests were the BNT and the Psycholinguistic Assessments of Language Processing in Aphasia (PALPA) (Kay et al., 1992). When invited to list up to five assessment procedures and tests they used, no functional assessments were listed by any group of therapists from the United States, Canada, Australia, or the United Kingdom (Katz et al., 1998). Hence, there appears to be no shift toward functional assessment in the acute care setting that presumably reflects a perception on the part of clinicians that assessment and treatment for communication impairments should be the focus of speech–language therapy in-hospital.

In this chapter, speech–language pathology practice in the acute care setting is reviewed in two ways. First, a new model of service delivery is explored that is based on the socioenvironmental approach. This approach has been advocated in other institutionalized settings such as rehabilitation facilities for people with traumatic brain injury (Ylvisaker et al., 1993) and in extended care facilities (Lubinski, 1981a; 1981b; 1991). The primary feature of this approach is the creation of a positive communication environment within the institution. By considering the role of communication in the delivery of acute care, the role of speech–language pathologists with in-patients is broadened considerably. This new role requires speech–language pathology to broaden its caseload within the hospital environment to include not only those with aphasia, dysarthria, cognitive communication disorders and so on, but also patients with sensory loss, and those whose illness or circumstances prevents communication. This conforms with Ringel and Chodzko-Zajkoet's model of the health disease continuum (Ringel & Chodzko-Zajko, 1988), with healthy ageing at one end of the continuum and pathological ageing at the other end. Hence, the distinction between those with a communication disability and those who are communicatively able becomes blurred. In addition, even those who are communicatively able may have difficulties in a hospital environment.

To expand the in-patient caseload when resources to speech–language pathology are diminishing is explained by linking speech–language pathology to a hospital-wide priority area of quality improvement. Communication plays a central, but often neglected, role in quality care in the acute setting. The approach described here has been developed in Australia where the acute health care context is focussed on consumer-driven quality improvement. In health-care contexts where quality improvement is not an integral part of the hospital culture and is not valued or resourced within the hospital, this approach may not be viable. It is, however, a consequence of the expansion of the conceptual framework of functional communication.

The second part of the review of speech–language pathology services in acute care, proposes that the World Health Organization's (WHO) biopsycho-social model of impairment, activity, and participation may provide a framework for clinicians working in the acute care setting. By focussing more on the dimensions of activity and participation, speech–language pathologists can utilize the limited resources available to them to meet the objectives of the acute care hospital and provide services that are relevant to patients with communication difficulties. One example of a hospital-based communication assessment in the activity dimension, is the In-patient Functional Communication Interview (IFCI) (Toffolo et al., 1995). The IFCI is being developed in Australia, and while it was originally developed for in-patients with speech and language impairments, it has been found to be useful in the assessment of the functional communication abilities of all hospital in-patients. The IFCI is used routinely with all patients who are referred to speech–language pathology. The speech–language pathologist conducts the IFCI as a structured interview to determine if the patient is having any communication difficulties. The IFCI can also be completed by nursing staff who use it to screen for communication difficulties. The IFCI can therefore be used as a functional communication assessment within a traditional speech–language pathology caseload or be used more widely using the institution-wide approach described in this chapter. The development of the IFCI is described.

### Communication in the Acute Care Hospital

Communicating well with patients results in more accurate diagnosis, more effective treatment and better compliance with treatment (Cleary et al., 1991). Outcome measures and quality indicators used to measure the performance of acute care facilities worldwide reflect the importance of communication. The United States has developed a vast range of quality indicator programs. For example, the Picker-Commonwealth Survey of Patient-Centered Care developed in the United States has been used in the United States, Canada, the United Kingdom, and Australia to investigate patients' perceptions of hospital care (Draper & Hill, 1995). It surveys patients on seven dimensions of care including respect for patient's values, preferences, and expressed needs; information, communication, and education; support and alleviation of fear and anxiety; and transition and continuity. Another example is the Consortium Research on Indicators of System Performance (CRISP) indicator set (Boyce et al., 1997). The CRISP indicator set is comprised of 11 categories of indicators, including quality of care, episode prevention, patient satisfaction, and efficiency (Boyce et al., 1997).

In the United Kingdom, the Department of Health has published The Patients Charter (Patients Charter Unit, 1996). While not a set of measures, The Patient's Charter outlines the responsibilities hospitals have to their patients. For example, hospitals must:

- give information about services, and specific information about quality;
- give patients full information about treatments and alternatives sufficiently in advance of decisions having to be made; and
- find out what patients think (Audit Commission, 1993, Appendix 1, p. 65).

In Australia, a standard set of quality and outcome indicators has been proposed for acute care facilities nationwide. These indicators relate to the dimensions of access, efficiency, safety, effectiveness, continuity, acceptability, technical proficiency, and appropriateness (Boyce et al., 1997). The dimension of acceptability encompasses consumer and customer perception, satisfaction, relevance, cultural appropriateness, and consumer involvement in health services.

Health-care providers in acute care hospitals are being encouraged through quality indicator programs to communicate with all in-patients in a timely, appropriate, and effective way. Speech–language pathologists working in acute care settings can use their expertise to ensure that in-patients with communication difficulties receive timely, appropriate, and effective communication throughout all aspects of their medical care. Clinicians can also be advocates for communicatively disadvantaged in-patients and ensure that their views are adequately sampled when in-patient satisfaction surveys are conducted.

## Potential Barriers to Communication in Acute Care Hospitals

The potential barriers to communication in hospital have been identified and described in varied ways. Consumer groups, hospitals, governments, and academia have all investigated the communication difficulties patients encounter. These difficulties are grouped into three categories; those related to patients, those related to hospital staff and those related to the hospital environment.

### Patient-Related Communication Difficulties

Elderly persons (65 years and over) constitute 13% of the U.S. population (U.S. Bureau of the Census, 1999), however, they accounted for 38% of all in-patient discharges from short stay non-Federal hospitals in the United States in 1996 (National Center of Health Statistics, 1999). The average length of in-patient stay for elderly people in the United States was 6.5 days compared with 5.2 days for all in-patients. Similar figures are reported in Australia, where 12% of the Australian population are elderly. In 1995–1996, the elderly in Australia accounted for 30% of the total number of admissions to public and private hospitals and 48% of total hospital patient days (Australian Institute of Health and Welfare, 1998). The average length of hospital stay for elderly patients was also higher, averaging 7.3 days compared with 4.5 days for all patients (Australian Institute of Health and Welfare, 1998). Given that the incidence of diseases that affect a person's ability to communicate and the prevalence of sensory impairments increase with age, many elderly patients are likely to face significant difficulties communicating effectively in-hospital.

Hearing and vision loss are distinctive among the many conditions associated with old age because they fundamentally alter an elderly person's perceptions, social interactions, and means of communication (McCallum et al., 1992). In the United States, significant hearing loss is reported in 23% of elders between 65 and 74 years and in 32% of elders over 75 years (Bello, 1996). In Australia, hearing loss affects 19% of people between 65 and 74 years of age, and 32% of people over 75 years (Australian Bureau of Statistics, Disability, Ageing and Carers Survey, 1993).

Visual impairment affects a person's ability to read and write but also limits the ability to attract attention and to utilize cues from lip reading, facial expressions and body language. It is estimated that nearly 14 million people in the U.S. suffer from a visual impairment and over two-thirds of these people are over 65 years of age (National Eye Institute, 1999). In Australia, over 5% of citizens aged between 65 and 74 years and 13.6% of people over 75 years have a visual disability (Australian Bureau of Statistics, Disability, Ageing and Carers Survey, 1993).

Based on projections from the Australian Bureau of Statistics, the National Centre for Ageing and Sensory Loss (1994) estimate that 49% of people between 65 and 74 and 68% of people over 75 will have a visual or hearing impairment. Elderly patients admitted to hospitals are not only trying to communicate despite an acute illness, but are also communicating in an unfamiliar environment and with unfamiliar people.

Patients who have communication difficulties as a result of disease or injury constitute the traditional speech–language pathology caseload. Several studies investigate the incidence of communication disorders, such as aphasia or dysarthria immediately after stroke and figures range from 37 to 74% (Harasty & McCooey, 1993). The effect on communication of right hemisphere damage, facial paresis, hemiplegia, apraxia and neglect, are however, typically not included in these incidence figures.

Hospital patients of all ages may experience communication difficulties as a result of their general medical condition. They may have impaired concentration, comprehension, and memory due to a combination of factors, such as acute pain, sleep deprivation, exhaustion, anxiety, and fear of death or disability (Dyer, 1996; Verity, 1996). This is especially so for the critically ill patient in the Intensive Care Unit (ICU), where medical intervention may create secondary communication problems. Patients who are intubated endotracheally or via tracheostomy, whether to facilitate ventilation or to protect the airway, are unable to communicate verbally. In addition, the restrictions of equipment or their disease process may limit their ability to move or see around them. They may have difficulty calling for a nurse when they need assistance, and this may further exacerbate their feelings of helplessness, isolation, and vulnerability especially when they are dependant on others for their most vital functions (Ashworth, 1987). Background noises, conversations, and the sound of equipment, all of which may not be fully understood, can increase levels of anxiety (Dyer, 1996). Sedatives are often administered to intubated or ventilated patients in an attempt to alleviate this anxiety, and may further diminish patients' perceptions of their immediate environment.

Finally, patients can adopt an overly passive and dependent role in-hospital. They may be reluctant to ask for information, out of deference to nursing and medical staff, fear of ridicule, not wanting to cause trouble, not knowing how to complain or feeling that staff are too busy (Field, 1992). Patients who are well known to hospital staff, for example, those who frequently need to use hospital services or who are residents of rural areas, have expressed concern about being labeled as troublemakers if they question hospital practices (Consumers' Health Forum, 1994). Yet encouraging patients to speak up has advantages. "Consumers who ask more questions are more likely to bring the significance of symptoms to the doctor, are more likely to draw attention to medication they already take and more likely to alert doctors and nurses to issues in treatment and medication" (Draper & Hill, 1995, p. 5).

Hence, if communication is viewed as a continuum from ability to disability, the distinction between people with a communication disability and people without a communication disability becomes blurred. Certainly, many hospital in-patients are not able communicators. It has been suggested that patients in hospital have a spectrum of communication difficulties due to sesnsory loss, acute illness, and increased dependency. While conventional practice in speech–language pathology defines the type of communication disorders that are referred, a closer inspection of communication abilities of in-patients reveals that many patients have unrecognized communication difficulties. A functional approach recognizes that there are many reasons why participation in hospital life is restricted. Patient-related communication difficulties have a major influence on participation in health care and many of these factors have been under-recognized within acute health care settings.

## Staff-Related Communication Difficulties

There has been considerable research into the amount and type of communication between staff and hospital patients. Nurse–patient communication has received the most attention, as nurses are the health professionals who have the most contact with the patient, and effective communication is considered to be an essential aspect of nursing care (Ashworth, 1984a). In a detailed study of communication between nurses and patients in ICUs, Ashworth (1980) concluded that much of the communication that occurred is automatic and routine. However, most everyday communication is automatic and routine and has an important social function. Therefore, nurses should be encouraged to value their communication with patients irrespective of its automaticity.

In addition, some patients are nonresponsive and this also requires special communication skills on behalf of the nursing staff. Ashworth (1980) found the length of time nurses engaged in communicating with patients and the number of utterances nurses produced were positively correlated with the patient's ability to communicate and give feedback. Communicating with a person who gives no verbal or nonverbal feedback is extremely difficult. Yet nonresponsive patients still may be completely aware of their surroundings. "These unresponsive patients are perhaps in greater need of information on which to structure their world since they cannot ask for information and are usually unable to open their eyes to see their surroundings" (Ashworth, 1980, p. 77).

Nurses may withdraw from communicating with patients to protect themselves from becoming overly involved (Field, 1992). Field (1992) reports that communicating with dying patients is partly influenced by a nurse's level of apprehension and their own attitudes and beliefs about how they should relate to patients and about death and dying.

The communication between nurses and patients on cancer units has also been investigated. The nurses sampled in Wilkinson's study (1991), for example, were generally poor communicators with cancer patients. "Whilst a few nurses were able to facilitate patients in discussing their worries or problems in detail at all stages of the disease, most nurses used a variety of blocking tactics to prevent patients divulging their problems" (p. 686). For example, the following extract is from a nursing interview with a patient readmitted with recurrence of prostate cancer:

*Nurse:*    Are you sleeping alright?
*Patient:*  I never do.
*Nurse:*    Appetite, is that O.K.?
*Patient:*  No, not really. I don't feel like food.
*Nurse:*    Good. Right then, you know what's going on, don't you? (p. 683).

Investigations of staff–patient communication from a patient's perspective have also revealed other staff-related problems. Patients' concerns mainly focus on the timeliness and appropriateness of the information they receive during their hospital stay (Draper & Hill, 1995). For example, results from the Picker Commonwealth survey conducted on 6455 patients across 62 hospitals in the United States found many patients reported not being told whom to ask for help, that tests were not explained, and that important side effects of medicines were not discussed in a way they could understand (Cleary et al., 1991). In other surveys, patients have reported a lack of information on the purpose of tests, inadequate explanations prior to being requested to sign consent forms, and a lack of information about medication (Draper & Hill, 1995). Information needs to be provided verbally and in written form for English speaking patients as well as in different languages for those from non-English-speaking backgrounds (Draper & Hill, 1995).

Patients from non-English-speaking backgrounds have also reported additional communication difficulties with staff. An acute care patient satisfaction survey conducted in Australia found patient satisfaction to be significantly lower among non-English-speaking patients (Department of Human Services, 1997). Specifically, these patients report difficulty understanding doctors' and nurses' answers to their questions, being limited in their involvement in decisions about their own care, and receiving inadequate information about impending surgery. While being extremely grateful for the interpreter services that are available, patients report a lack of specialized interpreter services (particularly in mental health) and serious breaches in confidentiality. These factors make patients reluctant to use interpreter services.

These are examples of staff-related institutionalized barriers to communication in a hospital. The role of the speech–language pathologist is to identify these barriers and work with quality improvement staff in the hospital to reduce the barriers. Patients who have experienced communication difficulties within the hospital will often report these difficulties to hospital staff who spend time listening to them. Speech–language pathologists often find themselves listening to patients, and in combination with their expertise in communication, are well placed to assist in the identification of communication breakdowns in the hospital setting.

### Environment-Related Communication Difficulties

There are many similarities between the communication-impaired environment that Lubinski (1981a; 1981b; 1991) describes as being typical of an extended-care facility, and the communication environment of an acute care facility. Similarities exist in the devaluing of communication in a nursing context that is primarily focused on physical aspects of care. There is also a similarity in the physical environments of both settings. A high level of background noise and a lack of privacy are examples of barriers to communication from the physical environment.

There is evidence that these communication barriers have already been identified in the acute care setting. A hospital's organizational structure has also been found to affect the quality of patient–staff communication. The leadership style of the senior nurse for example, may be influential in determining the degree to which nurses facilitate communication with their patients (Wilkinson, 1991). Senior nurses who shared the administrative load with other nurses and so had time for direct patient care are effective role models for other nursing staff. These senior nurses were more likely to give their nursing staff the autonomy to make independent decisions about their patient care. Nurses working with these head nurses were more likely to facilitate conversation and openly discuss the patient's illness with the patient (Wilkinson, 1991). Field (1992) also states that good communication needs to be seen as an important part of nursing care and valued as an integral component to nursing work.

Wilkinson (1991) concluded that the senior nurse and the structure of the ward were the *most* influential factors affecting the quality of communication patient's received. Finally, structures to support and help staff also need to be available for nurses and other health-care staff if they are to commit themselves to such a high level of patient care (Field, 1992; Jones, 1993).

In relation to the physical environment, the continuous background noise from equipment in ICU and the visual monotony of constant light in a very busy ward, can lead to disorientation in time (Dyer, 1996). Additionally in the ICU each patient bed is usually open to view from the nursing station, and close to other beds, and like other shared rooms there is little privacy, required for some conversations. Nurse call buttons can be difficult to see, to recognize, to reach, and to operate as they can require cognitive abilities and manual dexterity that is beyond many ill patients. Written information is often not available, accessible, or can be of poor quality (Audit Commission, 1993).

In summary, the potential barriers to good communication are numerous. Patients may experience communication difficulties in hospitals because of their medical conditions, language and cultural backgrounds, the attitudes of staff, and the infrastructure, and/or the physical environment of the hospital. Despite these potential difficulties, effective communication between patients and health providers is essential. Studies indicate effective communication results directly in better health outcomes for cardiac and surgical patients (Ashworth, 1984b; Mumford et al., 1982), and in better compliance and follow-up care (Cleary et al., 1991). Communicating well with patients is also one of the key factors in determining patient satisfaction with their stay in hospital (Department of Human Services, 1997).

The role of speech–language pathologists in facilitating better communication in hospitals has not been fully explored. It requires a paradigm shift from thinking that speech–language pathologists are only concerned with in-patients who have medical speech, language, voice, and swallowing impairments to considering the activity limitations and participation restrictions of communicatively disadvantaged in-patients. There is some evidence to suggest that a broad range of in-patients are disadvantaged in the communication process of hospitals. The role of speech–language pathology may be to facilitate communication throughout the institution and therefore become involved in the provision of quality improvement systems in the hospital. This expanded role may not be feasible in some health policy environments, however, in countries such as Australia where communication outcomes are being strongly addressed in some hospitals, this model can reinforce the centrality of communication in quality domains and emphasizes the speech–language pathologist's role in addressing communication.

## Impairment, Activity, and Participation in the Acute Care Setting

The International Classification of Impairment, Activities, and Participation (World Health Organization, 1997) may provide a useful framework for speech–language pathologists working in hospitals, to better understand the approaches that are available to them in the assessment and management of patients with communication disorders. In this section, the focus of attention returns to the traditional caseload of a speech–language pathologist in an acute care setting. This is the main target group of acute care hospitals and the approach advocated here is easier to understand when applied to conventional speech–language pathology cases. The ICIDH-2 framework, however, can be equally applied to the broader quality improvement focused model described previously.

Speech–language pathologists in the acute hospital setting primarily use conventional tests to assess and treat the patient's communication impairment (Katz et al., 1998). Identifying the type and degree of communication impairment is important in acute care. Differential diagnosis of the communication difficulty can contribute to the patient's medical diagnosis and provides the clinician with valuable information about the patient's strengths and weaknesses. However, the efficacy of impairment-based therapy in the acute phase has not been thoroughly investigated because most treatment efficacy studies in disorders such as aphasia, have deliberately used participants beyond the period of spontaneous recovery (Linebaugh et al., 1998). Nor does the type and degree of communication impairment necessarily predict the severity of the patient's communication activity limitations (disability) or participation restriction (handicap) (Frattali, 1992).

To understand the patient's activity limitations, the clinician must assess the patient's ability to communicate in hospital-specific situations. For example, the clinician may want to assess the patient's ability to describe his or her pain, call for help, ask the doctors and nurses questions, and comprehend and sign a consent form.

Similarly, to understand the patient's participation restriction in hospital, the clinician must assess the communicative disadvantage experienced by the patient, due to the hospital environment and/or interaction with hospital staff. The clinician may need to consider if the acoustics of the hospital ward or the background noise of medical equipment make it difficult for the patient to hear, if the patient can use the nurse call button, and whether the patient is involved in decisions about his or her medical care and discharge planning.

In a health-care climate that is restricting the amount of therapy a person with communication disorder receives, speech–language pathologists are in a position of having to prioritize the type of services that can be provided in the limited time available. The functional approach that focuses on activity limitations and participation restrictions must surely be accorded a high priority for the following reasons. It can make the hospital stay less bewildering and more effective if communication-disordered people are not disadvantaged in the hospital system. This approach has been described in the first part of this chapter. The second reason is that the functional approach can provide the degree of psychological and emotional support necessary for patients and their families in the days following hospitalization. This contrasts with an approach that places early impairment-based therapy as a higher priority than support. Third, the focus of assessment and intervention can be on preparing the patient for discharge. With the limited number of rehabilitation sessions available to speech–language pathologists, while the communication-disordered person is in hospital, these functional goals of intervention are achievable, realistic, and conform with current health-care policies such as early discharge from hospital, consumer-driven services, and high levels of client satisfaction.

Establishing treatment objectives on the basis of an assessment of the patient's communication activity limitations and participation restrictions in the hospital has several advantages. First, the clinician is helping the patient address the communication problems that exist now, so management can be directed toward practical outcomes that are relevant and meaningful to the patient and health-care staff. Second, as therapy aims will be based on the communication activities that occur on a regular basis, such as attracting a nurse's attention, they can be practiced regularly. Finally, with regular support from the therapist, the in-patient can immediately learn ways to minimize the communication disability, helping the patient discover how to compensate for communication impairments thereby overcoming some barriers to communication. This provides opportunities to experience some communicative success. Encouraging the use of communication alternatives also helps to minimize social isolation, increase control over the environment, and improve psychosocial adjustment.

With an understanding of the patient's communication impairment *and* the subsequent activity limitation and participation restriction, the therapist can plan treatment that is relevant and meaningful to the patient. One technique described by Holland (in press) to assist clinicians in linking specific treatment objectives to meaningful contexts is by using the phrase "in order to." For example, a comprehensive goal might read: "Mr. X will comprehend semantically related single words with 90% accuracy (a goal established from an assessment of the communication impairment), *in order to* understand different meal suggestions made by his wife (a goal established from an assessment of his communication activities), *in order to* maintain his involvement in planning the week's meals (a goal established from an assessment of his participation)." Impairment, activity, and participation are integrally linked and the clinician needs to understand the disorder from each perspective if treatment is to be ultimately effective in helping clients interact successfully in situations and with people who are important to them.

Assessment of the patient's communication activities and participation in hospital also has advantages for the health-care staff and assists the patient's general medical management. Speech–language pathologists can provide practical and relevant information to staff about the patient's ability to communicate at present (e.g., in attracting a nurse's attention, following instructions, and making requests). Nursing staff who do not know the patient, can check the speech–language pathologist's assessment to immediately find out how well the patient communicates his or her needs. For example, nurses may want to know if the patient is able to initiate a request for assistance or needs to be asked regularly, or if he or she can fill out a menu card independently. The patient should not have to work out ways to communicate with each change of shift (Ashworth, 1980). Documentation of the patient's communication disability may also prevent staff misinterpretations and subsequent mismanagement of a patient's behavior. A patient who consistently selects the wrong meal from the menu may become extremely frustrated. Without an understanding of the communication disability, this behavior could be misinterpreted as aggression. The clinician can also improve communication between staff and patient, by, for example, assisting nurses and doctors to modify the answers they give to a patient's questions to make them more understandable.

Finally, assessing a patient's communication activity limitations and participation restriction in hospital can also assist the clinician in identifying and reducing institutional and environmental barriers to communication. For example, if patients with vision impairments are unable to read medical consent forms, menu cards, and discharge information, there is good reason to produce large-print versions of these materials. Similarly, if patients do not have the manual dexterity to operate the nurse call button for communication in an emergency or communication of personal needs, then introducing less manually demanding call buttons may be required. These barriers to effective communication can only begin to be identified if we routinely assess and manage patients' communication activities and participation.

Reducing patients' communication difficulties can enhance every other aspect of their care in hospital and can improve patients' level of satisfaction with their hospital stay. The role of speech–language pathology needs to develop to meet the challenges of in-patient communication activities and participation in the acute hospital setting. Assessments specifically designed to assess in-patient communication activities and participation are required. One example of an in-patient communication activity interview is the IFCI (Toffolo et al., 1995). Development of the IFCI and its application in the acute hospital setting is illustrated to demonstrate one example of a functional approach.

## Development of the IFCI

An assessment of a patient's ability to cope with the communication activities in the acute hospital setting is currently under development. The measure could provide a valid and reliable assessment of a patient's ability to communicate in hospital activities. A functional communication assessment needs to meet several criteria described by Lomas et al. (1989) and Frattali (1992). Specifically, we wanted to ensure that:

1. the measure assessed communication needs unique to the hospital setting as perceived by staff and patients of the hospital;
2. communication needs were assessed within contexts of communication situations rather than isolated speech and language processes; and
3. the measure met psychometric standards.

Based on work by Beukelman et al. (1984), we needed to ask the following questions:

1. What are the communication needs of the hospital in-patient?
2. How successfully do the health caregiver and the in-patient communicate to meet those needs?

### Identifying Communication Needs in the Hospital

To identify the communication needs of patients in the hospital, groups of patients and staff were interviewed. Patient and staff groups were interviewed separately using the nominal group technique (Delbecq et al., 1975). This technique was used by Lomas et al. (1989) to develop the Communicative Effectiveness Index (CETI). Two groups of in-patients participated in the patient interviews. At least two members of each group had some type of communication impairment, including visual impairments, mild cognitive impairments, and dysarthria. Each patient group was asked the question: "In which hospital situations do you have to be able to get your meaning across to people and understand what they say?" The nominal group technique requires that each participant considers the question for 10 minutes on their own before being asked to offer a response (Lomas et al., 1989). One response is elicited from each participant in turn. This allows each person an equal opportunity to contribute (Lomas et al., 1989). The group then discusses each item to clarify its meaning further, so as to arrive at a final list.

The nominal group technique was repeated with four groups of hospital staff. Two groups comprised clinical staff including a doctor, physiotherapist, nurse, radiographer, and social worker. The two other staff groups were made up of nonclinical staff and included a ward clerk, volunteer, cleaner, and food monitor. Each staff group was asked the question: "In which hospital situations does a patient have to be able to get his or her meaning across to you or to understand what you say?"

At the completion of all the interviews there was a total of 82 hospital communication situations. The lists of communication situations were reviewed independently by three judges (the authors) to identify items that were redundant with other situations in the same list and to identify items that were not actually communication situations. For example, the situation "patient needs to understand what is being offered by (the) volunteer with (the) trolley, for example book, menu, clothing," was felt to be an object-recognition task rather than a communication task. All the judges agreed that 16 of the items were either repetitions of other items in the same list or not actually communication situations and were therefore removed. This reduced the list to 66 items.

A panel of seven speech–language pathologists experienced in adult hospital work then analyzed the data to determine if the communication situations generated in the interviews were representative and then sorted the situations into one of four categories that were modified from those used by Lomas et al. (1989). Each category was defined as follows:

1. "*Basic need*—communication that is required to meet basic needs (e.g., toileting, eating, grooming, positioning)" (Lomas et al., 1989, p. 123);
2. *Present health-care need*—communication that is needed for patients to get their current health needs met (e.g., stating where they have pain, explaining their medical problems, and cooperating with assessment and therapy);
3. *Future health-care need*—communication that is needed so patients may be involved in their future health management (e.g., describing their social or home situation, and being involved in their own discharge planning);
4. "*Social need*—communication that is primarily social in nature (e.g., communication with others as an end in and of itself such as dinner table conversation, playing cards, writing a letter to a friend)" (Lomas et al., 1989, p. 123).

An analysis of the situations according to communication category revealed that most situations in staff and patient groups related to basic needs and present health-care needs. Examples of basic needs included "patients need to be able to tell you they are hungry or thirsty" and "patients need to be able to tell you where things can be put." Present health-care needs were situations such as "patients need to be able to call for a nurse."

The speech–language pathologists as a group then analyzed the items generated across all of the interview groups to remove any further redundant items. The panel discussed each possibly redundant situation until a consensus was reached. This reduced the list to 35 items. Despite the different perspectives of patients and caregivers in-hospital, a high degree of similarity was found across the two groups.

Finally, to ensure that the final test items were true measures of patient performance in the hospital, the panel reviewed the remaining 35 items to ensure that each item met two criteria. First, each situation had to be one in which the patient's performance could be directly observed in a naturally occurring context. Second, the communication situation had to be relevant to an in-patient hospital setting. For example, the communication situation "the patient needs to be able to understand the principles of rehabilitation, i.e., increasing their independence, the importance of practice," was felt by the panel to be too complex an issue to be directly observable. Following this process, 23 hospital situations remained. These situations formed the basis of a hospital-based communication interview. The 23 communication activities are listed in Table 17–1.

### Assessing Patients' Ability to Meet Their Communicative Needs

The IFCI was developed to assess a patient-staff ability to communicate in the in-patient hospital context. It can be used as a screening tool by nursing staff to report in-patients with communication difficulties or by the speech–language pathologist to assess an in-patient's communication ability. Each of the 23 communication situations is assessed by the clinician through a partially structured bedside interview with the patient. This interview can be incorporated into the initial contact with the patient and many of the communication situations can also be assessed during a formal dysphagia or aphasia assessment. For example, if the patient requires assistance to move from bed to chair, then his or her ability to ask for help in this situation will be assessed. The clinician will ask, "Can you

Table 17–1.   Final 23 Communicative Activities for the IFCI

| | |
|---|---|
| 1A. | Responding to his/her name |
| 2A. | Asking for help with lifts/transfers |
| 3A. | Telling you where things can be put |
| 4B. | Telling you social, personal, and medical details |
| 5B. | Telling you about any pain or discomfort |
| 6B. | Giving information regarding progress |
| 7B. | Expressing satisfaction with care received |
| 8A. | Making a special request |
| 9A. | Indicating his/her emotional status |
| 10B. | Asking questions relating to his/her care |
| 11A. | Telling you if he/she is hungry or thirsty |
| 12A. | Asking for something he/she needs |
| 13A. | Filling in a menu card |
| 14A. | Telling you if he/she has had a shower/bath |
| 15A. | Reporting on toileting |
| 16A. | Following simple instructions |
| 17B. | Pointing to parts of his/her body |
| 18B. | Calling for a nurse |
| 19A. | Asking for washing to be done |
| 20A. | Asking for something to be bought from the shops |
| 21C. | Talking about himself/herself |
| 22C. | Asking for something to read |
| 23B. | Indicating when he/she does not understand |

A = Basic need; B = Present health-care need; C = Social need.

come over to this chair because we'll be doing some writing later?" without offering any assistance. If the patient attempts to move independently, he or she is stopped and asked, "Do you need help?" The patient is then scored as not asking for help to move when required. An interview script has been developed to guide the interviewer in eliciting the target responses. However, of primary importance is that the interview is seen by the patient as a genuine inquiry into his or her ability to manage with the communication demands of the hospital and not seen as a test of his or her communication abilities.

The patient and interviewer are scored on each item on a successful or unsuccessful basis, depending on their ability to communicate in each situation using any means they can. Research is currently being undertaken to determine the IFCI's psychometric properties.

## Case Study

The following case is presented as an illustration of testing the IFCI for its usefulness in identifying the level of communication disability of in-patients and in turn, minimizing the level of disability.

E.K. was a 76-year-old English-speaking woman admitted into the hospital following a left hemisphere stroke. Her medical assessment indicated that she had a dense right hemiplegia and left limb apraxia. Discussion with her husband revealed E.K. was visually impaired, but had adequate vision premorbidly to read and see at long distances with the two sets of glasses that were with her. There was no history of hearing loss. E.K. had a severe aphasia. Her level of auditory comprehension was difficult to gauge initially, as her verbal and gestural modalities were impaired by apraxia. Her verbal expression was limited to a "yes" response to all questions, comments, and instructions. Following some spontaneous recovery 3 days poststroke, she could indicate "no" by uttering a vowel sound and withholding the "yes" response. With a "yes" and "no" response, she demonstrated reliable auditory comprehension of biographical information only.

The IFCI was conducted. When asked if anything was worrying or upsetting her, E.K. responded "yes." Further questioning by the speech–language pathologist revealed that E.K. did not want to take the sedatives that were being given to her at night. The sedatives were withheld that evening. E.K. was more alert the following morning and could participate more fully in physiotherapy.

One treatment goal was as follows: E.K. will produce the CV single words "sore" and "here" in response to the questions "how are you feeling?" and "where is the pain?," respectively (a goal established from an assessment of her communication impairment) *in order to* say if she had pain and where (a goal established from the results of the IFCI), *in order to* have increased control over her pain management.

## Conclusion

Determining management aims on the basis of a patient's communication needs enables clinicians to make meaningful improvements in a patient's ability to communicate with his or her doctors, nurses, and other health caregivers. By approaching treatment in this way we are also informing hospital staff about the patient's communication abilities and identifying ways that staff can facilitate successful communication with the patient.

Indirectly we are also continually reinforcing the need for good communication for improving a patient's medical care and satisfaction with his or her hospital stay. Finally, we can begin to influence hospital procedures and policies, to change hospital structures, and even hospital design so that communicating well with patients is integral to quality care.

## Acknowledgments

Thanks to Ms. Jo Goodridge, Ms. Roslyn Janes, Professor Audrey Holland, and Dr. Peter Stow for their helpful comments on earlier drafts of this manuscript.

## References

American Speech–Language–Hearing Association. (1997). Omnibus survey results. Rockville, MD: Author.

Ashworth, P. (1980). Care to communicate. The Royal College of Nursing, London.

Ashworth, P. (1984a). Communicating in an intensive care unit. In A. Faulkner (ed): *Recent advances in nursing 7: Communication* (pp. 94–112). Edinburgh: Churchill Livingstone.

Ashworth, P. (1984b). Staff-patient communication in coronary care units. *Journal of Advanced Nursing, 9,* 35–42.

Ashworth, P. (1987). The needs of the critically ill patient. *Intensive Care Nursing, 3,* 182–190.

Audit Commission (1993). *What seems to be the matter: Communication between hospitals and patients.* London: National Health Services Report No. 12.

Australian Bureau of Statistics (1993). *Disability, ageing and carers survey: Australia users guide.* Catalogue no. 4431.0. Canberra: Author.

Australian Institute of Health and Welfare (1998). [http://www.aihw.gov.au].

Bello, J. (1996). *Communication facts: Prevalence of hearing loss in the Unites States.* Rockville, MD: ASHA.

Beukelman, D. R., Yorkston, K. M., & Lossing, C. A. (1984). Functional communication assessment of adults with neurogenic disorders. In A. S. Halpern, M. J. Fuhrer (eds): *Functional assessment in rehabilitation* (pp 101–115). Baltimore: Paul H Brookes.

Boyce, N., McNeill, J., Graves, D., & Dunt, D. (1997). *Quality and outcome indicators for acute health services.* Canberra: Australian Government Publishing Service.

Cleary, P. D., Edgman-Levitan, S., Roberts, M., Moloney, T. W., McMullen, W., Walker, J. D., & Delbanco, T. L. (1991). Patients evaluate their care: A national survey. *Health Affairs, 10,* 254–267.

Consumers' Health Forum (CHF) (1994). *Consumers' health forum casemix project: Final report.* CHF, Canberra.

Delbecq, A. L., Van de Ven, A. H., & Gustafson, D. H. (1975). *Group techniques for program planning—A guide to nominal and Delphi processes.* Boston: Glenview, Scott, Foresman and Co.

Department of Human Services (1997). *Patient satisfaction survey Victorian public hospitals.* Melbourne: Department of Human Services.

Draper, M., & Hill, S. (1995). *The role of patient satisfaction surveys in a national approach to hospital quality management.* Canberra: Australian Government Publishing Service.

Dyer, I. (1996). Intensive care unit syndrome. *Nursing Times, 92,* 58–59.

Field, D. (1992). Communication with dying patients in coronary care units. *Intensive and Critical Care Nursing, 8,* 24–32.

Frattali, C. M. (1992). Functional assessment of communication: Merging public policy with clinical views. *Aphasiology, 6,* 63–83.

Goodglass, H., & Kaplan, E. (1972). *The assessment of aphasia and related disorders.* Philadelphia: Lea and Febiger.

Harasty, J., & McCooey, R. (1993). The prevalence of communication impairment in adults. *Australian Journal of Human Communication Disorders, 21,* 81–95.

Holland, A. (in press). Functional outcomes in aphasia following stroke. In C. Frattali (ed): *Topics in Speech-Language Pathology.* Rockville: Aspen.

Jones, A. (1993). A first step in effective communication: Providing a supportive environment for counselling in hospital. *Professional Nursing, 8,* 501–505.

Kaplan, E., Goodglass, H., & Weintrub, S. (1983). *The Boston Naming Test*. Philadelphia: Lea & Febiger.

Katz, R. C., Hollowell, B., Code, C., Armstrong, E., Roberts, Pound, Katz. (1998). A multi-national comparison of aphasia management practices. Paper presented at the Clinical Aphasiology Conference. Ashville, N. Carolina, 1998.

Kay, J., Lesser, R., & Coltheart, M. (1992). *Psycholinguistic assessments of language processing in aphasia*. Hove: Erlbaum.

Kertesz, A. (1982). *Western Aphasia Battery*. New York: Grune & Stratton.

Linebaugh, C. W., Baron, C. R., & Corcoran, K. J. (1998). Assessing treatment efficacy in acute aphasia: Paradoxes, presumptions, problems and principles. *Aphasiology, 12,* 519–536.

Lomas, J., Pickard, L., Bester, S., Elbard, H., Finlayson, A., & Zoghaib, C. (1989). The communicative effectiveness index: Development and psychometric evaluation of a functional communication measure for adult aphasia. *Journal of Speech and Hearing Disorders, 54,* 113–124.

Lubinski, R. (1981a). Environmental language intervention. In R. Chapey (ed): *Language intervention strategies in adult aphasia* (pp. 223–245). Baltimore: Williams & Wilkins.

Lubinski, R. (1981b). Language and aging: An environmental approach to intervention. *Topics in Language Disorders, 1,* 89–97.

Lubinski, R. (1991). Environmental considerations for elderly patients. In R. Lubinski (ed): *Dementia and Communication* (pp. 256–278). Philadelphia: Mosby-Year Book.

McCallum, J., Mathers, C., & Freeman, E. (1992). Sensory loss and successful ageing: Australian evidence. *British Journal of Visual Impairment, 10,* 11–14.

Mumford, E., Schlesinger, H. J., & Glass, G. V. (1982). The effects of psychological intervention on recovery from surgery and heart attacks. *American Journal of Public Health, 72,* 141–151.

National Center for Health Statistics (1999). [http://www.cdc.gov/nchswww/faq/avglsl.htm].

National Centre for Ageing and Sensory Loss (NCASL) (1994). Late onset sensory loss. NCASL, Melbourne.

National Eye Institute (1999). [http://www.nei.nih.gov/publications/plan/NEIPlan/frm_toc.htm].

Patients Charter Unit (1996). Patients Charter [http://www.doh.gov.uk/pcharter/patientc.htm].

Ringel, R. L., & Chodzko-Zajko, W. J. (1988). Age, health and the speech process. *Seminars in Speech and Language, 9,* 95–107.

Toffolo, D., Code, C., & McCooey, R. (1995). A functional communication assessment for the hospital setting. Paper presented at the Australian Association of Speech and Hearing National Conference. Brisbane, Australia.

U.S. Bureau of the Census (1999). [http://www.census.gov/prod/1/pop/p23–190/p23190-f.pdf].

Verity, S. (1996). Communicating with sedated ventilated patients in intensive care: Focussing on the use of touch. *Intensive Critical Care Nursing, 12,* 354–358.

Wilkinson, S. (1991). Factors which influence how nurses communicate with cancer patients. *Journal of Advanced Nursing, 16,* 677–688.

Ylvisaker, M., Feeney, T. J., & Urbanczyk, B. (1993). A social-environmental approach to communication and behaviour after traumatic brain injury. *Seminars in Speech and Language, 14,* 74–87.

World Health Organization (1997). ICIDH-2 International Classification of Impairments, Activities, and Participation [http://www.who.ch/programmes/mnh/mnh/ems/icidh/icidh.htm].

18

# Assessment and Treatment of Functional Communication in an Extended Care Facility

### Deborah J. Pye
### Linda E. Worrall
### Louise M. H. Hickson

**The communicative opportunities of residents of extended care facilities are often restricted. A functional approach in this setting must encompass all levels of the ICIDH-2; however, there is a need for increasing emphasis on the Participation level. Australia, like many other countries of the world, describes participation of aged residents as an important outcome for extended care facilities. The importance of speech–language pathology embracing anti-ageist communication models in a functional approach is emphasized.**

## Introduction

With increasing numbers of older people living in extended care facilities, the role of the speech–language pathologist with this population has been expanding. The aims of this chapter are to describe the communication difficulties of the residents, the communication environment of the extended care facility, and the functional communication approach to management in such a setting. While swallowing disorders are another major concern in extended care facilities, the primary focus of this chapter is on communication. It is argued that the International Classification of Impairments, Activities, and Participation (ICIDH-2) is an appropriate model for work in the extended care facility and that management is necessary at all levels, but in particular at the level of participation.

## What is an Extended Care Facility?

An individual is usually admitted to an extended care facility when the family and community are no longer able to meet that person's needs. While these facilities are known by a number of names (e.g., nursing home, skilled nursing facility), all provide housing, medical, and custodial care to individuals with long-term disability or chronic illness (Lubinski, 1981a).

In addition to nursing staff providing 24-hour medical care, staff of extended care facilities may include social workers, occupational and physical therapists, speech–language pathologists and other health professionals. The employment of rehabilitation specialists reflects the commitment of some extended care facilities to the maintenance of a resident's maximal level of function (Extended Care Information Network, 1996–1997).

## The Extended Care Facility Population: Its Importance to the Speech–Language Pathologist

While most older individuals do not require long-term care, a significant number will require extended care services. In Australia, 6% of individuals aged over 65 are in residential care. This proportion is reflected in most western nations (France 6%, Denmark 6%, Sweden 6%, United Kingdom 5%, United States 5%, Germany 5%) (Australian Institute of Health and Welfare, 1997). However, among those aged 85 and over in Australia, 31% are residing in extended care facilities (Australian Institute of Health and Welfare, 1997). Similarly in the United States, approximately 35% of those aged 85 and over are in residential care facilities (Lubinski, 1995). The demand for extended care facilities is correlated with an increase in the number of dependent older persons (Lubinski & Frattali, 1993). The implications of this relationship are realized in light of the fact that an ageing population "is a defining characteristic of all developed and many developing nations in the latter part of the 20th century, and one which will continue into the 21st" (Australian Institute of Health and Welfare, 1997, p. 6).

While the ageing of the population is a continuous trend, the tendency is primarily evident among individuals over 80. It is among this age group that formal health care is organized, therefore the need for future health services is probably greater than if one concentrated on the growth in the total aged population alone (Australian Institute of Health and Welfare, 1997). Changes in age structure are therefore relevant in the consideration of health services provided in extended care facilities. On a larger scale, Zopf (1986) described the expanding proportion of older people in the global community as the basic fact shaping the human relationships and economic system of contemporary society.

The increase in the older population can be attributed largely to an increase in life expectancy, which is a result of a variety of public health measures including improved clinical treatment, enhanced environmental conditions, and positive changes in lifestyle (Commonwealth Department of Human Services and Health, 1994b). While an ageing population is obviously a significant factor impinging on the provision of services in extended care facilities, societal changes (e.g., higher divorce rates, greater proportion of women in the workforce) also impact on the type and level of support provided by extended care facilities.

In summary, the importance of speech–language pathology to the extended care facility is increasing as a result of the anticipated increase in chronic illness and long-term disability of an ageing population. The basis for the provision of speech–language pathology services to extended care facilities is further evident when one examines the prevalence of communication difficulties among residents and the nature of communicative interaction in extended care facilities (Lubinski, 1995). An understanding of communication in the extended care facility population is important in determining a holistic view of the role of the speech–language pathologist.

## Speech–Language Pathology: The Background to Our Role in the Extended Care Facility

A profile of the problematic nature of communication in the extended care facility population is emerging steadily in the literature, with discussion of the features inherent in establishing the need for speech–language pathology services. The prevalence of communication disorders in residents of extended care facilities has been reported as high as 98% (Worrall et al., 1994). This finding is in line with a previous Australian study that estimated that 90% of individuals in extended care present with some form of communication disorder (Geraldton Regional Hospital Speech Pathology Services, 1989).

Although the reported prevalence of communication impairment in residents of extended care facilities varies considerably, international research has established that a significant proportion of this population is likely to manifest a speech-, language-, hearing-, or communication-related disorder (Bryan & Drew, 1989; Chafee, 1967; Mueller & Peters, 1981; O'Connell & O'Connell, 1980; Sorin-Peters et al., 1989; Worrall et al., 1994). The prevalence figures range from 52.5% (Bryan & Drew, 1989) to 98% (Worrall et al., 1994). This reported high prevalence of communication disorders might be associated with Wilder's (1984) observation that the presence of a communication impairment was a significant indicator for an individual's placement in extended care.

The complexity of the issue of communication impairment in the extended care facility is increased by the multiplicity of communication disorders that are present. Residents generally present with several chronic illnesses (e.g., cardiovascular disease, arthritis, lung disease, and Parkinsonism), demonstrate poor mobility, and require a number of medications throughout each day (Lubinski, 1981b). Neurological disease, motor and sensory deficits, and mental illness are also frequently present in the extended care population (Le Dorze et al., 1994). In view of this profile, it is understandable that many residents have multiple communication disorders with various combinations of hearing impairment, dementia, pragmatic disorders, voice disorders, aphasia, and speech disorders (Geraldton Regional Hospital Speech Pathology Services, 1989; Worrall et al., 1994). Within the healthy ageing process, communication abilities are also variably affected depending on an individual's physical, mental, and social status. Communication changes associated with normal ageing generally occur over a prolonged period of time. The modifications that may be demonstrated in the speech, language, and sensory systems of a healthy older person have been described by a number of authors (Beasley & Davis, 1981; Huntley & Helfer, 1995; Maxim & Bryan, 1994; Mueller & Geoffrey, 1987; Von Leden, 1977; Weiss, 1971). While these communication changes differ from those of an individual with a disease-specific communication condition, they must also be considered as important when justifying the provision of speech–language pathology services to extended care facilities.

The knowledge base of the communication problems of residents of extended care facilities has been steadily expanding. In recent years, however, the literature has focused increasingly on the institutional features influencing the communicative health of an individual (Gravell, 1988; Lubinski, 1981a,b,c, 1991, 1995). The nature and quality of the communication environment in an extended care facility are both external determinants of a resident's communicative status.

Upon entry into an extended care setting, adjustment difficulties invariably arise as the individual copes with a new environment (Gravell, 1988). The concept of "environment" encompasses the physical background, the individual, and how that individual relates to others (Lubinski, 1991). The physical environment and the social environment (the opportunity for an individual to relate to others) are of particular interest in light of the nature of their effects on communication. The physical environment restricts communication in extended care facilities, with a scarcity of private areas for meaningful interaction to occur, and an atmosphere that is often sensory-depriving (Lubinski, 1991). Gravell (1988) similarly highlighted the problems of poor physical layout and acoustics in some residential care settings. For example, seats are frequently arranged in rows and hard floor coverings are typically used in communal areas.

Lubinski (1991) identified a variety of features that impair the communication environment by their effect on the quality of interaction in the extended care facility. Care staff frequently place limited value on the role of effective communication in a resident's quality of life. Residents also often think that they have very few meaningful contributions to make in conversation. Kaakinen (1995) suggested that unspoken restrictive rules contribute to a communication-impaired environment and that these rules primarily incorporated topic and partner restrictions (e.g., Do not complain about level of care; Do not speak to people of the opposite sex). Features such as few reasons to talk, limited accessibility to conversation partners, and socially stagnant surrounds, all add to the communication-impaired environment of the extended care facility (Lubinski, 1991).

A number of researchers have likewise identified features that negatively affect the social aspect of the communication environment. Wilder (1984) determined that residents were often unaware of their communication difficulties and avenues for optimizing communication. Parker (1987) commented that staff undervalued communication compared with other physical and medical aspects of care of the resident. Although Kato et al. (1996) found that staff desired more time communicating with residents, it was also evident that staff were often unaware of communication difficulties faced by residents. As Lubinski (1995) noted, research has revealed that there is likely to be minimal interaction in extended care facilities and if communication does occur, quality will be impoverished. This observed paucity in the communicative health of a resident could be attributed to a limited physical environment or a restricted social environment (Armstrong & Woodgates, 1996).

The importance of the environment to the communicative health of an individual is apparent when one considers the role of the speech–language pathologist in the extended care facility. Professional associations such as the American Speech–Language–Hearing Association (1988a,b) and the Speech Pathology Association of Australia (Australian Association of Speech and Hearing, 1993) have released position papers delineating the role of speech–language pathologists and audiologists working with older people. Traditional roles include the assessment, diagnosis, and treatment of impairments in speech, language, voice, fluency, hearing, and swallowing. Expansion of the speech–language pathologist's role beyond the traditional assessment and treatment of impairments is reflected in the outlined service delivery options. Further roles include group therapy, counseling, education, consultation, discharge planning, advocacy, referral, and environmental interventions (American Speech–Language–Hearing Association, 1988; Australian Association of Speech and Hearing, 1993).

Many authors recommend the extension of the role of the speech–language pathologist to optimizing the physical and social environments of the individual (American Speech–Language–Hearing Association, 1988a,b; Australian Association of Speech and Hearing, 1993; Armstrong & Woodgates, 1996; Kaakinen, 1995; Le Dorze et al., 1994; Lubinski, 1981a,b, 1991, 1995; O'Connell & O'Connell, 1980; Palmer & Henderson, 1993; Robertson, 1993; Sorin-Peters et al., 1989; Worrall & Hickson, 1993). The extension of the speech–language pathologist's role, beyond that of the individual and his or her disorder to holistic communication maintenance and enhancement, reflects a growing trend in the profession—the application of a functional approach in the management of communication.

## A Functional Approach in an Extended Care Facility: What is the Concept?

The concept of functional communication abilities extends beyond basic communication skills to the everyday abilities needed by an individual for optimal quality of life in his or her particular environment. A functional communication approach is best understood within the concepts of the World Health Organization's (WHO's) ICIDH (1980) and the more recent revision, the ICIDH-2 (1997). The emergence of the functional perspective and the development of the World Health Organization's ICIDH (1980) reflected a response to the established medical model in rehabilitation. The focus of the medical model is the identification of disease symptoms with the goal of removing or reducing these symptoms. Little attention is given within the model to the psychosocial and behavioral aspects of illness (Ramsberger, 1994). The psychosocial and behavioral aspects become more important in the context of the increasing prevalence of chronic illnesses. The foundation of the ICIDH (WHO, 1997) is an acknowledgment of these changing health experiences of the population. Health professionals are therefore becoming increasingly concerned with the disability and handicap that result from impairment (Badley, 1993).

A functional communication approach generally is not regarded as an alternative to other assessment or intervention paradigms; rather, it supplements more traditional diagnostic and treatment methods that may be based primarily on the medical model (Dekker, 1995; Frattali et al., 1995a; Hartley, 1992; Ramsberger, 1994). Traditional methods of diagnosis and treatment are insufficient in a setting where the population presents with chronic illness and a variety of factors clearly impinge upon their communication status. The clinician working within the extended care facility is an advocate for an individual coping with the persistent effects of illness on his or her communicative ability within a communication-impaired environment. The goals and procedures in the assessment and treatment of communication status therefore necessitate an approach that attaches particular emphasis on the disability and handicap of an individual—the ability to communicate sufficiently and appropriately within his or her environment to ensure optimal quality of life. While a complete concept of a functional diagnosis is evolving continually, the ICIDH-2 (WHO, 1997) provides an exceptional framework in which to incorporate these developments in our understanding of a functional approach (Dekker, 1995). The remainder of the chapter therefore describes a functional approach in extended care facilities within the framework of the ICIDH-2.

## The Level of Impairment

As previously noted, a functional approach acknowledges the potential presence of impairment, activity limitation and participation restriction. Within the extended care facility, the importance of assessing impairments relating to communication when using a functional approach is necessary for a number of reasons.

The organizational structure of an extended care facility is based on levels of nursing hierarchy. An extended care facility is primarily a nursing facility and therefore the medical model dominates the philosophy and culture of the institution. The medical model focuses care at the disease or disorder level and possibly at the impairment level. In contrast, the functional model also recognizes the importance of the loss of ability or social disadvantages that may reflect the effects of the disorder within an individual's particular environment. With such an emphasis on the medical model, the goals of the nursing staff tend to be related to the physical care of the resident. In staff–resident interactions, for example, studies have found that only 1 to 4% of nurses' time was spent in conversation with older patients (MacLeod, 1985). Oliver and Redfern (1991) report that 72% of the nurse–resident conversations observed during their study were concerned with the physical aspects of nursing care and that conversations were of short duration. Edwards et al. (1993) and Erber (1994) report that nurse–resident communication is typically brief, task orientated and primarily related to daily housekeeping. Hence, within this medical model, measurement of speech, language, swallowing, and hearing impairments are not only more readily understood by nursing staff, but are also recognized as important and generally acted upon by nursing staff.

The dominance of the medical model is also reflected in measures used to support funding in many extended care facilities. For example, the Australian Resident Classification Scale—RCS (Commonwealth Department of Health and Family Services, 1997) uses terminology that is clearly impairment-based in determining a resident's communication care needs. For example, the RCS manual states that "In assessing the care recipient's communication difficulties in relation to speech, take account of physical defects, speech defects and also language difficulties if relevant" (Commonwealth Department of Health and Family Services, 1997, pp. 5–6). In Australia, the measures that determine funding are so important to the life of the institution that speech–language pathologists are increasingly expected to provide services based upon the relative care needs of the resident as outlined by the RCS (Commonwealth Department of Health and Family Services, 1997). Because the measure is focused on impairments, speech–language pathology assessments need to incorporate measures of speech, language, hearing, and swallowing impairment. In Australia at least, the very presence of speech–language pathology in extended care facilities depends upon the ability of the speech–language pathologist to contribute to a profile of the resident that will maximize the funding that the institution receives from the government.

The importance of understanding the underlying impairments of individual residents is seen when one considers the high prevalence of speech, language, swallowing, and hearing impairments in these facilities. In addition, concomitant impairments are a distinguishing feature of older people in residential care (Worrall et al., 1994). That is, many older residents may have a hearing impairment as well as a visual impairment in addition to cognitive decline.

While it is important to assess at the impairment level, there are many difficulties associated with determining impairment levels in the extended care facility. In the first instance, there is often a lack of medical history information on admittance to the facility. Diagnoses are often broad and lacking results of investigations (e.g., computed tomography scans), which are generally expected within an acute setting. The multiplicity of impairments that a resident may present with often confound the results that may be found on a single impairment measure (Gravell, 1988). A common instance of this is the co-morbidity effect of the cognitive deficit associated with dementia on a test of language status. Other examples include the synergistic effect of sensory deficits on any communication task. That is, if an older person has a hearing loss, an added visual loss may greatly affect the persons' ability to recognize the speaker or to speech read. Added to this is a lack of age-appropriate normative data on impairment measures for this population. Sensory loss, reduced attention and motivation, fatigability, and medication (Gravell, 1988) similarly affect the success of direct individual intervention in an extended care facility.

Hence, within a functional approach it is still vital to be aware of the many impairments that affect everyday communication. It is also important to be conversant with the impairment of individuals in a setting that predominantly uses a medical model. The limitations of focusing solely at the impairment level have also been noted.

## The Disability (Activity Limitation) Level

The foundation and strength of a functional approach is derived from its consideration of communication in everyday life. While a functional approach acknowledges the need to assess and treat at the level of impairment, the focus of functional assessment and treatment is beyond the structure and function of the body (impairment) to the functioning of a whole person and that person's functioning within society. It recognizes the impact that context has on the functioning of speech, language, swallowing, and hearing mechanisms. A functional approach is relevant to the individual and the environment and because of its transparency to nonhealth professionals is favorable to clients, families, policy-makers, and payers. A functional approach creates a common language between health professionals and other key stakeholders in health care.

To assess functional communication at the disability (activity limitation) level in extended care facilities the nature, duration, and quality of everyday communicative activities in the facility needs to be assessed. Currently there is no assessment devised specifically to assess the everyday communicative needs of people in extended care facilities. Functional communication assessments such as the American Speech–Language–Hearing Association Functional Assessment of Communication Skills for Adults—ASHA FACS (Frattali et al., 1995a), the Communicative Abilities in Daily Living—CADL (Holland, 1980), and its second edition, the Communication Activities of Daily Living—CADL-2 (Holland et al., 1998), the Edinburgh Functional Communication Profile—EFCP (Skinner et al., 1984), and the Communicative Effectiveness Index—CETI (Lomas et al., 1989) have been psychometrically tested on individuals in aged care facilities, however, they were not developed specifically for the extended care facility population. Test items or situations in these assessment tools are subsequently often unrelated to life in an extended care facility (Le Dorze et al., 1994). Ethnographic studies are required to determine what communicative activities occur in extended care facilities, and then determine which activities key stakeholders (residents, family, staff, and payer) view as important enough to be included in an assessment specifically tailored for this setting.

The lack of tools specifically designed for extended care facilities perhaps is a reflection of the speech–language pathology profession's lack of recognition of the uniqueness of this population. Measures at the disability level have traditionally stemmed from acquired neurogenic disorders and have failed to recognize the specialized context of extended care facilities. Features particular to extended care facilities include the age and frailty of the population; care being provided by a multitude of health professionals rather than individual family members; and the limitations of daily activities because of the necessary schedule of nursing care. While the community-based population may enjoy a multitude of environments and considerable autonomy, the environment within the extended care facility is unchanging and comparatively stable. It is shared by all residents who have little choice in their communication environments.

Within the ICIDH-2 (WHO, 1997), there are two main areas of activity limitation that are relevant to speech–language pathologists: communication activities and interpersonal behaviors. In the activity dimension of the ICIDH-2 the speech–language pathologist's role in intervention is therefore to determine and provide assistance to enhance the performance of activities and extend the range of activities that residents can perform (e.g., reading books, expressing needs, making requests, drinking from a cup or glass without spilling, initiating conversation). Assistance can be in the form of personal assistance (e.g., "interpreting" needs for a communication-disordered residents) and nonpersonal assistance (e.g., providing a modified cup, using a communication book). Much of the speech–language pathologist's intervention at the activity level is building the components of communication in preparation for supporting greater participation of residents in the day-to-day life of the extended care facility.

## The Participation Restriction (Handicap) Level

Participation is essentially the outcome of the complex relationship between the health condition, the impairment, and any limitation to activities within the individual's own personal and environmental contexts (Madden & Hogan, 1997). According to the World Health Organization, there are seven domains of a person's involvement in life: participation in personal maintenance; participation in mobility; participation in exchange of information; participation in social relationships; participation in the areas of education, work, leisure, and spirituality; participation in economic life; and participation in civic and community life (WHO, 1997). It is evident that communication difficulties may have an impact on many of these domains.

The seven domains of participation remind us that residents in extended care facilities have a right to participate in areas such as civic and community life and economic life. Older age is often seen as a time of illness and withdrawal from community life (Becker & Kaufman, 1988). Speech–language pathologists have a specific role in facilitating the broader and socially just view of an individual in an extended care facility as remaining a vital member of the community. The extended care facility is the resident's home. It should not be thought of as a place merely to conduct therapy or a place where a resident's right to participate fully in all aspects of life is temporarily suspended.

Aged care policy and resource allocation vary considerably from country to country (Ribbe et al., 1997). In this chapter, examples will be drawn from the Australian aged care sector to illustrate the effect of policy and resource allocation on the practice of speech-language pathology. Like many other countries undergoing aged care reform, Australia has legislated the rights of residents in aged care facilities (Aged Care Act, 1997). These rights include *the right to full information about his or her own state of health and about available treatments, the right to personal privacy and the right to be consulted on, and to choose to have input into, decisions about the living arrangements of the residential care service* (Commonwealth Department of Human Services and Health, 1994a, p. 62). Linked to the rights of residents are outcome standards that are routinely monitored by the payer. The outcome standards ensure that extended care facilities in Australia are providing a standard of care consistent with the community's expectations of good care. The Australian outcome standards include the following language: *residents will be enabled and encouraged to make informed choices about their individual care plans and residents will be enabled to achieve a maximum degree of independence as members of society* (Commonwealth Department of Human Services and Health, 1994b, p. 62). The speech–language pathologist can identify and break down barriers that communication difficulty present to achieving these standards (Hamilton, 1993). In Australia, the actions of speech–language pathologists at this participation level are therefore the clinical interventions most likely to be recognized under Australian policy procedures. This does not appear to be the case in other countries, although it has been suggested that the primary aim of care in extended care facilities around the world should be to develop and optimize social and recreational programs appropriate to the resident's level of function and that provide significant involvement in their environment (Schroll et al., 1997). The role of the speech–language pathologist at the participation level can maximize this aim.

Implementing interventions that target participation restriction, the speech–language pathologist can have a substantial impact on the lives of *all* residents in the extended care facility. The extended care facility is the primary everyday social and physical world of the individuals residing there, and functions as the shared social system (Kaakinen, 1995). Subsequently, intervention at this level has the greatest potential to be time and cost-effective. Through modifying the community in which the residents live, the participation level of residents can be enhanced.

A number of service delivery models, currently perceived as part of the developing role for speech–language pathologists in extended care facilities, are targeted at the participation restriction level. Erber (1994) and Kaakinen (1995) describe a variety of ways to sustain effective conversational links between residents and reduce social isolation. These include matching talkers with talkers (e.g., in room sharing, dining room seating arrangement), establishing a buddy-mentoring system in which a resident takes time to orientate a new resident, and providing more resident-to-resident opportunities (e.g., recruiting age-related, peer volunteers). While these are practical ways to modify the social environment, alteration of the physical environment (e.g., changing topography to enhance privacy) and sensory environment (e.g., placing notices at eye-level) can also increase participation (Gravell, 1988; Kaakinen, 1995; Lubinski, 1991). These modifications may promote social interaction among residents more than many hours of impairment-based intervention or even activity-based intervention with each individual. In addition, counseling of family members (O'Connell & O'Connell, 1980) and education of nursing staff (e.g., training on the use of hearing-aids) (Gravell, 1988; Lubinski, 1995; O'Connell & O'Connell, 1980;) provide an indirect way to manipulate the structure and attitudes of the "society" of the extended care facility and increase participation levels of the majority of residents. Burgio and Scilley (1994) offer practical strategies to consider when conducting staff training in an extended care facility. A particular focus of education should be the training of conversational partners within the facility. This includes educating staff, family, volunteers, other residents, and outside supporting professionals (e.g., chaplains, solicitors, dentists) about maximizing the communicative potential of residents whom they encounter. Trained communication partners are described by Kagan and Gailey (1993) as "communication ramps" to society. Nowhere else is there a greater need for the communication ramps than in an extended care facility.

Traditionally, speech–language pathologists have provided education to staff using a deficit paradigm in which the multiple problems of communication with older people are emphasized. However, Chafetz and Wilson (1988) and McIntosh (1996) argue that stereotypical representations of interaction with the older population are often a reproduction of ageist views and may lead to behaviors such as elderspeak. Elderspeak was reported by Caporael (1981) to be a common form of communication in aged care facilities characterized by slower rate, increased loudness, greater repetition, high pitch, exaggerated intonation, reduced complexity of syntactic structure, and simplified vocabulary (Coupland et al., 1988). Such stereotypical accommodation may lead to fewer communication opportunities, reduced need for the elder person to initiate interaction, and reduction in the satisfaction gained from interaction (Ryan, 1991). In opposition to the deficit models, anti-ageist models of communication are gaining prominence. The Communication Accommodation Theory (Coupland et al., 1991) stands as an alternative basis for examining the interactions between individuals. The model is based on the premise that speakers and listeners accommodate to each other's individual communication patterns. Underaccommodation can occur if an interlocutor fails to recognize the cues of the other partner. Overaccommodation occurs when a partner has a stereotypical viewpoint and is particularly evident with older people. Behaviors such as shouting, simplified sentence instructions, and repetition of information is a reaction to the widespread belief that all older people have hearing and memory impairments. Ryan et al. (1995) have further developed the Communication Accommodation Theory into a model for educating conversational partners of older people. The Communication Enhancement Model (Ryan et al., 1995) identifies the steps involved in communicating effectively with older people (see Fig. 18–1). It is this model which may be more effective in educating conversational partners about maximizing their communication with older people.

In summary, if a speech–language pathologist chose to work at the participation level, he or she would need to determine the participation level of all residents in the extended care facility and not just focus on communicatively impaired residents. In addition, the speech–language pathologist would identify and minimize the barriers to participation within the institution. The influence of contextual factors, particularly environmental, in the extended care facility should not be underestimated.

There are some practical limitations of working at the participation level in extended care facilities. The role of the speech–language pathologist is often restricted to the medical model in extended care facilities because this is the preferred model of the facility. Many speech–language pathologists who are employed on a contractual basis are restricted to providing services at the impairment level. In addition, speech–language pathology training may perpetuate this medical approach through insufficient education about gerontological speech–

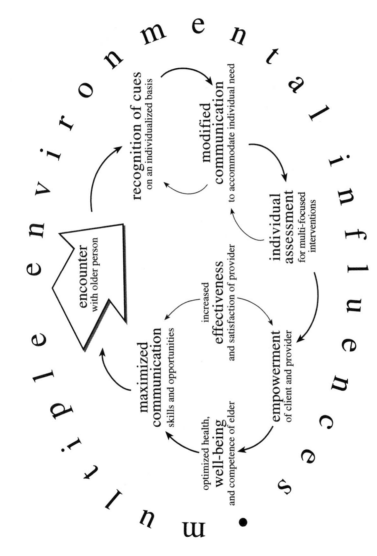

**Figure 18–1.** Communication enhancement model: Multiple environmental influences. (Reproduced with permission from Intl J Aging and Human Devlopment, 1995; 41:2, pp.89–107

language pathology (Brown, 1997). Finally, the finding that there are so few communication specialists in extended care facilities (Dahl, 1997; Lubinski, 1995) means that a collective of experienced practitioners is not developing models of best practice in the area.

## Conclusion

The extended care facility population presents an exciting challenge to the profession of speech–language pathology. Perhaps in no other setting is there such diversity in communication disorders, ready access to primary caregivers, shared environments across clients, and interplay of factors impinging on the communication abilities of an individual. However, the paucity of speech–language pathology research in the area, lack of speech–language pathology presence in extended care facilities, and limited staff awareness of the role of the speech–language pathologist in those facilities where one is employed, all indicate that this challenge has not as yet been adequately met by the profession.

One may argue that the lack of a recognized speech–language pathology role in extended care facilities is primarily the fault of the institution, the health-care culture, or many governments' increasingly strained health budget for the needs of the older population. If this is the case, the situation will remain status quo. It is our belief, however, that speech–language pathologists are currently presented with an opportunity to meet the needs of an increasing older population who reside in extended care facilities.

To ensure our continuing influence within a population that has been conclusively documented as warranting speech–language pathology management, the profession needs to take a broader role within the extended care facility. Positive outcomes need to be demonstrated at the level of the institution, not simply at the level of the individual. In Australia, this means that when an institution has a high compliance with outcome standards, speech–language pathologists must document their contribution to the institution's outcome standards. In addition, speech–language pathologists must play their part in assessing residents' communication status for institutional funding purposes. To achieve institutional recognition, the speech–language pathology profession needs to recognize and promote its role in the aged-care industry. Ageist attitudes may have been preventing the development of many initiatives that could have ensured an established place for the speech–language pathologist in the extended care facility. To combat this, attitudes need to be examined, undergraduate and graduate programs should prepare speech–language pathologists for work in this setting, and continued research and development of assessment/treatment instruments needs to be pursued.

The first step in meeting the challenge in extended care facilities lies in acknowledging that the assessment and treatment procedures long utilized in the medical model of the acute care hospital cannot be transferred for use in the extended care setting. The speech–language pathologist's role in this setting is maximized by first understanding, assessing, and treating the multitude of communication impairments. Second, extending the range and improving the quality of the communication activities is necessary. Finally, and most importantly, participation needs to be facilitated at the level of the individual within the context of the extended care environment—a place often considered home.

## References

American Speech–Language–Hearing Association (1988a). The roles of speech–language pathologists and audiologists in working with older persons. *American Speech–Language–Hearing Association, March,* 80–84.

American Speech–Language–Hearing Association (1988b). Provision of audiology and speech–language pathology services to older persons in nursing homes. *American Speech–Language–Hearing Association, March,* 72–74.

Armstrong, L., & Woodgates, S. (1996). Using a quantitative measure of communicative environment to compare two psychogeriatric day care settings. *European Journal of Disorders in Communication, 31,* 309–317.

Australian Association of Speech and Hearing (1993). The role of the speech pathologist working with older people. Melbourne: Australian Association of Speech Hearing.

Australian Institute of Health and Welfare (1997). *Aged and respite care in Australia: Extracts from recent publications.* Canberra: Australian Institute of Health and Welfare.

Badley, E. M. (1993). An introduction to the concepts and classifications of the international classification of impairments, disabilities, and handicaps. *Disease Rehabilitation, 15,* 161–178.

Beasley, D. S., & Davis, G. A. (Eds). (1981). *Aging: Communication processes and disorders.* New York: Grune & Stratton.

Becker, G., & Kaufman, S. (1988). Old age, rehabilitation, and research: A review of the issues. *Gerontologist, 28,* 459–468.

Brown, A. E. (1997). Geriatric communication disorders: Canadian University curriculum and clinical practice issues in speech–language pathology. Unpublished Masters thesis, The University of Western Ontario, Canada.

Bryan, K. L., & Drew, S. (1989). A survey of communication disability in an elderly population in an elderly population in residential care. *International Journal of Rehabilitation Research, 12,* 330–333.

Burgio, L. D., & Scilley, K. (1994). Caregiver performance in the nursing home: The use of staff training and management procedures. *Seminars in Speech and Language, 15,* 313–321.

Caporael, L. R. (1981). The paralanguage of caregiving: Baby talk to institutionalized aged. *Journal of Personality and Social Psychology, 40,* 876–884.

Chafee, C. (1967). Rehabilitation needs of nursing home residents: A report of a survey. *Rehabilitation Literature, 28,* 377–382.

Chafetz, P. K., & Wilson, N. L. (1988). Communicating effectively with elderly clients. *Seminars in Speech and Language, 9,* 177–182.

Commonwealth Department of Human Services and Health (1994a). *Your guide to residents' rights in nursing homes,* 2nd ed. Canberra: Australian Government Publishing Service.

Commonwealth Department of Human Services and Health (1994b). *Better health outcomes for all Australians: National goals, targets, strategies for better health outcomes into the next century.* Canberra: Australian Government Publishing Service.

Commonwealth Department of Health and Family Services (1997). *The residential care manual.* Canberra: Australian Government Publishing Service.

Coupland, N., Coupland, J., & Giles, H. (1991). *Language, society and the elderly: Discourse, identity and ageing.* Oxford: Blackwell.

Coupland, N., Coupland, J., Giles, H., & Henwood, K. (1988). Accommodating the elderly: Invoking and extending a theory. *Language and Society, 17,* 1–41.

Dahl, M. (1997). To hear again: A volunteer program in hearing health care for hard-of-hearing seniors. *Journal of Speech–Language Pathology and Audiology, 21,* 153–159.

Dekker, J. (1995). Application of the ICIDH in survey research on rehabilitation: The emergence of the functional diagnosis. *Disease Rehabilitation, 17,* 195–201.

Edwards, H. E., Weir, D., Clinton, M., & Moyle, W. Communication between residents and nurses in a dementia facility: An issue of quality of life. Paper presented at Alzheimer's Association Australia 3rd National Conference, Melbourne, May, 1993.

Erber, N. P. (1994). Conversation as therapy for older adults in residential care: The case for intervention. *European Journal of Disorders in Communication, 29,* 269–278.

Extended Care Information Network. (1996–1997). http://www.ElderConnect.com/ElderCare/HospMoreInfo.html. Extended Care Information Network, Inc.

Frattali, C. M., Thompson, C. K., Holland, A. L., Wohl, C. B., & Ferketic, M. M. (1995a). *ASHA Functional Assessment of Communication Skills for Adults (FACS)*. Rockville: American Speech–Language–Hearing Association.

Frattali, C. M., Thompson, C. K., Holland, A. L., Wohl, C. B., & Ferketic, M. M. (1995b). ASHA FACS: A functional outcome measure for adults. *American Speech–Language–Hearing Association, April*, 41–46.

Geraldton Regional Hospital Speech Pathology Services (1989). *Evaluation of the need for speech–language pathology services in nursing homes in Geraldton*. Geraldton: Geraldton Regional Hospital Speech Pathology Services.

Gravell, R. (1988). *Communication problems in elderly people: Practical approaches to management*. London: Croom Helm.

Hamilton, R. (1993). Paying for care in the nursing home industry. *Australian Communications Quarterly, Spring*, 12–15.

Hartley, L. L. (1992). Assessment of functional communication. *Seminars in Speech and Language, 13*, 264–279.

Holland, A. L. (1980). *Communicative abilities in daily living*. Baltimore: University Park Press.

Holland, A., Frattali, C., & Fromm, D. (1998). *Communication activities of daily living*. Austin, TX: Pro Ed.

Huntley, R. A., & Helfer, K. S. (eds.). (1995). *Communication in later life*. Boston: Butterworth-Heinemann.

Kaakinen, J. (1995). Talking among elderly nursing home residents. *Topics in Language Disorders, 15*, 36–46.

Kagan, A., & Gailey, G. F. (1993). Functional is not enough: Training conversation partners for aphasic adults. In A. L. Holland, M. M. Forbes (eds): *Aphasia treatment: World perspectives* (pp. 199–225). San Diego: Singular.

Kato, J., Hickson, L., & Worrall, L. (1996). Communication difficulties of nursing home residents. *Journal of Gerontological Nursing, 22*, 26–31.

Le Dorze, G., Julien, M., Brassard, C., Durocher, J., & Bovin, G. (1994). An analysis of the communication of adult residents of a long-term care hospital as perceived by their caregivers. *European Journal of Disorders in Communication, 29*, 241–267.

Lomas, J., Pickard, L., Bester, S., Elbard, H., Finlayson, A., & Zoghaib, C. (1989). The Communicative Effectiveness Index: Development and psychometric evaluation of a functional communication measure for adult aphasia. *Journal of Speech and Hearing Disorders, 54*, 113–124.

Lubinski, R. (1981a). Environmental language intervention. In R. Chapey (ed): *Language intervention strategies in adult aphasia* (pp. 223–245). Baltimore: Williams & Wilkins.

Lubinski, R. (1981b). Language and aging: An environmental approach to intervention. *Topics in Language Disorders, 1*, 89–97.

Lubinski, R. (1981c). Speech, language and audiology programs in home health care agencies and nursing homes. In D. Beasley, G. Davis (eds): *Aging: Communication processes and disorders* (pp. 339–356). New York: Grune and Stratton.

Lubinski, R. (1991). Environmental considerations for elderly patients. In R. Lubinski (ed): *Dementia and communication* (pp. 256–278). Philadelphia: Mosby-Year Book.

Lubinski, R. (1995). State-of-the-art perspectives on communication in nursing homes. *Topics in Language Disorders, 15*, 1–19.

Lubinski, R., & Frattali, C. (1993). The Resident Assessment Instrument. *American Speech–Language–Hearing Association, January*, 59–62.

McIntosh, I. (1996). Interaction between professionals and older people: Where does the problem lie? *Health Care in Later Life, 1*, 29–37.

MacLeod, C. J. (1985). The development of research in interpersonal skills in nursing. In C. M. Kagan (ed): *Interpersonal skills in nursing: Research and application* (pp. 9–21). London: Croom Helm.

Madden, R., & Hogan, T. (1997). The definition of disability in Australia: Moving toward national consistency. AIHW cat. No. DIS 5. Canberra: Australian Institute of Health and Welfare.

Maxim, J., & Bryan, K. (1994). *Language of the elderly*. London: Whurr.

Mueller, H. G., & Geoffrey, V.C. (eds). (1987). *Communication disorders in aging: Assessment and management*. Washington, DC: Gallaudet University press.

Mueller, P. B., & Peters, T. J. (1981). Needs and services in geriatric speech–language pathology and audiology. *American Speech–Language–Hearing Association, Sept.*, 627–632.

O'Connell, P. F., & O'Connell, E. J. (1980). Speech–language pathology services in a skilled nursing facility: A retrospective study. *Journal of Communication Disorders, 13*, 93–103.

Oliver, S., & Redfern, S. (1991). Interpersonal communication between nurses and elderly patients: Refinement of an observational schedule. *Journal of Advanced Nursing, 16*, 30–38.

Palmer, F., & Henderson, N. (1993). The role of the private speech pathologist in the private nursing home sector. *Australian Communications Quarterly, Spring,* 17–19.

Parker, R. A. (1987). *The elderly and residential care: Australian lessons for Britain.* Aldershot: Gower.

Ramsberger, G. (1994). Functional perspective for assessment and rehabilitation of persons with severe aphasia. *Seminars in Speech and Language, 15,* 1–15.

Ribbe, M. W., Ljunggren, G., Steel, K., Topinkova, E., Hawes, C., Ikegami, N., Henrard, J., & Johnson, P. (1997). Nursing homes in 10 nations: A comparison between countries and settings. *Age and Ageing, 26,* S3.

Robertson, C. (1993). Speech pathology services in a state government residential facility: A descriptive account. *Australian Communications Quarterly, Spring,* 18–19.

Ryan, E. B. (1991). Attitudes and behaviors toward older adults in communication contexts. Paper presented at the Fourth International Conference on Language and Social Psychology, Santa Barbara.

Ryan, E. B., Meredith, S. D., MacLean, M. J., & Orange, J. B. (1995). Changing the way we talk with elders: Promoting health using the Communication Enhancement Model. *International Journal of Aging and Human Development, 41,* 87–105.

Schroll, M., Jonsson, P. V., Mor, V., Berg, K., & Sherwood, S. (1997). An international study of social engagement among nursing home residents. *Age & Ageing, 26,* 55–59.

Skinner, C., Wirz, S., Thompson, I., & Davidson, J. (1984). Edinburgh Functional Communication Profile. United Kingdom: Winslow Press.

Sorin-Peters, R., Tse, S., & Kapelus, G. (1989). Communication screening program for a geriatric continuing care unit. *Journal of Speech–Language Pathology and Audiology, 13,* 63–70.

Von Leden, H. (1977). Speech and hearing problems in the geriatric patient. *Journal of the American Geriatric Society, 15,* 422–426.

Weiss, C. E. (1971). Communicative needs of the geriatric population. *Journal of the American Geriatric Society, 19,* 640–645.

Wilder, C. N. (1984). Normal and disordered speech and voice. In C. N. Wilder, B. E. Weinstein (eds): *Aging and communication: Problems in management* (pp. 21–29). New York: Haworth.

World Health Organization (1980). International Classification of Impairments, Disabilities and Handicaps. Geneva: Author.

World Health Organization (1997). ICIDH-2 International Classification of Impairments, Activities and Participation. [http://www.who.ch/programmes/mnh/ems/icidh/introduction.htm].

Worrall, L., & Hickson, L. (1993). Speech pathology services for Australia's ageing population. *Australian Communications Quarterly, Spring,* 15–16.

Worrall, L., Hickson, L., & Dodd, B. (1994). Screening for communication impairment in nursing homes and hostels. *Australian Journal of Human Communication Disorders, 21,* 53–64.

Zopf, P. (1986). *America's older population.* Houston: Cap and Gown Press.

# SECTION 5

# *Future Directions and Research Needs*

# 19

# Future Directions and Research Issues in Functional Communication Assessment and Treatment

## Linda E. Worrall

This volume has described functional approaches from different perspectives and with different populations. This concluding chapter brings together the major issues and challenges that have arisen. The challenges include the need for consensus on a conceptual model, the influence of health-care policy on functional approaches, and the need to extend the functional approach to a range of communication disorders and clinical settings. Future research topics are identified to ensure that the study of functional communication flourishes in the next millenium.

## Introduction

The field of functional communication has come of age. Over the past three decades, the functional approach has steadily gained acceptance due to pioneers such as Martha Taylor Sarno and Audrey Holland. Theoretical models of disablement such as the ICIDH-2 have focused speech-language pathologists' attention on the conceptual framework, payers have emphasized the need for speech-language pathologists to examine functional outcomes and the diversity of assessment and treatment approaches in various populations testify to a strengthening area of research and clinical practice in speech-language pathology. This chapter discusses these themes in greater depth and distills some of the issues into research questions within the field of functional communication. Hence, a major aim of this chapter is to extract some of the themes of this volume and promote further discussion so that outstanding issues are resolved. A further aim is to encourage research into the many aspects of functional communication.

### New Versus Old Approaches in Functional Communication

Holland (1998a) coined the term the "new" functionalism that refers to a social approach to communication disorders. By implication, the "old" functional approach could be described as the traditional activity-based approach (see Davidson & Worrall in Chapter 2 for a description). In this volume, the social approach or the new functional approach is described in the chapters by Parr and Byng (Chapter 4), Lyon (Chapter 9), and Simmons-Mackie (Chapter 10). See also the Hirsch and Holland chapter (Chapter 3) for a review of measures associated with this approach. The new functional approach could be said to describe the Participation and Quality of Life dimensions of the ICIDH-2. However, some advocates of the social model of disability do not consider that their approach is encompassed within the functional approach. The phrase "functional is not enough" first used by Kagan and Gailey (1993) has been re-iterated by Parr & Byng in Chapter 4. This conceptual disagreement must be resolved.

It is suggested here that functional is predominantly a medical term applied in rehabilitation settings and because of that, the term is inappropriate for use in community settings where the social approach is used (see Byng et al., in press). In this volume, functional communication has been said to encompass both Activity and Participation dimensions of the ICIDH-2. Hence, both the old and new functional approaches have been encompassed under the one term of functional communication. To add further complexity, the functional approach has also been described as targeting any of the ICIDH-2 dimensions "in order to" achieve a goal based in either the Activity or Participation dimensions. It is timely to consider whether the terms "functional communication" or the "functional approach" are adequate to describe the breadth of the concepts described in the chapters of this volume. More sophisticated terminology is required to describe the diversity of approaches within the functional approach and the ICIDH-2 provides the most suitable terminology and conceptual framework.

There are essentially two forms of functional treatment and both need to be recognized, particularly in the terms used to describe the concepts within them. The first is an indirect approach to improving communication for everyday life by first improving the component skills necessary for everyday communication. This is sometimes called component skills training (Ylvisaker & Holland, 1985) and relies on the generalization of component skills to everyday life. Hence, the functional approach may target the speech, language, voice, or swallowing impairment in order to accomplish Activity-based or Participation-based goals. The second type of functional intervention is the direct approach that specifically targets communication and its use in everyday life. Hence, the functional approach may also focus directly on communication activities, participation, or quality of life issues within the ICIDH-2. Speech-language pathologists need to differentiate between these concepts and it is recommended that the ICIDH-2 terms be used rather than the generic term of functional communication. For example, rather than stating a goal of therapy as functional communication, the goal should be stated in the terms of the ICIDH-2. An example of this might be to state that the goal of intervention is to enhance a person's ability to use the telephone (an Activity level goal) or to enable someone to return to work (a Participation goal). As Byng et al. (in press) state, functional communication is an overused and confusing term. The ICIDH-2 terms add more detail and greater sophistication to the term of functional communication, because it encompasses both the Activity and Participation domains. It is noted however, that the terms Impairments, Activities, and Participation are also confusing to many speech-language pathologists and clarity of terminology may take some time. However, the argument that "functional is not enough" becomes obsolete when the term functional is replaced with the ICIDH-2 terminology. The social model of disability is encompassed within the ICIDH-2, hence both old and new functional approaches are represented in the most recent WHO conceptual framework.

Byng et al. (in press) rightly argue for a dynamic intervention approach that focuses on the needs of the client at a particular time in his or her rehabilitation, and present an argument for a portfolio of intervention options that are made available to all clients. This holistic view of intervention presents as a vision to be aspired to and one that the profession must ultimately embrace. It remains however that there are few developed services that adequately target participation and quality of life issues for people with communication and related disorders. The focus of the profession remains on impairment-based assessment, therapy, and research. Hence, there is an argument for retaining the term functional communication to focus the attention of the profession on this relatively neglected area of service. When Activity and Participation domains become as prominent in the profession as Impairments, then the need for the collective term of functional communication may diminish.

While there is agreement that a holistic approach to intervention must be the goal, there is no consensus about the theoretical model that will serve as an overarching framework for speech-language pathology so that such a holistic approach can be achieved. Petheram and Parr (1998) argue that there is a need for a meta-theory in aphasiology because of the diversity of theoretical positions within the area. They describe a meta-theory as "a coherent approach to assessment and treatment, which draws on different theoretical constructions of aphasia in accord with the perceived needs of the client" (Petheram & Parr, 1998, p. 441). The selection of the approach to suit the client's needs becomes explicit and the meta-theory approach thereby encourages clinical diversity. Worrall (1999) argued that a meta-theory is required for speech-language pathology as a whole. The aims of the meta-theory are to encompass all theoretical and intervention approaches, guide clinical decision-making, and describe the scope of the profession to others (Worrall, 1999). The ICIDH-2 was suggested as a meta-theory for speech-language pathology. Advocates of a social approach to communication disorders however may be concerned that the ICIDH-2 does not adequately reflect the social model of disablement. This was, however, a major focus of the revision of the original version of the ICIDH. The inclusion of the social model in the new version is one of its greatest strengths. The ICIDH-2 therefore attempts to provide a "synthesis that offers a coherent view of different dimensions of health at both biological and social levels" (WHO, 1997 p. 4). This is termed a "biopsychosocial" approach to disablement. In speech-language pathology terms, this might be termed an holistic approach to disablement.

To demonstrate the inclusion of the social model in the ICIDH-2, not only are the terms disability and handicap revised to the neutral terms of Activity and Participation, but there are also numerous references to the social model of disability in the extensive documentation supporting the ICIDH-2. For example, the stated social policy implications of the ICIDH-2 include:

- support for endeavors to provide equal opportunity,
- maximization of participation of people with disabilities,
- identifying enabling responses of society to increase independence and choice,
- improvement in the living conditions and quality of life of people, and
- awareness of and changes in social practices (e.g., rejection of discrimination and stigmatization) (WHO, 1997, p. 4).

A lack of a scientific or theoretical foundation, lack of accepted common terminology, and a lack of research has dogged the study and practice of functional approaches to assessment and treatment in the field. The ICIDH-2 is a robust framework for functional communication because it addresses these issues. Many are included in the aims of the ICIDH-2, specifically:

- to provide a scientific basis to understand and study the consequences of health conditions,
- to establish a common language for describing consequences of health conditions in order to improve communications between health care workers, other sectors and disabled people/people with disabilities,
- to permit comparison of data across countries, health care disciplines, services and time,
- to stimulate research on the consequences of health conditions (WHO, 1997, p. 5).

One of the greatest strengths of the ICIDH-2 for speech-language pathology is that it facilitates communication across professions. It also expands the repertoire of concepts and methodologies available to speech-language pathologists because it represents a consensus framework among many disciplines. It is an attempt to provide a meta-theory for many health and welfare professions around the world. Why should the small profession of speech-language pathology not embrace it?

The ICIDH and the ICIDH-2 aim to be all things to all people. This might be considered to be a disadvantage of the WHO models. Since its inception in 1980 ICIDH has been used for various purposes, for example:

- as a statistical tool—in the collection and recording of data (e.g., in demography, population studies and surveys or in management information systems),
- as a research tool—to measure outcomes, quality of life or environmental factors,

- as a clinical tool—in needs assessment, matching treatments with specific conditions, vocational assessment, rehabilitation, and outcome evaluation,
- as a social policy tool—social security planning, compensation systems, policy design and implementation,
- as an educational tool—curriculum design, identification of needs for awareness and social actions.

However, if ever there was a meta-theory that encompasses the diversity of approaches within speech-language pathology (Petheram & Parr, 1998), the current WHO model of disablement must be it. The WHO models are consensus-driven working documents responding to feedback from the international scientific, clinical and disabled community. Field trails of the Beta version of the ICIDH-2 continue to refine the classification scheme and it is expected that the final version will be put to the governing bodies of the World Health Organization for ratification in the year 2000. Publication of the Beta-2 draft of the ICIDH-2 is proposed for May, 2000 (Halbertsma, 1999).

Advocates of the "new" functional approach must not lessen the need for functional outcomes by devaluing other longer established functional approaches. Holland (1998b) has suggested that the phrase "in order to" could be used to link impairment oriented outcomes to functional outcomes. Hence an impairment-based goal may be targeted in therapy "in order to" improve an everyday communication activity "in order to" optimize participation in a life role. It is also suggested that Impairment-based and Activity-based interventions may form the building blocks toward enhanced Participation in some cases of communication disorder. Another approach strongly advocated here, is to ask the client what outcomes are important to him or her. This consumer-driven approach will often yield goals in different dimensions of the ICIDH-2 framework and the dynamic nature of intervention as described by Byng et al. (in press) becomes apparent as the needs of the individual change over time. Some individuals choose impairment-based goals (e.g., to speak better), others activity-based goals (e.g., to be able to withdraw money from the bank) while yet others wish to target participation goals (e.g., to resume their role as treasurer of the local lawn bowls association). Intervention may focus directly on these goals hence participation may be facilitated without addressing the impairment or activity limitations at all. Certainly the relationships among the dimensions need to be explored further in research and the ICIDH-2 model needs to be trialed by speech-language pathologists. Further, interventions that are based on the "in order to" or indirect approach (e.g., treating word-finding in order to go shopping in order to enhance autonomy) that actively promote generalization need to be rigorously evaluated. In addition, the direct approach to achieving client's functional goals by providing functional treatment that specifically targets the functional goals of the client (e.g., functional skills training such as practicing to use the telephone) also needs to be evaluated. Certainly, the effectiveness of the social approach to functional communication needs to be evaluated as much as the activity based functional approach.

In summary, a debate based on the phrase "Functional is not enough" has emerged in the literature. A new paradigm of intervention has emerged that is based firmly within the social approach. Proponents of this approach suggest that the older functional activity-based approach is not sufficient for many people seeking the services of speech-language pathologists. Before the argument about new versus old functional approaches takes hold however, there has been a move to find a meta-theory that encompasses the diversity of all approaches (Petheram & Parr, 1998). It is argued here that the ICIDH-2 meets the criterion for a meta-theory because it is a consensual document representing the views of people with disabilities and the scientific and clinical communities of the world.

## The Influence of Health and Social Policy on Functional Communication

The health care climate is changing in many countries of the world. The United States in particular has experienced dramatic changes to health care funding that are having a profound effect on speech-language pathology services. Frattali (Chapter 5) describes the impact that the current health care policies in the United States have had on speech-language pathology services. A positive approach to these changes is suggested by a set of recommendations that speech-language pathologists can follow to begin to manage the changes.

A similar positive approach to managing change in other countries is taking hold. Policy changes in Australia for example, have led to some innovative functional approaches being trialed. In the aged care sector, a policy shift to monitoring outcomes in extended care facilities has meant that a greater focus on participation outcomes is highly valued in these settings (Pye et al., in Chapter 18). Similarly, an emphasis on consumer satisfaction in some Australian acute care hospitals has encouraged a combined social and environmental approach (McCooey et al., Chapter 17) that aims to improve communication for all communicatively disadvantaged patients hospital-wide. Hence, policy changes have galvanized speech-language pathologists into developing innovative approaches that link intervention to current policies in their workplace.

A frequent conflict in policy direction is whose views are most valued—the payer's, the provider's or the consumer's? Lyon (Chapter 9) argues strongly for speech-language pathologists to retain their particular perspective of communication disorders and the treatments that are most effective for those disorders. He argues that the provider's view should not give way to the payer's view and result in the withdrawal of effective services for people with communication disorders due to lack of payer support. Lyon is therefore arguing for the retention of effective services for people who require them.

Two issues emerge. The first is whether the policy changes are having a negative impact on clients or whether they are merely changing service provision? The second is who should pay for the provision of services?

Frattali (Chapter 5) describes the criteria commonly used by payers in the U.S. to decide who receives care and for how long care is provided. Functional goals are a feature of the criteria. Larkins et al. (Chapter 12) summarize the features of functional intervention that the major New Zealand insurer promotes and emphasizes that the economic viability of the "no fault" New Zealand scheme is dependent upon a return to work for head injured clients. It is therefore apparent that payers are demanding that health services, including speech-language pathology services, consider "value for money" issues and functional outcomes play a major role in these considerations. The influence of policy on functional communication has become even greater since Frattali's seminal article on the topic in 1992. Will the payer's emphasis on functional outcomes improve client services in speech-language pathology? Few speech-language pathologists would question that practical and real-life benefits of treatment are important. The argument seems to be based on how these outcomes should be gained. Payers want these gains to be made as efficiently as possible; speech-language pathologists have a diversity of opinions about how these outcomes can be achieved; consumers are often left without services at all. There is an urgent need for leadership, collaboration and research that can progress this debate so that optimal outcomes are achieved.

The research opportunities that this presents are now discussed. First, there is a research opportunity to measure the impact that policy changes have on service delivery. Speech-language pathologists have long been concerned about the quality of their services, particularly in terms of the access to speech-language pathology services by people with communication and or swallowing disorders. Communication disordered clients are marginalized as consumers and their "invisible" disabilities are often overlooked. Access to speech-language pathology services has not been a major focus of research despite the on-going concern of speech-language pathologists that clients are not receiving services or are not identified initially as requiring services. Now is the time to study trends in access as a result of policy changes.

Second, Lyon (Chapter 9) urges speech-language pathologists to take steps toward life-altering interventions and rightly states that it is the profession's responsibility to ensure that consumers' needs continue to be met, despite changes in health care policies. There are many opportunities to develop functional communication assessments and treatments that meet these needs. Evaluation of the effectiveness and efficiency of intervention programs that make a real difference to people's lives are indeed a priority.

The issue of who should pay for the range of speech-language pathology services is more complex. Funding systems for speech-language pathology services vary considerably around the world, however, the trend toward community-based options such as Living with Aphasia, Inc. or the Aphasia Centres in North York, Ontario and City University, London is increasing and funding for these services poses a new challenge for speech-language pathologists and the community in general. These centers currently gain funding from a variety of sources: charities, governments, universities, and private health care insurers, however ongoing and adequate levels of funding is an issue for many.

Speech-language pathologists have long operated within the medical model and hence funding for services has emanated from the same model, mostly from with health care budgets of governments. In its endeavor to meet functional goals, speech-language pathology is increasingly turning to social models of intervention. Funding for such services must therefore come from society as a whole and communities more specifically. It is time to focus on non-government sources to ensure that clients continue to receive services. As Lyon notes, this is not a time to shirk our professional responsibility and relevant services must continue to be delivered.

Within the acute care setting, there are some real questions that need answering. First, how can a relevant service be provided to communication disordered clients when the balance of service has shifted to patients with dysphagia? Both Sonies (Chapter 15) and McCooey et al. (Chapter 17) note that dysphagia referrals have multiplied considerably in recent years. A shift in emphasis in speech-language pathology practice is required for acute-stage communication disordered patients. Certainly, the emphasis must remain on the early identification of communication disorders, support and information for both the patient and family, facilitation of communication within the hospital, and preparation for appropriate discharge from the hospital. These are predominantly functional aims, however, the focus of treatment in the acute phase is directed at the impairment. How effective is early impairment-based treatment?

Linebaugh et al. (1998) examine the paradox that while most efficacy studies of aphasia have involved participants with chronic, stable aphasia, most treatment occurs during the period of spontaneous recovery. While studies of efficacy use chronic, stable participants to control for the effect of spontaneous recovery, it remains that there are few studies of the efficacy of acute-stage treatment. This paradox is not unique to aphasia. The effectiveness of impairment-based intervention in the acute stage would seem a priority given the restriction to rehabilitation services generally. The efficiency of providing impairment-based therapy as the predominant form of intervention to communication disordered clients with little evidence that functional goals are being achieved requires considerable debate in the profession.

### Extending the Functional Approach Beyond Aphasia

The field of aphasiology has one of the richest traditions in functional communication. There has been over three decades of research reported in the literature in aphasiology since Martha Taylor Sarno's seminal publication in 1965 (Taylor, 1965). Aphasiology has witnessed a recent explosion of interest in functional outcomes. Other communication and swallowing disorders are also being examined in terms of functional outcomes, but the aphasiology literature continues to lead the field in the discussion of functional approaches. It is suggested in this section that the unique impairments of swallowing; motor speech disorders; and cognitive-communication disturbance resulting from right hemisphere damage, traumatic brain injury and dementia should not be assumed to have the same impact on Activities and Participation as aphasia. Hence, assessments and interventions that are sensitive to these differences need to be developed.

The current emphasis on outcome measurement in health care may drive this development. Alternatively, it may also be driven by a realization by speech-language pathologists that methods developed for aphasia are not meeting the needs of other speech and language disordered clients. It is suggested that both will create the required interest in functional approaches in impairments other than aphasia. Both these sources of interest will now be explored.

Frattali (1993) suggests that the growing interest in functional communication is not so much a clinical interest but a result of increased pressure from the payers of health care. There has been a surge of interest in the literature about the concept of functional outcome measures used by speech-language pathologists (see Frattali, 1998 and a clinical forum by Hesketh & Sage, 1999a; Enderby, 1999; Frattali, 1999; Holland, 1999; LaPointe, 1999; Onslow; 1999; Worrall, 1999; Hesketh & Sage, 1999b). Rating scales that purport to measure function are being used to measure the outcome of speech-language pathology service provision, and in the future funding may be linked to these outcomes. Hence the need to implement simple, reliable, valid and sensitive ratings of function has become a high priority for many speech-language pathology facilities. The need for functional outcome measures has heightened the priority of functional communication in speech-language pathology.

While payers are demanding outcome data in many countries, a recent survey of Australian speech-language pathologists (Worrall, 1998) suggests that speech-language pathologists themselves are driving the implementation of facility level functional outcome measurement. In the survey of 249 speech-language pathology facilities, 26% reported that the incentive to measure outcomes was from their employer while 46% stated that the speech-language pathologists themselves initiated outcome measurement in their facility. The conclusion was that speech-language pathologists had developed a strong sense of clinical inquiry and professional accountability. Hence, the drive to implement functional outcome measures may not be entirely due to pressure exerted by the payers.

The recent increase in interest in functional communication may also reflect the growth and maturity of the discipline's research base. Now that the profession understands more fully the underlying nature of impairments such as aphasia, dysarthria, dysphagia, and the cognitive communication impairments associated with right hemisphere damage, dementia and traumatic brain injury, it is now able to tackle the complexities of measuring and treating the long-term consequences of impairments, that is, the activity limitations and participation restrictions that may result. Professional maturity is reflected in the way that debates in the literature have moved away from whether functional communication should be assessed at all, to the present situation of exploring ways in which the balance between all approaches can be redressed (Byng et al., in press; Petheram & Parr, 1998). Whether functional assessment has become routine clinical practice has yet to be determined, although surveys of the use of assessments (Katz et al., 1998; Smith-Worrall & Burtenshaw, 1990) would suggest that standardized functional communication assessments are still not part of the clinician's routine assessment battery.

The current focus on the conceptual basis of functional communication has meant that a diversity of functional assessments and treatments have expanded the horizons of clients as well as speech-language pathologists. The profession's knowledge base is expanding beyond the impairment level, which uses the basic sciences such as physiology, linguistics, and psychology, toward a discipline-specific research base that characterises communicative activities and participation and which now links speech-language pathology with other rehabilitation professions. In areas other than aphasia however, functional communication and functional swallowing are struggling to obtain an identity and hence, there is much to be done in terms of research and practice development.

An overriding theme in the chapters describing the functional approach in cognitive communication disorders such as traumatic brain injury and right hemisphere damage (Cherney & Halper in Chapter 16; Larkins et al., in Chapter 12) is that the uniqueness of the impairments demands a functional assessment and treatment approach that is separate and different from that used with aphasia. Within the disorders associated with traumatic brain injury and right hemisphere damage, there are also major differences. For example, communicative activities that are popular with younger people need to be sampled more in functional communication assessments of traumatic brain injury. The uniqueness of these populations has yet to be reflected in functional assessments and treatment approaches designed specifically for these populations.

The burgeoning popularity of outcome scales for dysphagia is evident in Sonies' review of functional outcome scales (see Chapter 15). The nature of the functional approach to swallowing however is just emerging. The need to examine difficulties in eating and drinking in terms of the conceptual framework of the ICIDH-2 are an essential pre-requisite to the development of valid functional outcome measures for dysphagia. Debate about service issues can then occur once the desired outcomes are articulated. For example, the goal of maintained or heightened quality of life is an important outcome in the functional approach. Quality of life issues are certainly important in many cases where dysphagia becomes a chronic condition. These have been considered as ethical issues for the profession, however, the ICIDH-2 provides a theoretical basis for asking research questions such as the effect of a modified diet on quality of life for people with chronic dysphagia, or the effectiveness of interventions that directly target eating and drinking activities and social participation.

Lubinski and Orange (Chapter 11) embrace the notion of enhancing well being in people with dementia. The Wellness to Opportunity framework of assessment and intervention described by Lubinski and Orange recognizes the difficulty of achieving cognitive and linguistic improvement in dementia and therefore the focus is placed strongly on promoting communicative wellness, enhancing communication skills, emphasizing effectiveness of communication and increasing opportunities for communication. This is recognition of the progressive nature of dementia, a feature that it doesn't share with stroke-related aphasia and hence a specific functional approach separate from non-progressive aphasia has been advanced for this disorder.

Enderby (Chapter 14) presents data on how the dysarthrias associated with different aetiologies (e.g., cerebral palsy, Parkinson's disease, head injury, stroke) have different effects on communicative activity limitations (disabilities) or participation restrictions (handicaps). For example, the start scores on the Therapy Outcome Measures (i.e., pre-treatment ratings of impairment, disability, handicap and well-being) vary across the aetiologies with disorders such as cerebral palsy having less impact on handicap or well-being than more recent-onset disorders such as stroke or head injury. While the effect of a communication disorder on an individual and their role in society varies considerably, further research in this area may provide insights into the differing intervention approaches that are needed for these populations.

The chapters by McCooey et al. and Pye et al. also suggest that the communication environment plays a major role in functional assessment and management. When considering that context or environmental issues are a major factor in the functional approach, the notion that the functional approach can be applied at the institutional level should not be surprising. Lubinski (1981) has long been championing an environmental approach to communication in nursing homes and Ylvisaker et al. (1993) have described the socioenvironmental approach for residents with traumatic brain injuries. Similarly, communication within the institution of the acute care hospital has been the focus for the chapter by McCooey et al.

## Research Directions

Other disciplines have much to offer speech-language pathology as it considers how to optimize rehabilitation efforts with people with communication and swallowing disorders. The field of gerontology has embraced the concept of successful ageing (Baltes & Baltes, 1990; Day, 1991). Much research is being conducted to determine why some people grow old with few health difficulties and retain a good quality of life. As some older people live past 100 years, these centenarians have become a focus of study. Many speech–language pathologists know of people with long-standing communication disorders who enjoy their life to the full. Why have they overcome or adjusted to the potentially debilitating effect of aphasia or dysarthria? How can the collective experiences of these people help guide rehabilitation professionals? What can we learn from those who have the unique experience of having lived their life with a communication disorder? Methodologies from the gerontological field of inquiry into successful ageing are relevant to this research question.

The paradigm shift from expert clinician to pupil does not come easily to professions. The process whereby professional values are debated within a profession has much to offer the discipline as a whole. In Chapter 11, some values from the social work profession were discussed. Values such as shared decision-making have a profound influence on the everyday practice of a profession. It is suggested that proponents of the functional communication approach have a different value system to those who advocate impairment-based approaches exclusively. In reality, many clinicians use a combination of both. The professional values of speech-language pathologists are another topic of future research. The link between preferred treatment approach and professional values of speech-language pathologists might unearth a rich vein of inquiry.

In summary, there is considerable research to be done in reflecting the unique features of people with a range of disorders of communication and swallowing. It is envisaged that if the current trend in functional approaches continues, the development of the functional approach with all disorders will dramatically change the way rehabilitation services are offered.

In conclusion, a paradigm shift is occurring in speech-language pathology. The shift is not exclusively toward the functional approach, but in partnership with other methods. It is imperative that the clients' voice be heard. As this occurs, the long awaited "equal billing" of the functional approach will happen. For equal billing to occur, many more speech-language pathologists need to value the functional approach. It might be suggested that many clinicians who use a functional approach have experienced impairment-based therapy, but many clinicians who use impairment-based therapy have not had experience of a functional approach. Professional values must be examined.

The ICIDH-2 continues to provide a robust framework for the functional approach in neurogenic communication disorders. It is also a potential meta-theory for speech-language pathology intervention generally. While theoretical frameworks are important to professionals, they are simply guides to potential interventions that professionals can offer. For clinicians, the challenge is to know the client's needs and goals and relate these to a sound theoretical framework.

## References

Baltes, P. B., & Baltes, M. M. (Eds.) (1990). *Successful aging: Perspectives from the behavioral sciences.* Cambridge: Cambridge University Press.

Byng, S., Pound, C., & Parr, S. (in press). Living with aphasia: A framework for therapy interventions. In I. Papathanasiou (ed): *Acquired Neurological Communication Disorders: A Clinical Perspective.* London: Whurr Publishers.

Day, A. T. (1991). *Remarkable survivors: Insights into successful aging among women.* Washington, DC: Urban Institute Press.

Enderby, P. (1999). For richer for poorer: Outcome measurement in speech and language therapy. *Advances in Speech-Language Pathology, 1*(1), 63–65.

Frattali, C. M. (1993). Perspectives on functional assessment: Its use for policy making. *Disability and Rehabilitation, 15,* 1–9.

Frattali, C. M. (Ed). (1998). *Measuring Outcomes in Speech-Language Pathology.* New York: Thieme Medical Publishers.

Frattali, C. M. (1999). Measuring outcomes "for the better." *Advances in Speech-Language Pathology, 1*(1), 47–49.

Halbertsma, J. (Ed). (1999). ICIDH Revision News. RIVM Newsletter, WHO Collaborating Centre for the ICIDH, Department of Public Health Forecasting, National Institute of Public Health and the Environment, The Netherlands.

Hesketh, A., & Sage, K. (1999a). For better, for worse: Outcome measurement in speech and language therapy. *Advances in Speech-Language Pathology, 1*(1), 37–45.

Hesketh, A., & Sage, K. (1999b). Reply—outcome measurement: In sickness and in health. *Advances in Speech-Language Pathology, 1*(1), 67–69.

Holland, A. (1998a). Aphasia treatment in the next decade: The new functionalism. Paper presented at the 8th International Aphasia Rehabilitation Conference. Kwa Maritane, South Africa. 26–28 August, 1998.

Holland, A. (1998b). Functional outcomes in aphasia following left hemisphere stroke. *Seminars in Speech and Language, 19*(3), 249–260.

Holland, A. (1999). Consumers and functional outcomes. *Advances in Speech-Language Pathology, 1*(1), 51–52.

Kagan, A., & Gailey, G. (1993). Functional is not enough: Training conversation partners for aphasic adults. In A. Holland, M. Forbes (eds): *Aphasia Treatment: World Perspectives.* San Diego: Singular Publishing Group.

Katz, R. C., Hollowell, B., Code, C., Armstrong, E., Roberts, P., Pound, C., Katz, L. (1998). A multinational comparison of aphasia management practices. Paper presented at the Clinical Aphasiology Conference. Ashville, N. Carolina.

LaPointe, L. L. (1999). An enigma: Outcome measurement in speech and language therapy. *Advances in Speech-Language Pathology, 1*(1), 57–58.

Linebaugh, C. W., Baron, C. R., & Corcoran, K. J. (1998). Assessing treatment efficacy in acute aphasia: Paradoxes, presumptions, problems and principles. *Aphasiology, 12, (7/8),* 519–536.

Lubinski R. (1981). Environmental language intervention. In R. Chapey (ed): *Language Intervention Strategies In Adult Aphasia* (pp. 223–245). Baltimore: Williams & Wilkins.

Onslow, M. (1999). Science and antiscience: Outcome measures in speech-language pathology. *Advances in Speech-Language Pathology, 1*(1), 59–61.

Petheram, B., & Parr, S. (1998). Diversity in aphasiology: Crisis or increasing competence. *Aphasiology, 12,*(6), 435–487.

Smith-Worrall, L., & Burtenshaw, E. J. (1990). Frequency of use and utility of aphasia tests *Australian Journal of Human Communication Disorders, 18*(2), 53–67.

Taylor, M. L. (1965). A measurement of functional communication in aphasia. *Archives of Physical Medicine and Rehabilitation, 46,* 101–107.

WHO: ICIDH-2 International Classification of Impairments, Activities, and Participation [http://www.who.ch/programmes/mnh/mnh/ems/icidh/icidh.htm] 1997.

Worrall, L. (1998). A national survey of speech pathology outcome measures. Paper presented at the Speech Pathology Australia conference, Freemantle, Western Australia.

Worrall, L. (1999). Keynote address: Speech Pathology: Giving people a say in life? Conference Proceedings of the Speech Pathology Australia National Conference, Sydney, Australia.

Worrall, L. (1999). Outcome measurement: How to play the game. *Advances in Speech-Language Pathology, 1*(1), 53–55.

Ylvisaker. M., Feeney, T. J., & Urbanczyk, B. (1993). A social-environmental approach to communication and behaviour after traumatic brain injury. *Seminars in Speech and Language, 14*(1),

Ylvisaker, M., & Holland, A. L. (1985). Coaching, self coaching and rehabilitation of head injury. In D. F. Johns (ed): *Clinical Management of Neurogenic Communicative Disorders* (pp. 243–257). Boston: Little Brown & Co.

# Index

Page numbers in *italics* indicate figures. Page numbers followed by "t" indicate tables.